High-Yield Histopathology

High-Yield Histopathology

Ronald W. Dudek, Ph.D.
Full Professor
Department of Anatomy and Cell Biology
East Carolina University School of Medicine
Brody School of Medicine
Greenville, North Carolina

 Wolters Kluwer | Lippincott Williams & Wilkins
Health
Philadelphia · Baltimore · New York · London
Buenos Aires · Hong Kong · Sydney · Tokyo

Acquisitions Editor: Crystal Taylor
Developmental Editor: Kathleen H. Scogna
Project Editor: Bridget H. Meyer
Marketing Manager: Valerie Sunders
Designer: Terry Mallon
Compositor: International Typesetting and Composition
Printer: DRC

Printed in the United States of America

Library of Congress Cataloging-in-Publication Data

Dudek, Ronald W., 1950-
    High-yield histopathology / Ronald W. Dudek.
        p.; cm.
    Rev. ed. of: High-yield histology / Ronald W. Dudek. 3rd ed. c2004.
    Includes bibliographical references and index.
    ISBN–13: 978-0-7817-6959-4 (alk. paper)
    ISBN–10: 0-7817-6959-0 (alk. paper)
    1. Histology, Pathological—Outlines, syllabi, etc.   I. Dudek, Ronald
W., 1950- High-yield histology.   II. Title.
    [DNLM: 1. Histology—Outlines.   2. Pathology—Outlines.   QS 518.2
D845h 2008]
    RB32.DB3 2008
    611'.018076—dc22

                                                    2007008561

To purchase additional copies of this book, call our customer service department at (800) 638-3030 or fax orders to (301) 223-2320. International customers should call (301) 223-2300.

Visit Lippincott Williams & Wilkins on the Internet: http://www.LWW.com. Lippincott Williams & Wilkins customer service representatives are available from 8:30 am to 6:00 pm, EST.

Lippincott Williams & Wilkins, a Wolters Kluwer business

07 08 09 10 11
1 2 3 4 5 6 7 8 9 10

I would like to dedicate this book to my mother, Lottie Dudek, who was born on November 11, 1918. Through the years my mother raised her children, maintained a loving marriage, and worked 40 hours per week. In the year 2004, society would describe such a person as a "liberated woman" or "supermom." I would like to acknowledge that my mother was a "supermom" 20 years before the word was fashionable. A son cannot repay a mother. My hope is that "I love you and thank you" will suffice.

Preface

The fourth edition of *High-Yield Histology* has been renamed *High-Yield Histopathology* in order to give the student a more accurate indication of the book's contents. *High-Yield Histopathology* does more than just review histology. As you may know, the questions on the USMLE Step 1 cross traditional course boundaries, making it difficult to identify a question that is "strictly histology." Many USMLE Step 1 questions fall into categories such as histopathology, histophysiology, histomicrobiology, and histobiochemistry. To write a review book on basic, traditional histology would not be helpful to the student preparing for the USMLE Step 1 since there are no basic traditional histology questions on the exam. In this regard, *High-Yield Histopathology*, 4th ed, reviews important histology concepts and then extends the discussion to pathology, physiology, microbiology, and pharmacology of clinically relevant topics.

In addition, many students have commented that cell biology topics have been well represented on the USMLE Step 1. To this end, I have included Chapter 1 (Nucleus), Chapter 2 (Cytoplasm and Organelles), and Chapter 3 (Cell Membrane) with up-to-date and clinically relevant information.

I would, appreciate any comments or suggestions concerning *High-Yield Histopathology*, 4th ed, especially after you have taken the USMLE Step 1 that you think might improve the book. You may contact me at dudekr@ecu.edu

Contents

Chapter 1

Nucleus

❶ Nuclear Envelope.

The nuclear envelope is a two-membrane structure. The **inner membrane** is associated with a network of **intermediate filaments (lamins A, B, C)** called the **nuclear lamina,** which plays a role in the disassembly of the nuclear envelope during prometaphase of mitosis by phosphorylation of the lamins by **lamin kinase** and reassembly of the nuclear envelope during telophase. The **outer membrane** is studded with ribosomes and is continuous with the rough endoplasmic reticulum (rER). The inner and outer membranes are separated by a **perinuclear cisterna.** The nuclear envelope contains many pores that allow passage of molecules between the nucleus and cytoplasm (Table 1-1). The pores are associated with a **nuclear pore complex,** which consists of many different proteins arranged in octagonal symmetry with a central channel.

TABLE 1-1	MOLECULAR TRANSPORT BETWEEN NUCLEUS AND CYTOPLASM	
	Direction of Movement	Mechanism
Ions Small molecules (<5,000 daltons) Proteins (<60,000 daltons)	Nucleus → cytoplasm Nucleus ← cytoplasm	Passive transport (diffusion) No ATP hydrolysis
mRNA tRNA rRNA	Nucleus → cytoplasm	Active transport Requires ATP hydrolysis Requires binding of RNA to proteins with a signal sequence of 4–8 amino acids for recognition by the nuclear pore complex
Proteins (>60,000 daltons) nucleoplasmin, steroid receptors, DNA and RNA polymerases, gene regulatory proteins, RNA-processing proteins	Nucleus ← cytoplasm	Active transport Require ATP hydrolysis Requires a signal sequence of 4–8 amino acids for recognition by the nuclear pore complex

Ⅱ Apoptosis.

Apoptosis is **programmed cell death ("cell suicide")** that is characterized by **DNA fragmentation** with chromatin clumping into a distinct crescent pattern along the inner margins of the nuclear envelope and then into a dense body; **decrease in cell volume; loss of mitochondrial function; cell membrane blebbing;** and **formation of apoptotic bodies,** which are rapidly phagocytosed without an inflammatory response. The chromatin is eventually cleaved by a specific endonuclease into DNA fragments that generate a distinctive **180-bp ladder** that is pathognomonic of apoptotic cell death. Apotosis is related to a family of proteases called **caspases (procaspases** are the inactive precursors), which are found in all cells and cleave target proteins at specific aspartic acid sites. Caspases are activated either by extracellular death signals (e.g., killer lymphocytes produce **Fas ligand,** which binds to the **Fas death receptor** on the target cell; **tumor necrosis factor (TNF)** binds to the **TNF death receptor** on the target cell) or intracellular death signals (e.g., mitochondria release **cytochrome c** into the cytoplasm where it activates **Apaf-1 adaptor protein** that in turn activates caspases). The **Bcl-2 family of proteins** is a main regulator of apoptosis. *Bcl-2* and *Bcl-X$_L$* are apoptosis inhibitors, whereas *Bad, Bax,* and *Bak* are apoptosis promoters. In addition, the **IAP family of proteins** is also a main regulator of apotosis. IAP proteins are all apoptosis inhibitors. Apoptosis occurs in hormone-dependent involution of cells during the menstrual cycle, embryogenesis, toxin-induced injury (e.g., diphtheria), viral cell death (e.g., Councilman bodies in yellow fever); and cell death via cytotoxic T cells or other immune cells. Apoptosis does not elicit an inflammatory response.

Ⅲ Nucleolus (Figure 1-1)

A. **GENERAL FEATURES.** The nucleolus consists of portions of five pairs of chromosomes (i.e., 13, 14, 15, 21, and 22) that contain about **200 copies of ribosomal RNA (rRNA)** genes per haploid genome which code for **rRNA.** The genes are arranged in clusters called **nucleolar organizers** and within the nucleolar organizers the genes are arranged in a **tandem series.** In humans, **RNA polymerase I** catalyzes the formation of **45S rRNA.** Another set of rRNA genes located outside of the nucleolus are transcribed by **RNA Polymerase III** to form **5S rRNA.** The nucleolus also contains **small nucleolar RNAs (snoRNAs)** that direct site-specific base modifications in rRNA. The **C/Dbox snoRNAs** direct the 2′-O-ribose methylation in rRNA. The **H/ACA snoRNAs** direct site-specific pseudouridylation (uridine is isomerized to pseudouridine) of rRNA.

B. **ULTRASTRUCTURE.** By electron microscopy, three regions of the nucleolus can be distinguished.
   1. The **dense fibrillar component** is dense-staining and contains **transcriptionally active DNA, RNA polymerase I,** and **45S RNA.**
   2. The **granular component** contains maturing ribosomal precursors, i.e., **45S RNA, 5S RNA, ribosomal proteins, RNA-binding proteins, and snRNPs.**
   3. The **fibrillar center** is pale-staining and contains **transcriptionally inactive DNA.**

Ⅳ Chromatin. Chromatin is double-helical DNA associated with histones and nonhistone proteins.

A. **HETEROCHROMATIN** is condensed chromatin and is **transcriptionally inactive.** In electron micrographs, heterochromatin is electron dense (i.e., very black). An example of heterochromatin is the **Barr body,** which is found in female cells and represents the inactive X chromosome. Heterochromatin comprises ~10% of the total chromatin. **Constitutive heterochromatin** is always condensed (i.e., transcriptionally inactive)

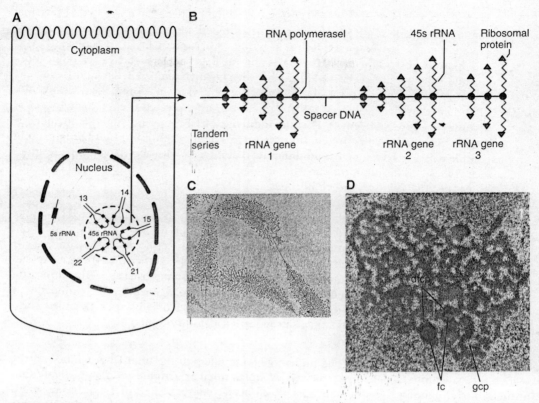

● **Figure 1-1 Organization of the nucleolus. (A)** Schematic diagram of a cell showing the non–membrane-bound (dotted lines) nucleolus containing DNA loops from chromosomes #13, #14, #15, #21, and #22. The rRNA genes are organized on these DNA loops as nucleolar organizers (thick lines). Note that 5S rRNA is transcribed from genes located outside the nucleolus. **(B)** Schematic of the nucleolar organizer. A closer look at the nucleolar organizer shows three rRNA genes in a tandem series separated by spacer DNA. During transcription of rRNA genes, a Christmas tree pattern is observed ultrastructurally. A particle corresponding to RNA polymerase I, varying lengths of 45S rRNA, and a particle corresponding to ribosomal proteins involved in early packaging can be observed. **(C)** EM of an rRNA gene undergoing transcription demonstrating the Christmas tree pattern. **(D)** EM of the nucleolus shows dense fibrillar component (dfcp) in a half-moon shape, granular component (gcp), and fibrillar center (fc).

and consists of repetitive DNA found near the centromere and other regions. **Facultative heterochromatin** can be either condensed (i.e., transcriptionally inactive) or dispersed (i.e., transcriptionally active). An example of facultative heterochromatin is the **XY body,** which forms when both the X and Y chromosome are inactivated for ~15 days during male meiosis.

B. EUCHROMATIN is dispersed chromatin and comprises ~90% of the total chromatin. Of this 90%, 10% is transcriptionally active and 80% is transcriptionally inactive. When chromatin is transcriptionally active, there is weak binding to the H1 histone protein and **acetylation** of the H2A, H2B, H3, and H4 histone proteins.

C. NUCLEOSOME. The most fundamental unit of packaging of DNA is the nucleosome. A nucleosome consists of a histone protein octamer (two each of **H2A, H2B, H3, and H4 histone proteins)** around which 146 bp of DNA is coiled in 1.75 turns. The nucleosomes are connected by spacer DNA, which results in a 10-nm diameter fiber that resembles a "beads-on-a-string" appearance by electron microscopy. Histones are small proteins containing a high proportion of **lysine** and **arginine** that impart a positive charge to the proteins that enhance it, binding to negatively charged DNA. Histones bind to DNA in A-T rich regions of DNA. Histone proteins have exposed N-terminal amino acid tails that are subject to modification and are crucial in regulating nucleo-some structure. **Histone acetylation** of lysine by **histone acetyltransferases (HATs)** and **histone deacetylases (HDACs)** is the most investigated histone modification. Histone acetylation reduces the affinity between histones and DNA. An increased acety-lation of histone proteins will make a DNA segment more likely to be transcribed into RNA; hence, any genes in that DNA segment will be expressed (i.e., ↑ **acetylation of histones = expressed genes**). **Histone methylation** of lysine and arginine by **methyl-transferases** also occurs. In addition, ATP-dependent **chromatin remodeling protein complexes,** which contain **bromodomains** that interact with acetylated lysine residues in histones and **chromodomains** that interact with methylated lysine residues in his-tones alter the affinity between histones and DNA.

D. **30-NM CHROMATIN FIBER.** The 10-nm nucleosome fiber is joined by **H1 histone protein** to form a **30-nm chromatin fiber.** Loops of the 30-nm chromatin fiber (~20–100 kb) are attached to a central **scaffold** consisting of notable **topoisomerase II** (an enzyme that can pass on DNA double helix through another by cutting a gap and then repairing it). During interphase of mitosis, chromosomes exist as 30-nm chromatin fibers organized as **extended chromatin.** (*Note*: when the general term "chromatin" is used, it refers specifically to the 30-nm chromatin fiber organized as extended chro-matin.) The extended chromatin also can form **secondary loops.**

V **Chromosomes** (Figure 1-2). The human genome refers to the total DNA content in the cell, which is divided into two genomes: the very complex **nuclear genome** and the relatively sim-ple **mitochondrial genome.** The human nuclear genome consists of 24 different chromosomes (22 autosomes; X and Y sex chromosomes). The human nuclear genome codes for **~30,000 genes** (the precise number is uncertain), which make up **~2% of human nuclear genome.** There are **~27,000 protein-coding genes** and **~3,000 RNA-coding genes.** The fact that the ~30,000 genes make up only ~2% of the human nuclear genome means that **~2% of the human nuclear genome consists of coding DNA** and **~98% of the human nuclear genome consists of non-coding DNA.**

A. **GENES.** A gene is a region of DNA that produces a functional RNA molecule. A gene contains two distinct regions.
    1. **Noncoding regions (called introns; intervening sequences)** make up a majority of the nucleotide sequences of a gene.
    2. **Coding regions (called exons; expression sequences)** make up a minority of the nucleotide sequences of a gene.

B. **NUCLEIC ACIDS.** A **nucleoside** consists of a nitrogenous base and a sugar. A **nucleotide** consists of a nitrogenous base, a sugar, and a phosphate group. DNA and RNA consist of a chain of nucleotides that are composed of the following components:
    1. **Nitrogenous bases. Purines (adenine and guanine)** and **pyrimidines (cytosine, thymine, uracil** [present in RNA only]).
    2. **Sugars.** Deoxyribose and ribose (present in RNA only).
    3. **Phosphate (PO_4^{2-})**

C. **SPECIAL DNA NUCLEOTIDE SEQUENCES**
    1. **Centromere.** A centromere is a specialized nucleotide DNA sequence that binds to the mitotic spindle during cell division. A major component of centromeric DNA is **a satellite DNA,** which consists of a 171-bp repeat unit. **β-satellite DNA**

A

Nitrogenous Bases

Purines

Adenine (A)   Guanine (G)

Pyrimidines

Cytosine (C)   Uracil (U)   Thymine (T)

Sugars

Ribose   Deoxyribose

Phosphate

Nucleoside
Nucleoside monophosphate
Nucleoside diphosphate   } Nucleotides
Nucleoside triphosphate

C

Polynucleotide chain

5' end

Adenine

Cytosine

Guanine

Thymine

3´, 5´-Phosphodiester bond

3' end

B

Base	Nucleoside (Base+sugar)	Nucleotide (Base+sugar+phosphate)			Nucleic Acid
		Monophosphate	Diphosphate	Triphosphate	
Purines					
Adennine	Adenosine	AMP	ADP	ATP	RNA
	Deoxyadenosine	dAMP	dADP	dATP	DNA
Guanine	Guanosine	GMP	GDP	GTP	RNA
	Deoxyguanosine	dGMP	dGDP	dGTP	DNA
Pyrimidines					
Cytosine	Cytidine	CMP	CDP	CTP	RNA
	Deoxycytidine	dCMP	dCDP	dCTP	DNA
Thymine	Thymidine	TMP	TDP	TTP	RNA
	Deoxythymidine	dTMP	dTDP	dTTP	DNA
Uracil	Uridine	UMP	UDP	UTP	RNA
	Deoxyuridine	dUMP	dUDP	dUTP	DNA

● **Figure 1-2 (A) Structure of the biochemical components of DNA and RNA (purines, pyrimidines, sugars, and phosphate).** Diagram depicting the chemical structure of the various components of DNA. **(B)** Table indicating the nomenclature of the nucleosides and nucleotides **(C)** Diagram of a DNA polynucleotide chain. The biochemical components (purines, pyrimidines, sugar, and phosphate) form a polynucleotide chain through a 3′, 5′-phosphodiester bond.

(a 68-bp repeat unit) and **satellite 1 DNA** (a 25- to 48- bp repeat unit) are also components of centromeric DNA. A centromere is also associated with a number of centromeric proteins, which include: **CENP-A, CENP-B** (which binds to a 17-bp sequence in a satellite DNA), **CENP-C,** and **CENP-G.** Chromosomes have a single centromere, which is observed microscopically as a **primary constriction,** the region that sister chromatids are joined. During prometaphase, a pair of protein complexes called **kinetochores** forms at the centromere where one kinetochore is attached to each sister chromatid. Microtubules produced by the **centrosome** of the cell attached to the kinetochore (called **kinetochore microtubules**) and pull the two sister chromatids toward opposite poles of the mitotic cell.

2. **TELOMERE.** The human telomere is a 3- to 20-kb repeating nucleotide sequence **(TTAGGG)** located at the end of a chromosome. The 3- to 20-kb $(TTAGGG)_n$ array is preceded by 100–300 kb of telomere–associated repeats before any unique sequence is found. The telomere allows replication of linear DNA to its full length. Since DNA polymerases can *not* synthesize in the $3' \rightarrow 5'$ direction or start synthesis *de novo*, removal of the RNA primers will always leave the 5' end of the lagging strand shorter than the leading strand. If the 5' end of the lagging strand is not lengthened, a chromosome would get progressively shorter as the cell goes through a number of cell divisions. This would lead to cell death and some investigators believe this may be related to the aging process in humans. This problem is solved by a special **RNA-directed DNA polymerase or reverse transcriptase** called **telomerase** (which has a RNA and protein component). The RNA component of telomerase carries a **CCCUAA** sequence (antisense sequence of the TTAGGG telomere), recognizes the TTAGGG sequence on the leading strand, and adds many repeats of TTAGGG to the leading strand. After the repeats of TTAGGG are added to the leading strand, **DNA polymerase α** uses the TTAGGG repeats as a template to synthesize the complementary repeats on the lagging strand. Thus, the lagging strand is lengthened. **DNA ligase** joins the repeats to the lagging strand and a **nuclease** cleaves the ends to form double helix DNA with flush ends. Telomerase is present in human germline cells (i.e., spermatogonia, oogonia) and stem cells (e.g., in skin, bone marrow, and gut), but is absent from most other somatic cells. When a somatic cell without telomerase divides, the telomere length decreases by ~50–100 bp per cell division. Most somatic cells in prolonged culture reach a point of **senescence** where they stop dividing. However, some somatic cells that are deficient in tumor suppressor genes (e.g., p53 or Rb; see Chapter 14) can continue beyond senescence and hit a **crisis point** where most cells die but a few cells survive that have gross chromosomal abnormalities, acquire telomerase, and therefore become **immortalized cells.**

VI   Chromosome Replication (Figure 1-3).

A. The replication process starts when **topoisomerase** nicks (or breaks) a single strand of DNA, which causes DNA unwinding.

B. Chromosome replication begins at specific nucleotide sequences located throughout the chromosome called **replication origins.** Eukaryotic DNA contains **multiple replication origins** to ensure rapid DNA synthesis. If human chromosome 1 contained only one replication origin, the rate of cell division would be severely decreased. Assume that human chromosome 1 contains 260,000,000 base pairs, the replication origin is located in the exact *center* of the chromosome, and DNA synthesis occurs at a rate of 100 base pairs/second. Two replication forks form (one at each end of the replication bubble) so that each replication fork will replicate 130,000,000 base pairs since the replication origin is located in the center of chromosome 1. Therefore, the total time to replicate chromosome 1 is 1,300,000 seconds or about **15 days** (1,300,000 base pairs ÷ 100 base pairs/second = 1,300,000 seconds). Normally, the S phase of the mammalian cell cycle is **8 hours.** If the single replication origin was located *off-center* (to one end of the chromosome), the total time to replicate chromosome 1 would be even longer than 15 days since now one replication fork would have to do most of the replication by itself.

C. **DNA HELICASE** recognizes the replication origin and opens up the double helix at that site forming a **replication bubble** with a **replication fork** at each end. The stability of the replication fork is maintained by **single-stranded binding proteins.**

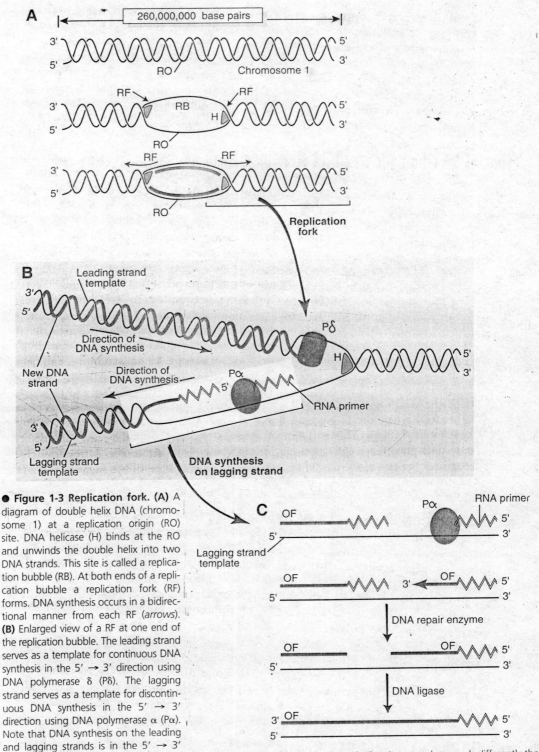

● **Figure 1-3 Replication fork. (A)** A diagram of double helix DNA (chromosome 1) at a replication origin (RO) site. DNA helicase (H) binds at the RO and unwinds the double helix into two DNA strands. This site is called a replication bubble (RB). At both ends of a replication bubble a replication fork (RF) forms. DNA synthesis occurs in a bidirectional manner from each RF (*arrows*). **(B)** Enlarged view of a RF at one end of the replication bubble. The leading strand serves as a template for continuous DNA synthesis in the 5′ → 3′ direction using DNA polymerase δ (Pδ). The lagging strand serves as a template for discontinuous DNA synthesis in the 5′ → 3′ direction using DNA polymerase α (Pα). Note that DNA synthesis on the leading and lagging strands is in the 5′ → 3′ direction but physically are running in opposite directions. **(C)** DNA synthesis on the lagging strand proceeds differently than on the leading strand. DNA primase synthesizes RNA primers. DNA polymerase α uses these RNA primers to synthesize DNA fragments called Okazaki fragments (OF). Okazaki fragments end when they run into a downstream RNA primer. Subsequently, DNA repair enzymes remove the RNA primers and replace it with DNA. Finally, DNA ligase joins all the Okazaki fragments together.

D. A replication fork contains a:
1. **Leading strand** that is synthesized continuously by **DNA polymerase δ (delta)**.
2. **Lagging strand** that is synthesized discontinuously by **DNA polymerase α (alpha)**. **DNA primase** synthesizes short RNA primers along the lagging strand. DNA polymerase α uses the RNA primer to synthesize DNA fragments called **Okazaki fragments**. Okazaki fragments end when they run into a downstream RNA primer. To form a continuous DNA strand from the Okazaki fragments, a **DNA repair enzyme** erases the RNA primers and replaces it with DNA. **DNA ligase** subsequently joins all the DNA fragments together.

VII Types of DNA Damage and DNA Repair.

Chromosomal breakage refers to breaks in chromosomes due to sunlight (or ultraviolet) irradiation, ionizing irradiation, DNA cross-linking agents, or DNA damaging agents. These insults may cause **depurination of DNA, deamination of cytosine to uracil**, or **pyrimidine dimerization** which must be repaired by DNA repair enzymes. In general, DNA repair involves **DNA excision** of the damaged site, **DNA synthesis** of the correct sequence, and **DNA ligation**. The normal response to DNA damage is to stall the cell in the G_1 phase of the cell cycle until the damage is repaired. The system that detects and signals DNA damage is a multiprotein complex called **BASC (BRCA1-associated genome surveillance complex)**. Some of the components of BASC include: **ATM (ataxia telangiectasia mutated) protein** where one region resembles a Pl-3 kinase and another region resembles a DNA repair enzyme/cell cycle checkpoint protein; **nibrin**; **BRCA1 protein**; and **BRCA2 protein**. The clinical importance of DNA repair enzymes is illustrated by some rare inherited diseases that involve genetic defects in DNA repair enzymes, such as xeroderma pigmentosa (XP), ataxia-telangiectasia, Fanconi anemia, Bloom syndrome, and hereditary nonpolyposis colorectal cance.

A. DEPURINATION. About 5,000 purines (As or Gs) per day are lost from DNA of each human cell when the N-glycosyl bond between the purine and deoxyribose sugar-phosphate is broken. This is the most frequent type of lesion and leaves the deoxyribose sugar-phosphate with a missing purine base. To begin repair, **AP endonuclease** recognizes the site of the missing purine and nicks the deoxyribose sugar-phosphate. A **phosphodiesterase** excises the deoxyribose sugar-phosphate. **DNA polymerase** and **DNA ligase** restores the correct DNA sequence.

B. DEAMINATION OF CYTOSINE OF URACIL. About 100 cytosines (C) per day are spontaneously deaminated to uracil (U). If the U is not corrected back to a C, then upon replication instead of the occurrence of a correct C-G base pairing, U-A base pairing will occur instead. To begin repair, **uracil-DNA glycosidase** recognizes uracil and removes it. This enzyme does not remove thymine since thymine is distinguished from uracil by a **methyl group on carbon 5**. An **AP endonuclease** recognizes the site of the missing base and nicks the deoxyribose sugar-phosphate. A **phosphodiesterase** excises the deoxyribose sugar-phosphate. **DNA polymerase** and **DNA ligase** restore the correct DNA sequence.

C. PYRIMIDINE DIMERIZATION. Sunlight (UV radiation) can cause covalent linkage of adjacent pyrimidines forming for example, **thymine dimers**. To begin repair, **uvrABC enzyme** recognizes the pyrimidine dimer and excises a 12-residue oligonucleotide that includes the dimer. **DNA polymerase** and **DNA ligase** restore the correct DNA sequence.

VIII Clinical Importance of DNA Repair.

Breakages are breaks in chromosomes due to sunlight (or ultraviolet) irradiation, ionizing irradiation, DNA cross-linking agents, or DNA damaging agents. These insults may cause **depuration of DNA, deamination of cytosine to uracil**, or **pyrimidine dimerization,** which must be repaired by DNA repair enzymes. The clinical importance of DNA repair enzymes is illustrated by some rare inherited diseases that involve genetic defects in DNA repair enzymes such as the following.

A. **XERODERMA PIGMENTOSUM (XP)** is an autosomal recessive genetic disorder in which the affected individuals are hypersensitive to **sunlight (UV radiation).** XP is characterized by: acute sun sensitivity with sunburn-like reaction, severe skin lesions around the eyes and eyelids, and malignant skin cancers (basal and squamous cell carcinomas and melanomas) whereby most individuals die by 30 years of age. XP is caused by the inability to remove pyrimidine dimers due to a genetic defect in one or more of the **nucleotide excision repair enzymes.** There are seven complementation groups in XP (**XPA-XPG**). The seven genes involved in the cause of XP include: **XPA gene** located on chromosome 9q22.3 which encodes for a DNA repair enzyme; **ERCC3 gene** located on chromosome 2q21, which encodes for TFIIH basal transcription factor complex helicase; **XPC gene** located on chromosome 3p25, which encodes for a DNA repair enzyme; **ERCC2 gene** located on chromosome 19q13.2, which encodes for TFIIH basal transcription factor complex helicase; **DDB2 gene** located on chromosome 11p12, which encodes for DNA damage binding protein 2; **ERCC4 gene** located on chromosome 16p 13.3, which encodes for a DNA repair enzyme; **ERCC5 gene** located on chromosome 13q33, which encodes for DNA repair enzyme. There is an XP variant gene (**XPV gene or hRAD30 gene**), which encodes for DNA polymerase eta that is involved in error-free replication of DNA damaged by UV radiation.

B. **ATAXIA-TELANGIECTASIA (AT)** is an autosomal recessive genetic disorder involving a gene locus on chromosome 11q22-q23 in which the affected individuals are hypersensitive to **ionizing radiation.** AT is characterized by: cerebellar ataxia with depletion of Purkinje cells; progressive nystagmus; slurred speech; oculocutaneous telangiectasia initially in the bulbar conjunctiva followed by ear, eyelid, cheeks, and neck immunodeficiency; and death in the second decade of life. AT is caused by genetic defects in **DNA recombination repair enzymes.** The **ATM gene (AT mutated)** is involved in the cause of AT. The ATM gene located on chromosome 11q22 encodes for a protein where one region resembles a **Pl-3 kinase** (phosphatidylinositol-3 kinase) and another region resembles a **DNA repair enzyme/cell cycle checkpoint protein.**

C. **FANCONI'S ANEMIA (FA;** the most common form of congenital aplastic anemia) is an autosomal recessive genetic disorder involving gene loci on chromosomes 16q24, 9q22, and 3p26 in which affected individuals are hypersensitive to **DNA cross-linking agents.** FA is characterized by: short stature, hypopigmented spots, café-au-lait spots, hypogonadism, microcephaly, hypoplastic or aplastic thumbs, renal malformation including unilateral aplasia or horseshoe kidney, acute leukemia, progressive aplastic anemia, head and neck tumors, and medulloblastoma. FA is caused by genetic defects in **DNA recombination repair enzymes** used to repair chromosome defects that occur during homologous recombination. There are eleven complementation groups in FA (**FA-A to FA-L**). To date, eight of the genes have been cloned. The **FA-A gene** (involved in 65% of FA cases) located on chromosome 16q24 encodes for a protein that normalizes cell growth, corrects sensitivity to chromosomal breakage in the presence of mitomycin C, and generally promotes genomic stability. Several of the FA genes form a nuclear-protein complex that interacts with **BRCA1 and BRCA2** (breast cancer susceptibility genes 1 and 2) as the final common pathway. In this regard, BRCA2 has been found to be identical to FANC-D1.

D. BLOOM SYNDROME (BS) is an autosomal recessive genetic disorder involving a gene locus on chromosome 15q26 in which affected individuals are hypersensitive to a **wide variety of DNA-damaging agents.** BS is characterized by: long, narrow face; erythema with telangiectasias in a butterfly distribution over the nose and cheeks; high-pitched voice; small stature; small mandible; immunodeficiency with decreased IgA, IgM, and IgG levels; predisposition to several types of cancers; and increased frequency in the Ashkenazi Jewish population. BS is caused by genetic defects in enzymes involved in DNA repair. The **BLM gene** is involved in the cause of BS. The BLM gene located on chromosome 15q26 encodes for a protein that has strong homology to the **RecQ helicases** (a subfamily of DExH box-containing DNA and RNA helicases).

E. HEREDITARY NONPOLYPOSIS COLORECTAL CANCER (HNPCC) is an autosomal-dominant genetic disorder that accounts for 3%–5% of all colorectal cancers. HNPCC is characterized by: onset of colorectal cancer at a young age; high frequency of carcinomas proximal to the splenic flexure; multiple synchronous or metachronous colorectal cancers; and presence of extracolonic cancers (e.g., endometrial and ovarian cancer; adenocarcinomas of the stomach, small intestine, and hepatobiliary tract). HNPCC is caused by genetic defects in **DNA mismatch repair enzymes** that recognize single nucleotide mismatches or loops that occur in microsatellite repeat areas. The **MLH1, MSH2, MSH6, PMS1, and PMS2 genes** are involved in the cause of HPNCC. These genes are the human homologues to the *Escherichia coli* **mutS** and **mutL** genes that code for DNA mismatch repair enzymes.

IX Cell Cycle

A. PHASES OF THE CELL CYCLE (Table 1-2)
1. **G_0 (gap) phase.** The G_0 phase is the resting phase of the cell where the cell cycle is suspended.
2. **G_1 (gap) phase.** The G_1 phase is the gap of time between mitosis (M phase) and DNA synthesis (S phase). The G_1 phase is the phase in which **RNA, protein, and organelle synthesis** occurs. The G_1 phase lasts about **5 hours** in a typical mammalian cell with a 16-hour cell cycle.
3. **S (synthesis) phase.** The S phase is the phase in which **DNA synthesis** occurs. The S phase lasts about **7 hours** in a typical mammalian cell with a 16-hour cell cycle.
4. **G_2 (gap) phase.** The G_2 phase is the gap of time between DNA synthesis (S phase) and mitosis (M phase). The G_2 phase is the phase in which **ATP synthesis** occurs. The G_2 phase lasts about **3 hours** in a typical mammalian cell with a 16-hour cell cycle.
5. **M (mitosis) phase.** The M phase is the phase in which **cell division** occurs. The M phase is divided into six stages called **prophase, prometaphase, metaphase, anaphase, telophase,** and **cytokinesis.** The M phase lasts about **1 hour** in a typical mammalian cell with a 16-hour cell cycle.

B. CONTROL OF THE CELL CYCLE (Figure 1-4)
1. **Cdk–cyclin complexes.** The two main protein families that control the cell cycle are **cyclins** and the **cyclin-dependent protein kinases (Cdks).** A cyclin is a protein that regulates the activity of Cdks and are named because cyclins undergo a cycle of synthesis and degradation during the cell cycle. The cyclins and Cdks form complexes called **Cdk–cyclin complexes.** The ability of Cdks to phosphorylate target proteins is dependent on the particular cyclin that complexes with it.

Table 1-2

G$_0$ Phase

Resting phase
Cell cycle suspended

G$_1$ Phase

Lasts 5 hours
RNA, protein, and organelle synthesis
Cdk2-cyclin D and Cdk2-cyclin E synthesis

p53

⊖

Cdk2-cyclin D
Cdk2-cyclin E

⊕ → G$_1$ checkpoint

S Phase

Lasts 7 hours
DNA synthesis
RNA and histone synthesis
Centrosome (MTOC) duplicates but remains together as a complex on one side of the
    nucleus
Methotrexate (Folex), 5-fluorouracil (Adrucil), Cytarabine (cytosine arabinoside), 6-mer
    captopurine, Doxorubicin (Adriamycin), Daunorubicin (Cerubidine) are S phase
    specific

← Etoposide prevents entry into G$_2$ phase

G$_2$ Phase

Lasts 3 hours
ATP synthesis
Cdk1-cyclin A and Cdk1-cyclin B synthesis
Bleomycin (Blenoxane) is G$_2$ phase specific

Cdk1-cyclin A
Cdk1-cyclin B

⊕ → G$_2$ checkpoint

Interphase
Lasts 15 hours

PROPHASE

Chromatin condenses to form well-defined chromosomes
Centrosomes (MTOC) move to opposite poles
Mitotic spindle (microtubules) forms between the centrosomes

PROMETAPHASE

Nuclear envelope dis-assembles
Nucleolus disappears
Kinetochores assemble at each centromere
Kinetochore, polar, and astral microtubules are apparent

METAPHASE

Chromosomes align at the metaphase plate
Cells can be arrested in this phase by microtubule inhibitors (e.g., colchicine)
Cells can be isolated for karyotype analysis

ANAPHASE

Cyclins are inactivated by polyubiquitination
Kinetochores separate and chromosomes move to opposite poles

TELOPHASE

Chromosomes decondense to form chromatin
Nuclear envelope re-assembles
Nucleolus reappears

CYTOKINESIS

Cytoplasm divides by a process called cleavage
A cleavage furrow forms around the middle of the cell
A contractile ring (actin and myosin) forms at the cleavage furrow

M Phase
Lasts 1 hour
Vinblastin (Velban), Vincristine (Oncovin), and Pazlitaxel (Taxol) are M phase specific

● **Figure 1-4 Diagram of the cell cycle with checkpoints and signaling mechanisms.** Note the location of the four stop signs. → = activation; — = inactivation.

    a. **Cdk2–cyclin D and Cdk2–cyclin E:** mediate the $G_1 \rightarrow S$ **phase** transition at the G_1 **checkpoint.**

    b. **Cdk1–cyclin A and Cdk1–cyclin B:** mediate the $G_2 \rightarrow M$ **phase** transition at the G_2 **checkpoint.**

  2. **Checkpoints.** The checkpoints in the cell cycle are specialized signaling mechanisms that regulate and coordinate the cell response to **DNA damage** (e.g., dimers,

mismatches, base modifications [oxidative damage, aberrant methylation, depurination], intrastrand cross-links, interstrand cross-links, single-strand breaks, and double-strand breaks) and **replication fork blockage.** When the extent of DNA damage or replication fork blockage is beyond the steady-state threshold of DNA repair pathways, a checkpoint signal is produced and a checkpoint is activated. The activation of a checkpoint slows down the cell cycle so that DNA repair may occur and/or blocked replication forks can be recovered. This prevents DNA damage from being converted into inheritable mutations producing highly transformed, metastatic cells.

The **ATR kinase** (a member of the PI-3-kinase–like kinase family) and its associated proteins **ATRIP, Rad17, Rad9, Rad1,** and **Hus1** respond to the **sustained presence of single-stranded DNA (ssDNA)** because ssDNA is generated in virtually all types of DNA damage and replication fork blockage by activation (i.e., phosphorylation) of **Chk1 kinase** and **p53.** The ATR response also requires additional proteins that include: **BRCA1, claspin, TopBP1,** and **Mdc1.** The **ATM kinase** (a member of the PI-3-kinase–like kinase family) responds particularly to **double-stranded DNA breaks** by activation (i.e., phosphorylation) of **Chk2 kinase** and **p53.** The ATM response also requires additional proteins that include: **53BP1** and **Mdc1.**

3. **Control of the G_1 checkpoint.** There are three pathways that control the G_1 checkpoint, which include:

   a. Depending on the type of the DNA damage, **ATR kinase** and **ATM kinase** will activate (i.e., phosphorylate) **Chk1 kinase** or **Chk2 kinase,** respectively. The activation of Chk1 kinase or Chk2 kinase causes the inactivation of **CDC25A phosphatase** (a tyrosine phosphatase that normally activates Cdk2–cyclin D and Cdk2–cyclin E by removing inhibitory tyrosine phosphorylation). The inactivation of CDC25A phosphatase causes the downstream stoppage at the G_1 checkpoint. The downstream pathways is as follows: Cdk2–cyclinD and Cdk2–cyclinE phosphorylates the E2F–RB complex, which causes phosphorylated RB to disassociate from E2F. E2F is a transcription factor that causes the expression of gene products that stimulate the cell cycle.

   b. Depending on the type of the DNA damage, **ATR kinase** and **ATM kinase** will activate (i.e., phosphorylate) **p53,** which allows p53 to disassociate from **Mdm2** (a ubiquitin ligase that inhibits p53 action through protein degradation). The activation of p53 causes the transcriptional upregulation of **p21.** The binding of p21 to the Cdk2–cyclin D and Cdk2–cyclin E inhibits their action and causes downstream stoppage at the G_1 checkpoint. The downstream pathway is as follows: Cdk2–cyclinD and Cdk2–cyclinE phosphorylates the E2F–RB complex, which causes phosphorylated RB to disassociate from E2F. E2F is a transcription factor that causes the expression of gene products that stimulate the cell cycle.

   c. Depending on the type of the DNA damage, **ATR kinase** and **ATM kinase** will activate (i.e., phosphorylate) **p16,** which inactivates **Cdk4/6–cyclin D** (a Cdk–cyclin complex that normally activates RB) and thereby causes downstream stoppage at the G_1 checkpoint. The downstream pathways is as follows: Cdk4/6–cyclinD phosphorylates the E2F–RB complex, which causes phosphorylated RB to disassociate from E2F. E2F is a transcription factor that causes the expression of gene products that stimulate the cell cycle.

4. **Control of the G_2 checkpoint.** Depending on the type of the DNA damage, **ATR kinase** and **ATM kinase** will activate (i.e., phosphorylate) **Chk1 kinase** or **Chk2 kinase,** respectively. The activation of Chk1 kinase or Chk2 kinase causes the inactivation of **CDC25C phosphatase** (a tyrosine phosphatase that activates Cdk1–cyclin

A and Cdk1–cyclin B at the G_2 checkpoint by removing inhibitory tyrosine phosphorylation). The deactivation of CDC25C phosphatase will cause the downstream stoppage at the G_2 checkpoint.

5. **Inactivation of cyclins.** Cyclins are inactivated by **protein degradation** during **anaphase of the M phase.** The cyclin genes contain a homologous DNA sequence called a **destruction box.** A specific **recognition protein** binds to the amino acid sequence coded by the destruction box that allows **ubiquitin** (a 76-amino acid protein) to be covalently attached to lysine residues of cyclin by the enzyme **ubiquitin ligase.** This process is called **polyubiquitination.** Polyubiquitinated cyclins are rapidly degraded by proteolytic enzyme complexes called **protesomes.** Polyubiquitination is a widely occurring process for marking many different types of proteins (cyclins are just a specific example) for rapid degradation.

X Proto-Oncogenes, Oncogenes, and Tumor-Suppressor Genes

A. DEFINITIONS

1. **A proto-oncogene** is a normal gene that encodes a protein involved in **stimulation of the cell cycle.**
2. **An oncogene** is a mutated proto-oncogene that encodes for an **oncoprotein** (that produces abnormalities in the cell cycle leading to the induction of cancer.
3. A **tumor-suppressor gene (or anti-oncogene)** is a normal gene that encodes a protein involved in **suppression of the cell cycle.**

B. THE HISTORY OF PROTO-ONCOGENES AND ONCOGENES.

In the 1960s, it was discovered that some animal cancers (e.g., leukemias and lymphomas) were caused by DNA or RNA viruses. A non–cancer-causing RNA virus contains three transcription units: *gag*, which encodes internal proteins; *pol*, which encodes a polymerase; and *env*, which encodes envelope proteins. However, a cancer-causing RNA virus contains one extra gene called the oncogene, which is responsible for the cancer-causing (or transforming) properties of the virus. This discovery received unparalleled publicity at the time since most scientists thought that all the human cancers would soon be explained by infection with oncogene-containing viruses. However, the excitement was soon dashed when it was realized that oncogenes were nothing more that copies of normal cellular genes (called proto-oncogenes) that had been accidentally incorporated into the RNA virus. We know now that the vast majority of human cancers are not caused by viruses. The majority of human cancers are caused by activation of proto-oncogenes by a number of mechanisms discussed below.

1. **Amplification.** Cancer cells may contain hundreds of extra copies of proto-oncogenes. These extra copies are found as either small paired chromatin bodies separated from the chromosomes (double minutes) or insertions within normal chromosomes. Amplification in cancer cells can be studied by comparative genomic hybridization.
2. **Point mutation.** A point mutation of a proto-oncogene leads to the formation of an oncogene that encodes for an oncoprotein that produces abnormalities in the cell cycle leading to the induction of cancer.
3. **Translocation.** A translocation results from breakage and exchange of segments between chromosomes. This may result in the formation of an oncogene (also called a fusion gene or chimeric gene) that encodes for an oncoprotein (also called a fusion protein or chimeric protein). A good example is seen in chronic myeloid leukemia (CML). CML **t(9;22) (q34;q 11)** is caused by a reciprocal translocation between band q34 on chromosome 9 and band q11 on chromosome 22. This is

referred to as the **Philadelphia chromosome.** This results in a fusion of the **ABL gene** on chromosome 9q34 with the **BCR gene** on chromosome 22q11, thereby forming the *abl/bcr* **oncogene.** The **Abl/Bcr oncoprotein** (a tyrosine kinase) has enhanced tyrosine kinase activity that transforms hematopoietic precursor cells.

4. **Translocation into a transcriptionally active region.** A translocation results from breakage and exchange of segments between chromosomes. This may result in the formation of an oncogene by placing a gene in a transcriptionally active region. A good example is seen in Burkitt lymphoma. **Burkitt lymphoma t(8;14) (q24; q32)** is caused by a reciprocal translocation between band q24 on chromosome 8 and band q32 on chromosome 14. This results in placing the **MYC gene** on chromosome 8q24 in close proximity to the **IGH gene** locus (i.e., an immunoglobulin gene locus) on chromosome 14q32, thereby putting the MYC gene in a transcriptionally active area in B lymphocytes (or antibody-producing plasma cells).

C. **MECHANISM OF ACTION OF THE *RAS* PROTO-ONCOGENE** (Figure 1-6). The *ras* proto-oncogene encodes a normal G-protein with GTPase activity. The G protein is attached to the cytoplasmic face of the cell membrane by a lipid called **farnesyl isoprenoid.** When a hormone binds to its receptor, the G protein is activated. The activated G protein binds GTP, which stimulates the cell cycle. After a brief period, the activated G protein splits GTP into GDP and phosphate such that the stimulation of the cell cycle is terminated. If the *ras* proto-oncogene undergoes a mutation, it forms the *ras* oncogene. The *ras* oncogene encodes an abnormal G protein (Ras oncoprotein) where a glycine is changed to a valine at position 12. The Ras oncoprotein binds GTP, which stimulates the cell cycle. However, the Ras oncoprotein can **not** split GTP into GDP and phosphate, so the stimulation of the cell cycle is never terminated.

D. **TUMOR SUPPRESSOR GENES**
1. **Mechanism of action of the RB tumor-suppressor gene (retinoblastoma)** (Figure 1-7). The RB tumor-suppressor gene is located on chromosome 13q14 and encodes for **normal RB protein** that will bind to **E2F** (a gene regulatory protein) such that there will be no expression of target genes whose gene products stimulate the cell cycle. Therefore, there is suppression of the cell cycle. A mutation of the RB tumor-suppressor gene will encode an **abnormal RB protein** that can not bind to a gene regulatory protein (GRP) such that there will be expression of target genes whose gene products stimulate the cell cycle. Therefore, there is no suppression of the cell cycle. This leads to the formation of a **retinoblastoma** tumor. Even though retinoblastoma is a rare type of cancer, the RB tumor-suppressor gene is involved in many types of human cancer. Retinoblastoma occurs in childhood and develops from precursor cells in the immature retina. There are two types of retinoblastomas:
   a. **Hereditary retinoblastoma.** The individual inherits one mutant copy of the RB gene from his parents. A mutation of the second copy of the RB gene may occur later in life within **many** cells of the retina leading to **multiple tumors in both eyes.**
   b. **Nonhereditary retinoblastoma.** The individual does **not** inherit a mutant copy of the RB from his parents. Instead, two subsequent mutations of both copies of the RB gene may occur within **one** cell of the retina leading to **one tumor in one eye.**
2. **Mechanism of action of the p53 tumor-suppressor gene** (Figure 1-7). The p53 tumor-suppressor gene is located on chromosome 17p13 and encodes for **normal p53 protein (a zinc finger gene regulatory protein)** that will cause the expression of target genes whose gene products suppress the cell cycle at **G1** by inhibiting

Cdk–cyclin D and **Cdk–cyclin E.** Therefore, there is suppression of the cell cycle. A mutation of p53 tumor-suppressor gene will encode an **abnormal p53 protein** that will cause no expression of target genes whose gene products suppress the cell cycle. Therefore, there is no suppression of the cell cycle. The normal role of p53 is to arrest cells with damaged DNA (e.g., by γ-irradiation) in G1 of the cell cycle. The p53 tumor-suppressor gene is the **most common target** for mutation in human cancers. The p53 tumor-suppressor gene plays a role in **Li-Fraumeni syndrome,** which is an inherited susceptibility to a variety of cancers where 50% of the affected individuals develop cancer by age 30 and 90% by age 70.

● **Figure 1-5 Diagram of *ras* oncogene action.**

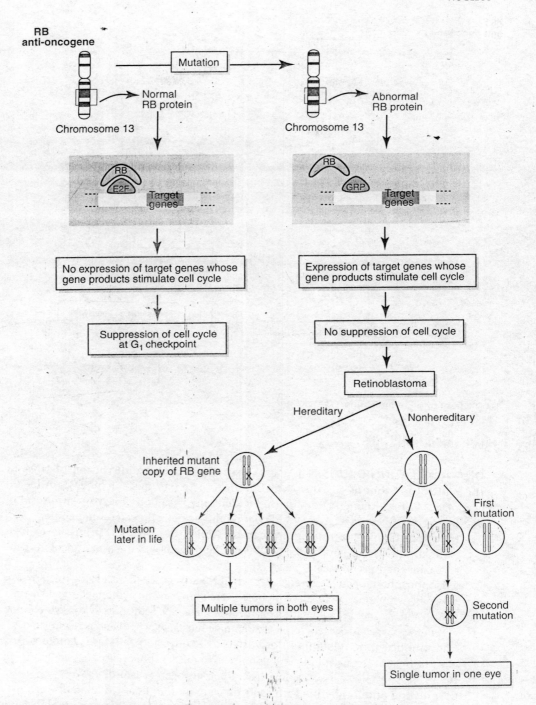

● **Figure 1-6 Diagram of Rb tumor-suppressor action.** E2F = gene regulatory protein.

● **Figure 1-7** Diagram of p53 tumor-suppressor action.

XI Cancer Chemotherapy

A. **DNA ALKYLATING DRUGS.** The mechanism of action is via **alkylation of DNA at the 7-nitrogen atom of guanine,** which leads to base pair mismatching, DNA breakage, or DNA cross-linking. Dose-limiting toxicity involves **bone marrow suppression** and **hemorrhagic cystitis.** All DNA alkylating drugs are **cell cycle nonspecific.**

1. **Mechlorethamine (a nitrogen mustard; Mustargen)** is used primarily to treat Hodgkin disease as part of the MOPP regime (**m**echlorethamine, **o**ncovin, **p**rocarbazine, and **p**rednisone).

2. **Cyclophosphamide (a nitrogen mustard; Cytoxan)** is used to treat Hodgkin and non-Hodgkin lymphomas, Burkitt lymphoma, childhood acute lymphoblastic leukemia (ALL), and Wegner granulomatosis. It requires metabolic activation by the cytochrome P_{450} mono-oxygenase system to phosphoramide mustard (active) and acrolein (toxic).

3. **Chorambucil (phenylalanine derivative of a nitrogen mustard; Leukeran)** is used to treat Waldenstrom macroglobulinemia and chronic lymphocytic leukemia (CLL). It is the slowest-acting and least toxic nitrogen mustard.

4. **Carmustine and lomustine (nitrosoureas)** are used to treat Hodgkin disease, primary brain tumors, astrocytomas, and meningeal leukemia. They are lipophilic and therefore cross the blood-brain barrier.

5. **Busulfan (an alkyl sulfonate; Myleran)** is used to treat chronic myeloid leukemia (CML).

6. **Dacarbazine** is used to treat malignant Hodgkin disease as part of the ABVD regime (**a**driamycin, **b**leomycin, **v**inblastine, and **d**acarbazine) and malignant melanoma. It requires metabolic activation by the cytochrome P_{450} mono-oxygenase to diazomethane and carbonium ions (active compounds).

7. **Cisplatin (Platinol)** is used to treat testicular carcinoma as part of the VBC regime (**v**inblastine, **b**leomycin, and **c**isplatin) and bladder carcinoma. It is a platinum coordination complex which enters the cell by diffusion and alkylates DNA.

B. **ANTIMETABOLITE DRUGS.** The mechanism of action is interference with normal metabolic pathways by competing for enzymatic active sites. All antimetabolite drugs are **cell cycle specific for the S (DNA synthesis) phase.**

1. **Methotrexate (Folex, Mexate)** is a folic acid analogue that competitively inhibits dihydrofolate reductase (DHFR) and therefore inhibits DNA synthesis. It is used for maintenance of remission of childhood ALL Leucovorin (folinic acid) is used to rescue normal cells from methotrexate toxicity (i.e., leucovorin rescue).

2. **5-Fluorouracil (Adrucil)** is a pyrimidine analogue that is converted to F-deoxyuridine monophosphate (5F-dUMP), which covalently binds to thymidylate synthetase and tetrahydrofolate (i.e., forms a tertiary complex). This blocks the conversion of dUMP to deoxythymidine monophosphate (dTMP) so that no thymidine is formed ("thymidineless death") and DNA synthesis stops. It is used to treat metastatic colorectal carcinoma, basal cell carcinoma, and breast carcinoma.

3. **Cytarabine (cytosine arabinoside)** is a pyrimidine nucleoside analogue (the deoxyribose sugar is replaced by arabinose) that is converted intracellularly to arabinose deoxycytidine triphosphate (Ara-dCTP). Ara-dCTP inhibits DNA polymerase and alters function of newly synthesized DNA. It is used to treat acute myeloid leukemia (AML).

4. **6-Mercaptopurine** is a purine analogue of hypoxanthine that is converted to thioinosine monophosphate (tIMP) by hypoxanthine-guanine phosphoribosyltransferase (HGPRT). tIMP blokcs the conversion of IMP to adenosine monophosphate (AMP) and guanosine monophosphate (GMP). It is used to treat childhood ALL and AML.

C. **VINCA PLANT ALKALOIDS** are derived from the periwinkle plant and bind to tubulin, which is the protein component of microtubules, thereby inhibiting microtubule assembly (i.e., polymerization; a spindle poison). Vinca plant alkaloid are **cell-cycle–specific for the M (mitosis) phase.**

1. **Vinblastine (Velban)** is used to treat testicular carcinoma (part of **V**BC regime) and Hodgkin disease (part of ABVD regime).

2. **Vincristine (Oncovin)** is used to treat Hodgkin disease (part of M**O**PP regime)

3. **Paclitaxel (Taxol)**

D. **EPIPODOPHYLLOTOXIN (ETOPOSIDE)** is derived from the myapple plant and inhibits DNA topoisomerase II. It is cell cycle specific for the S phase $\rightarrow$ G_2 phase (i.e., prevents entry into the G_2 phase).

E. **ANTIBIOTICS**

1. **Dactinomycin (Actinomycin; Cosmegen)** is used to treat Wilms' tumor as part of the VAC regime (**v**incristine, **a**ctinomycin, **c**yclophosphamide). It inhibits DNA-dependent RNA polymerase and is cell cycle non-specific.

2. **Doxorubicin (Adriamycin) and daunorubicin (Cerubidine)** are used to treat AML and ALL. They are anthracycline antibiotics and are cell-cycle–specific for the S phase although at low doses cells may proceed to the G_2 phase and die.

3. **Bleomycin (Blenoxane)** is used to treat testicular carcinoma (part of the VBC regime). It produces free radicals that cause DNA fragmentation and is cell cycle specific for the G_2 phase.

F. **ENDOCRINE AGENTS**

1. **Glucocorticoids (Prednisone)** binds to the glucocorticoid receptor and inhibits T-cell proliferation and induces T-cell apoptosis.

2. **Tamoxifen (Novaldex)** competitively inhibits the binding of estrogen to the estrogen receptor. It is used to treat breast carcinoma.

3. **Flutamide (Euflex)** is an androgen receptor antagonist. It is used to treat prostatic carcinoma along with leuprolide.

4. **Leuprolide (Lupron)** is gonadotropin-releasing hormone (GnRH) analogue that inhibits the release of FSH and LH from the hypophysis when administered in a continous fashion.

G. **IMMUNOMODULATOR DRUGS.** These drugs are used mainly in conjunction with chemotherapy to heighten the immune response.

1. **Granulocyte-colony stimulating factor (G-CSF) and granulocyte-macrophage colony stimulating factor (GM-CSF)** are recombinant G-CSF and GM-CSF that stimulate the proliferation and activation of neutrophils (G-CSF) or granulocytes/macrophages (GM-CSF), respectively.

2. **Levamisole** stimulates delayed hypersensitivity and T-cell–mediated immunity.

3. **Bacillus Calmette-Guerin (BCG; Theracys)** is an attenuated strain of *Mycobacterium bovis* that activates T cells and natural killer cells.

4. **Alesleukin (Proleukin)** is a recombinant IL-2 that promotes differentiation of lymphocytes into cytotoxic T cells and natural killer cells.

XII Oncofetal Antigens and Tumor Markers (Table 1-3)

TABLE 1-3

Antigen	Associated Tumor
α-Fetoprotein (AFP)	Hepatocellular carcinoma, germ cell neoplasms, yolk sac or endodermal sinus tumors of the testicle or ovary
AAT	Hepatocellular carcinoma, yolk sac or endodermal sinus tumors of the testicle or ovary
Carcinoembryonic antigen (CEA)	Colorectal cancer, pancreatic cancer, breast cancer, and small cell cancer of the lung; bad prognostic sign if elevated preoperatively
β_2-Microglobulin	Multiple myeloma (excellent prognostic factor), light chains in urine (Bence Jones protein)
CA 125	Surface derived ovarian cancer
CA 15-3	Breast cancer
CA 19-9	Pancreatic cancer (excellent marker)
Neuron-specific enolase (NSE)	Small cell carcinoma of the lung, seminoma, neuroblastoma
Prostate-specific antigen (PSA)	Prostate cancer
hCG	Trophoblastic tumors; hydatidiform mole (benign); choriocarcinoma (malignant)
Bombesin	Small cell carcinoma of the lung, neuroblastoma
LDH	Hodgkin's disease
S-100	Melanoma
Placental alkaline phosphatase	Seminoma
CD1	Histiocytosis
Synaptophysin	Carcinoid tumors
Calcitonin	Medullary carcinoma of the thyroid
Catecholamines	Pheochromocytoma, neuroblastoma

CA = cancer antigen.

XIII Transcription

Transcription in Protein Synthesis (Figure 1-8). In protein synthesis, RNA polymerase II produces an RNA transcript that is further processed into mRNA by a complex process that involves a number of **general transcription factors** called **TFIIs** (transcription factors for RNA polymerase II). **TFIID** binds to the TATA box, which then allows the adjacent binding of **TFIIB**. The next step involves **TFIIA, TFIIE, TFIIF,** and **TFIIH,** and **RNA polymerase II** engaged to the promoter forming a **transcription initiation (TI) complex.** The TI complex must gain access to the DNA template strand at the transcription start site. This is accomplished by TFIIH, which contains a **DNA helicase.** In addition, TFIIH, also contains a **protein kinase** that phosphorylates RNA polymerase II so that RNA polymerase II is released from the TI complex. However, the TI complex will produce only a **basal level of transcription** or **constitutive expression.** Other factors called **cis-acting DNA sequences** and **trans-acting proteins** are necessary.

● **Figure 1-8 Transcription in protein synthesis.** TFIIs = transcription factors for RNA polymerase II; TI = transcription initiation complex; TATA = TATA box (a repeated DNA sequence of thymine and adenine); P = phosphate group.

XIV **Processing the RNA Transcript into mRNA** (Figure 1-9). A cell involved in protein synthesis will use RNA polymerase II to transcribe a protein-coding gene into a **RNA transcript** that must be further processed into mRNA. This processing involves:

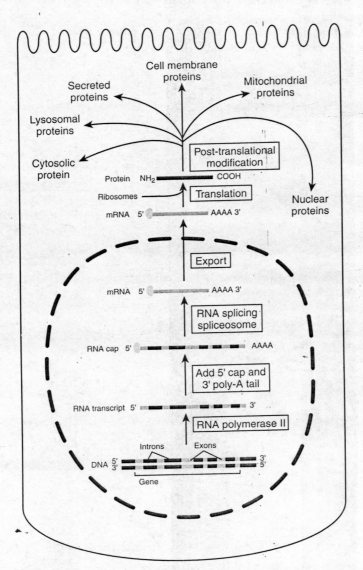

● **Figure 1-9 Transcription and processing of RNA into mRNA.** All eucaryotic genes contains non-coding regions (introns) separated by coding regions (exons). During transcription, RNA polymerase II transcribes both intron and exon sequences into a RNA transcript. A 5′-cap and a 3′-polyA tail are added. The introns are spliced out of the RNA transcript by a spliceosome, so that all the exons are joined in sequence. The mRNA with the 5′-cap and 3′-polyA tail is then able to exit the nucleus through the nuclear pore complex into the cytoplasm for subsequent translation into protein. Proteins then undergo post-translational modifications and are directed to various regions of the cell.

A. RNA CAPPING is the addition of a **7-methylguanosine** to the first nucleotide at the **5′ end** of the RNA transcript. RNA capping functions: to protect the RNA transcript from exonuclease attack, facilitate transport from the nucleus to the cytoplasm, facilitate RNA splicing, and attach the mRNA to the 40S subunit of the ribosome.

B. RNA POLYADENYLATION is the addition of a **poly-A tail** (about 200 repeated AMPs) to the **3′ end** of the RNA transcript. The **AAUAAA sequence** is a **polyadenylation signal sequence,** which signals the 3′ cleavage of the RNA transcript. After 3′ cleavage, polyadenylation occurs. RNA polyadenylation functions to protect against degradation, facilitate transport from the nucleus to the cytoplasm, and enhance recognition of the mRNA by the ribosomes.

C. RNA SPLICING is a process whereby all **introns (noncoding regions; intervening sequences)** are removed from the RNA transcript and all **exons (coding regions; expression sequences)** are joined together within the RNA transcript. RNA splicing requires that the intron/exon boundaries (or **splice junctions**) be recognized. In most cases, introns start with a GT (GU at the RNA level) sequence and end with a GU sequence (called the **GT-GU rule**). RNA splicing is carried out by a large RNA–protein complex called the **spliceosome,** which consists of **five types of small nuclear RNA (i.e., U1snRNA, U2snRNA, U4snRNA, U5snRNA, and U6 snRNA)** and more than **50 different proteins.** Each snRNA is complexed to specific proteins to form **small nuclear ribonucleoprotein particles (snRNPs).** The RNA portion of the snRNPs hybridizes to a nucleotide sequence that marks the intron site (GT-GU rule), whereas the protein potion cuts out the intron and rejoins the RNA transcript. This produces **mRNA** that can leave the nucleus and be translated in the cytoplasm. There are two types of splicesomes: the **major GU-AG spliceosome,** which splices GT-GU introns, and the **minor AU-AC spliceosome,** which splices the rare class of AT-AC introns. Systemic lupus erythematousus (SLE) is a chronic autoimmune disease that causes rashes, arthritis, and kidney disease caused by autoantibodies frequently against components of the nucleus (e.g., snRNPs).

XV Selected Photomicrographs

A. Nucleus, nuclear envelope, nuclear pore complex, and apoptosis (Figure 1-10)

B. Chromatin, nucleosome, and metaphase chromosome (Figure 1-11).

● **Figure 1-10 The nucleus. (A)** EM of a nucleus shows predominately euchromatin (E), peripherally located heterochromatin (H), and conspicuous nucleolus (NL). **Inset:** Nuclear envelope with nuclear pores (large arrows) is shown. **(B)** Diagram shows the interconnections between the nuclear envelope and the rough endoplasmic reticulum. **(C)** Diagram of a model of the nuclear pore complex. **(D)** A freeze-fracture replica of the nuclear envelope shows a nuclear pore complex (*arrow 1*) and the outer membrane of the nuclear envelope that has been stripped away (*arrow 2*), exposing the perinuclear cisterna **(E)** EM of nucleoplasmin labeled with colloidal gold particles. Nucleoplasmin is a large protein synthesized in the cytoplasm and transported into the nucleus. *Brackets* denote a nuclear pore complex. Note that the gold particles are localized specifically at the nuclear pore complex as nucleoplasmin moves from the cytoplasm to nucleus. **(F, G, H)** Apoptosis. Human T cells treated with a lipid hydroperoxide that is toxic to cells and induces apoptosis. **(F)** EM shows the chromatin of an apoptotic cell condensed into a distinctive crescent-shaped pattern along the inner margins of the nuclear envelope. **(G)** EM shows chromatin clumping and mitochondrial changes (*arrows*). **(H)** EM shows various apoptotic bodies.

● **Figure 1-11 DNA. (A)** EM of DNA containing the gene for ovalbumin hybridized with ovalbumin mRNA. Linear regions of the gene (bracket 1) that hybridize to mRNA are called **exons** because the processed mRNA "exits" the nucleus into the cytoplasm to participate in translation. Looped regions of the gene (*arrow 2*) that do *not* hybridize to mRNA are called **introns. (B)** Electron micrograph of DNA isolated and subjected to treatments that unfold its native structure. This "beads-on-a-string" appearance is the basic unit of chromatin packing called a **nucleosome.** The globular structure ("bead") (*arrow 1*) is a histone octamer that is composed of specific proteins (H2A, H2B, H3, and H4). The linear structure ("string") (*arrow 2*) is DNA. **(C)** A diagram of a nucleosome demonstrating the histone octamer (arrow 1) and DNA (arrow 2). **(D)** Electron micrograph of a mitotic cell in metaphase showing the metaphase chromosomes (arrows) aligned at the metaphase plate. **(E)** Electron micrograph of an isolated metaphase chromosome. **(F)** Diagram of a metaphase chromosome showing the centromere **(C).**

Chapter 2

Cytoplasm and Organelles

I **Cytoplasm.** The cytoplasm has a wide composition that includes:

A. **ENZYMES** involved in various biochemical pathways: **glycolysis** (e.g., hexokinase, phosphofructokinase), **fatty acid synthesis** (e.g., fatty acid synthase), three reactions of the **urea cycle (using argininosuccinate synthetase, argininosuccinate lyase, and arginase),** **glycogen synthesis** (e.g., glycogen synthase), **glycogen degradation** (e.g., glycogen phosphorylase), and **protein synthesis** (e.g., aminoacyl-tRNA synthetase, peptidyl transferase).

B. **PROTEOSOMES** are proteolytic enzyme complexes that are involved in the rapid degradation of a **ubiquitinylated protein** (i.e., addition of **ubiquitin** to the lysine amino acid of a protein by **ubiquitin ligase**). For example, **cyclins** are inactivated by this process during anaphase of mitosis. In addition, **endogenous antigens** (produced by intracellular viruses or bacteria) undergo proteosomal degradation by proteosomes to form antigen peptide fragments that become associated with **Class I MHC** and are transported and exposed on the cell surface of the infected cell.

C. **INTERMEDIATES OF METABOLISM.**

D. **COFACTORS (E.G., NAD, NADH).**

E. **STEROID HORMONE RECEPTORS** (Figure 2-1). Steroid hormone receptors are composed structurally of a polypeptide with a zinc atom that is bound to four cysteine amino acids, which falls into the classification of a **zinc finger protein**. A zinc finger protein has a **hormone-binding region** and a **DNA-binding region** that activates gene transcription. Steroid hormone receptors include the **estrogen receptor, glucocorticoid receptor, progesterone receptor, thyroid hormone (T3 and T4) receptor, retinoic acid receptor, 1,25-dihydroxyvitamin D$_3$ receptor.**

II **Ribosomes.**
Ribosomes are large RNA–protein complexes that consist of a **40S (small) subunit** and a **60S (large) subunit,** both of which contain rRNA and various proteins. The 40S subunit (consisting of 18S rRNA and ~30 ribosomal proteins) **binds to mRNA and tRNA** and **finds the start codon AUG.** The 60S subunit (consisting of 5S rRNA, 5.8S rRNA, 28S rRNA, and ~50 ribosomal proteins) **binds to the 40S subunit** after it finds the start codon and has **peptidyl transferase activity.** Ribosomes provide the structural framework for the **translation of mRNA** into an amino acid sequence (i.e., **protein synthesis**) to occur. The RNA components are predominantly responsible for the catalytic function of the ribosome. Ribosomes may cluster along a strand of mRNA to form a **polyribosome (or polysome)** that is involved in the **synthesis of cytoplasmic proteins** (e.g., actin, hemoglobulin). Or, ribosomes may be directed to the endoplasmic reticulum to form rER if

● **Figure 2-1 Mechanism of steroid hormone action.** An inactive steroid hormone receptor is found in the cytoplasm where it is bound to **heat shock proteins (hsp 90 and hsp 56).** When a steroid hormone (e.g., 17b-estradiol) diffuses across the cell membrane and binds to the hormone-binding regions of the receptor, hsp 90 and hsp 56 are released and the DNA-binding region is exposed. Subsequently, the steroid hormone–receptor complex is transported into the nucleus, where it binds to DNA and activates the transcription of a small number of specific genes within approximately 30 minutes **(primary response).** The gene products of the primary response activate other genes to produce a **secondary response.** Steroid hormone receptors are actually gene regulatory proteins.

the nascent protein contains a hydrophobic **signal sequence** at its amino terminal end, which is cleaved in the rER lumen by **signal peptidase.**

Ⅲ **Rough Endoplasmic Reticulum (rER).** This membranous organelle contains ribosomes attached to its cytoplasmic surface by the binding of **ribophorin I and II** to the **60S subunit** of the ribosome. The rER is the site of **synthesis of secretory proteins** (e.g., insulin), **cell membrane proteins** (e.g., receptors), and **lysosomal enzymes.** The rER is the site of **co-translational modification** of proteins which includes:

A. **N-LINKED GLYCOSYLATION** (addition of sugars to asparagines begins in the rER and is completed in the Golgi complex)

B. **HYDROXYLATION OF PROLINE AND LYSINE** during collagen synthesis

C. **CLEAVAGE** of the signal sequence

D. **FOLDING** of the nascent protein into three-dimensional configuration

E. **ASSOCIATION** of protein subunits into multimeric complex

IV   Translation (Figure 2-2) is the mechanism by which only the centrally located **nucleotide sequence of mRNA** is translated into the **amino acid sequence of a protein** and occurs in the **cytoplasm.** The end or flanking sequences of the mRNA (called the **5′ and 3′ untranslated regions; 5′UTR** and **3′UTR**) are not translated. Translation decodes a set of **three** nucleotides (called a **codon**) into **one** amino acid (e.g., GCA codes for alanine, UAC codes for tyrosine, etc.). The code is said to be **redundant,** which means that more than one codon specifies a particular amino acid (e.g., GCA, GCC, GCG, GCU all specify alanine and UAC, UAU both specify tyrosine).

A. Translation uses **transfer RNA (tRNA),** which has two important binding sites. The first site of tRNA called the **anticodon** binds to the complementary codon on the

● **Figure 2-2 Translation.** This diagram joins the process of translation at a point where three amino acids have already been linked together (amino acid 1, 2, and 3). The process of translation is basically a three-step process that is repeated over and over during the synthesis of a protein. The enzyme aminoacyl-tRNA synthetase links a specific amino acid with its specific tRNA. In step 1, the tRNA and amino acid complex 4 binds to the A site on the ribosome. Note that the direction of movement of the ribosome along the mRNA is in a 5′ → 3′ direction. In step 2, the enzyme peptidyl transferase forms a peptide bond between amino acid 3 and amino acid 4 and the small subunit of the ribosome reconfigures so that the A site is vacant. In step 3, the used tRNA 3 is ejected and the ribosome is ready for tRNA and amino acid complex 5.

mRNA and demonstrates **tRNA wobble** whereby the normal A-U and G-C pairing is required only in the first two base positions of the codon but variability or wobble occurs at the third position. The second site of tRNA is the **amino acid-binding site** on the acceptor arm, which covalently binds the amino acid to the 3′ end of tRNA.

B. Translation uses the enzyme **aminoacyl-tRNA synthetase,** which links an amino acid to tRNA. **tRNA charging** refers to the fact that the amino acid–tRNA bond contains the energy for the formation of the peptide bond between amino acids. There is a specific aminoacyl-tRNA synthetase for each amino acid. Since there are 20 different amino acids, there are 20 different aminoacyl-tRNA synthetase enzymes.

C. Translation uses the enzyme **peptidyl transferase,** which participates in forming the peptide bond between amino acids of the growing protein.

D. Translation requires the use of **ribosomes,** which are large RNA-protein complexes that consist of a 40S subunit (consisting of 18S rRNA and ~30 ribosomal proteins) and a 60S subunit (consisting of 5S rRNA, 5.8 rRNA, 28S rRNA, and ~50 ribosomal proteins). The ribosome moves along the mRNA in a **5′ → 3′ direction** such that the **NH2-terminal end** of a protein is synthesized **first** and the **COOH-terminal end** of a protein is synthesized **last.**

E. Translation begins with the **start codon AUG** that codes for **methionine** (the optimal initiation codon recognition sequence is **GCACCAUGG**) so that all newly synthesized proteins have methionine as their first (or NH2-terminal) amino acid, which is usually removed later by a protease.

F. Translation terminates at the **stop codon (UAA, UAG, UGA).** The stop codon binds **release factors** that cause the protein to be released from the ribosome into the cytoplasm.

G. **β° Thalassemia** is a genetic disease whereby the affected individuals are unable to synthesize the **β-globin protein** and thus produce far too little hemoglobin. Adult hemoglobin consists of two **α-globin proteins** and two **β-globin proteins.** The **β-globin gene** has three exons and two introns. The introns contain a **G-T sequence** that are responsible for correct RNA splicing to occur and form normal β-globin mRNA. In β° thalassemia, the G-T sequence is mutated to A-T such that correct RNA splicing does *not* occur and the defective β-globin mRNA cannot be translated into β-globin protein. β° thalassemia produces severe anemia in the affected individuals.

ⓥ Golgi Complex. The Golgi complex is a stack of membranous cisternae with a *cis-face* **(convex)** that receives vesicles of newly synthesized proteins from the rER and a *trans-face* **(concave)** that releases condensing vacuoles of posttranslationally modified proteins. The functions of the Golgi complex include:

A. POSTTRANSLATIONAL MODIFICATION of proteins, which includes: **completion of N-linked glycosylation** that began in the rER; **O-linked glycosylation** (addition of sugars to serine, threonin, or hydroxylysine by glycosyltransferase); **sulfation; phosphorylation** (of tyrosine, serine, or threonine by kinases/phosphatases); **methylation** (of lysine by methylases/demethylases); **acetylation** (of lysine by acetylases/deacetyleses); **carboxylation** (of glutamate by Y-carboxylase); **addition of GPI** (a glycolipid added to aspartate); **myristoylation** (addition of a C_{14} fatty acyl group to glycine); **palmitoylation** (addition of a C_{16} fatty acyl group to cysteine); **farnesylation** (addition of a C_{15} prenyl group to cysteine); **granylgeranylation** (addition of a C_{20} prenyl group to cysteine).

B. **PROTEIN SORTING AND PACKAGING. Secretory proteins** (e.g., insulin) are packaged into **clathrin-coated vesicles. Cell membrane proteins** (e.g., receptors) are packaged into nonclathrin-coated vesicles. **Lysosomal enzymes** are packaged into **clathrin-coated vesicles** after phosphorylation of mannose to form **mannose-6-phosphate.**

C. **MEMBRANE RECYCLING.**

VI Smooth Endoplasmic Reticulum (sER). This membranous organelle contains no ribosomes and is involved in:

A. **SYNTHESIS OF MEMBRANE PHOSPHOLIPIDS** (phosphatidylcholine, sphingomyelin, phosphatidylserine, phosphatidylthanolamine), **cholesterol, and ceramide.**

B. **SYNTHESIS OF STEROID HORMONES** in testes, ovary, adrenal cortex, and placenta.

C. **DRUG DETOXIFICATION USING CYTOCHROME P$_{450}$ MONO-OXYGENASE,** which is a family of heme proteins (also called **mixed function oxidase system**) that catalyzes (**Phase I reactions**) the biotransformation of drugs by hydroxylation, de-alkylation, oxidation, and reduction reactions. For example, cytochrome P$_{450}$ mono-oxygenase catalyzes the hydroxylation of barbiturates, phenytoin, or benzopyrene (a carcinogen found in cigarette somke), which makes them more soluble in water and allows excretion into the urine. Activation of cytochrome P$_{450}$ by one agent enhances the detoxification of other agents, which has clinical implications. In **chronic alcoholics** or **newborns,** large amounts of anesthesia are needed (which may be dangerous) because cytochrome P$_{450}$ has been activated by detoxifying either alcohol or breakdown products of fetal hemoglobin, respectively.

D. **DRUG DETOXIFICATION USING GLUCURONYL TRANSFERASE** that catalyzes (**Phase II reactions**) the conjugation of glucuronic acid to a variety of drugs using **UDP-glucuronic acid** as the glucuronide donor.

E. **GLYCOGEN DEGRADATION.** The enzyme glucose-6-phosphatase is an integral membrane protein of the sER.

F. **FATTY ACID ELONGATION**

G. **LIPOLYSIS** begins in the sER with the release of a fatty acid from triacylglyceride.

H. **LIPOPROTEIN ASSEMBLY**

I. **CALCIUM FLUXES** associated with muscle contraction

VII Mitochondria

A. **FUNCTION.** Mitochondria are involved in the production of acetyl coenzyme A (CoA), the tricarboxylic acid cycle, fatty acid b-oxidation, amino acid oxidation, and oxidative phosphorylation [which causes the **synthesis of adenosine triphosphate (ATP)** driven by electron transfer to oxygen].
  1. Substrates are metabolized in the mitochondrial matrix to produce **acetyl CoA,** which is oxidized by the tricarboxylic acid cycle to carbon dioxide.
  2. The energy released by this oxidation is captured by reduced nicotinamide adenine dinucleotide (NADH) and flavin adenine dinucleotide (FADH$_2$). NADH and FADH$_2$ are further oxidized, producing **hydrogen ions** and **electrons.**

3. The electrons are transferred along the **electron transport chain,** which is accompanied by the outward pumping of hydrogen ions into the intermembrane space **(chemiosmotic theory).**

4. The **F_0 subunit of ATP synthase** forms a transmembrane hydrogen ion pore so that hydrogen ions can flow from the intermembrane space into the matrix, where the **F_1 subunit of ATP synthase** catalyzes the reaction **$ADP + P_i \rightarrow ATP$.**

B. **COMPONENTS AND CONTENTS** are listed in Table 2-1.

C. **CLINICAL CONSIDERATIONS**
   1. **Leber's hereditary optic neuropathy (LHON).** The characteristic dysfunction is **progressive optic nerve degeneration** that results clinically in **blindness.** Approximately 50% of all cases of LHON involve the **ND4 gene** located on mtDNA when a missense mutation changes an **arginine to histidine.** The ND4 gene encodes for a protein called **subunit 4 of the NADH dehydrogenase complex,** which functions in the **electron transport chain** and the **production of ATP.** A mutation of the ND4 gene decreases production of ATP such that the demands of a very active neuronal metabolism can not be met.
   2. **Kearns-Sayre syndrome** is characterized by ophthalmoplegia (degeneration of the motor nerves of the eye), pigmentary degeneration of the retina, and complete heart block, short stature, and cerebellar ataxia.
   3. **Myoclonic epilepsy with ragged red fibers syndrome.** The syndrome is characterized by myoclonus (muscle twitching), seizures, cerebellar ataxia, and mitochondrial myopathy. The most consistent pathologic finding in mitochondrial myopathy is abnormal mitochondria within skeletal muscle that impart an irregular shape and blotchy red appearance to the muscle cells, hence the term ragged red fibers.

TABLE 2-1	COMPONENTS AND CONTENTS OF MITOCHONDRIA
Components	**Contents**
Outer membrane	Porin (a transport protein that increases permeability to metabolic substrates)
Intermembrane space	H^+ ions
Inner membrane (folded into cristae)	Electron transport chain (NADH dehydrogenase, succinate dehydrogenase, ubiquinone-cytochrome c oxidoreductase, cytochrome oxidase)
	ATP synthase (found on elementary particles)
	ATP-ADP translocator (moves ADP into the matrix and ATP out of the matrix)
	Various transporters or translocators
Matrix compartment	TCA cycle enzymes (except succinate dehydrogenase)
	Fatty acid b-oxidation enzymes
	Amino acid oxidation enzymes
	Pyruvate dehydrogenase complex
	Carbamoylphosphate synthetase I*
	Ornithine transcarbamoylase*
	Monoamine oxidase (MAO; oxidation of catecholamines)
	Desmolase, 18-methyloxidase, 11β-hydroxylase**
	DNA, mRNA, tRNA, rRNA
	Granules containing Ca^{2+} and Mg^{2+}

*Part of the urea cycle; other enzymes of urea cycle are located in the cytoplasm.
**Involved in steroid hormone synthesis.
TCA = tricarboxylic acid cycle (Krebs cycle).

4. **Cyanide, carbon monoxide,** and **antimycin A** inhibit the electron transport chain and thus block ATP synthesis.

5. **Oligomycin** and **venturicidin** are antibiotics that bind to ATP synthase and thus block ATP synthesis.

6. **Isocarboxazid (Marplan), phenelzine (Nardil),** and **tranylcypromine (Parnate)** are monoamine oxidase (MAO) inhibitors used in the treatment of depression. MAO is a mitochondrial enzyme that oxidatively deaminates catecholamines (i.e., epinephrine, norepinephrine, and serotonin). MAO inhibitors reversibly or irreversibly inhibit MAO, which results in the accumulation of catecholamines in the presynaptic neuron and synaptic cleft. A side effect of these drugs is a hypertensive crisis that can be eliminated by avoiding foods (e.g., cheese and wine) that contain tyramine.

VIII **Lysosomes.** Lysosomes are membrane-bound organelles that contain lysosomal enzymes (also called **acid hydrolase enzymes**) including cathepsin B and L (proteases), nuclease, 5-nuclelotidase, β-galactosidase, β-glucuronidase, glycosidase, aryl sulfatase, lipase, esterase, and acid phosphatase that function at **pH 5.** Most lysosomes function intracellularly; however, some cells (e.g., neutrophils, osteoclasts) release their lysosomal contents extracellularly.

A. **LYSOSOMAL ACTION** occurs as follows: **Golgi hydrolase vesicles** bud from the Golgi complex and contain inactive acid hydrolase enzymes. The Golgi hydrolase vesicles fuse with an **endosome,** which contains an H^+-ATPase in its membrane that produces a pH 5 environment, and activates the acid hydrolases. This forms an **endolysosome.** An endolysosome may fuse with a **phagocytic vacuole** forming a **phagolysosome,** which degrades material phagocytosed by the cell. Or, an endolysosome may fuse with an **autophagic vacuole** forming an **autophagolysosome,** which degrades cell organelles. **Residual bodies** contain undigestible material and may accumulate within a cell as **lipofuscin pigment.** In addition, **exogenous protein antigens** are phagocytosed by antigen-presenting cells (APCs or macrophages) and undergo lysosomal degradation in endolysosomes to form antigen peptide fragments that become associated with **Class II MHC** and are transported and exposed on the cell surface of the APC.

B. **CLINICAL CONSIDERATIONS.** There are a number of genetic diseases that involve mutations of genes for various lysosomal enzymes (acid hydrolases; Table 2-2).

TABLE 2-2	LYSOSOMAL STORAGE DISEASES	
Disease	Enzyme Involved	Major Accumulating Metabolite
Hurler disease	L-Iduronidase	Heparan sulfate Dermatan sulfate
Sanfilippo A	Heparan sulfamidase	Heparan sulfate
Tay Sachs disease	Hexosaminidase A	GM2 ganglioside
Gaucher disease	β-Glucosidase	Glucosylceramide
Niemann-Pick disease	Sphingomyelinase	Sphingomyelin
Pompe's disease	α-1, 4-Glucosidase (acid maltase)	Glycogen
I-Cell disease	Phosphotransferase	Mucopolysaccharide
Krabbe's disease	β-Galactosidase	Galactosylceramide

IX **Peroxisomes.** These are membrane-bound organelles.

A. **CONTENTS OF PEROXISOMES** include:

1. **Amino acid oxidase** and **hydroxyacid oxidase** that use molecular (O_2) to oxidize organic substances, producing hydrogen peroxide ($R\text{-}H_2 + O_2 \rightarrow R + H_2O_2$). About 25% of all ethanol we drink is oxidized in peroxisomes (sometimes called the **microsomal ethanol oxidizing system**) to **acetaldehyde** by this reaction. The remaining 75% of ethanol is handled outside the peroxisomes by being converted to acetaldehyde by alcohol dehydrogenase which is then converted to either **acetate** (which enters the TCA cycle to be converted to $CO_2 + H_2O$) or **acetyl CoA** (which enters fatty acid synthesis).

2. **Catalase** and **other peroxidases** that decompose hydrogen peroxide to water and oxygen

$$(H_2O_2 \rightarrow H_2O + O_2).$$

3. **Fatty acid ß-oxidation enzymes** that oxidize long-chain fatty acids (>20 carbons) to short-chain fatty acids, which are transferred to mitochondria for complete oxidation.

4. **Enzymes for bile acid synthesis.**

5. **Urate oxidase** that breaks down purines.

B. **CLINICAL CONSIDERATION. Adrenoleukodystrophy** is a genetic disease that involves mutation of genes for various peroxisomal enzymes used in fatty acid b-oxidation that results in **abnormal accumulation of lipid** in the brain, spinal cord, and adrenal gland and leads to **dementia** and **adrenal failure.**

X **Cytoskeleton**

A. **FILAMENTOUS ACTIN (F-ACTIN)** is a **6-nm diameter microfilament** arranged in a helix of polymerized **globular monomers of actin (G-actin)**. F-actin is in dynamic equilibrium with a cytoplasmic pool of G-actin such that a polymerization end (plus end) and a depolymerization end (minus end) are present on each actin filament. The functions of F-actin include: exocytosis, endocytosis, cytokinesis, locomotion of cells forming lamellipodia, and movement of cell membrane proteins. **Cytochalasin** is a toxic fungal alkaloid that causes F-actin to depolymerize. **Phalloidin is** a toxic substance derived from the *Amanita* mushroom that binds to F-actin, thereby inhibiting polymerization/depolymerization.

B. **INTERMEDIATE FILAMENTS** are 10 **to 12-nm–diameter filaments.** Intermediate filament function as a cytoplasmic link among the extracellular matrix, cytoplasm, and nucleus. Intermediate filaments demonstrate specificity for certain cell types/tumors, and therefore can be used as markers for pathologic analysis (Table 2-3).

C. **MICROTUBULES** are **25-nm diameter tubules** that consist of 13 circularly arranged proteins called **a- and b-tubulin.**

1. Microtubules are in dynamic equilibrium with a cytoplasmic pool of a- and b-tubulin such that a polymerization end (plus end) and a depolymerization end (minus end) are present on each microtubule.

2. Microtubules are always associated with **microtubule-associated proteins (MAPs).** MAPs include:

a. **Kinesin** has ATPase activity for movement of vesicles along microtubules toward the plus end **(anterograde transport).**

TABLE 2-3	SPECIFICITY OF INTERMEDIATE FILAMENTS FOR CELL TYPES OR TUMORS
Cytokeratin	Epithelial cells Epithelial tumors (e.g., squamous carcinoma, adenocarcinoma)
Vimentin	Endothelial cells, vascular smooth muscle, fibroblasts, chondroblasts, and macrophages Mesenchymal tumors (e.g., fibrosarcoma, liposarcoma, angiosarcoma, chondrosarcoma, osteosarcoma)
Desmin	Skeletal muscle, nonvascular smooth muscle Muscle tumors (e.g., rhabdomyosarcoma)
Neurofilament	Neurons Neuronal tumors
Glial fibrillar acidic protein (GFAP)	Astrocytes, oligodendroglia, microglia, Schwann cells, ependymal cells, and pituicytes Gliomatous tumors
Lamins A, B, C	Inner membrane of nuclear envelope

   b. **Dynein** has ATPase activity for movement of vesicles along microtubules toward the minus end **(retrograde transport).**
   c. **Dynamin** has ATPase activity for elongation of nerve axons.
3. Microtubule functions include: maintenance of cell shape (polarity), movement of chromosomes (karyokinesis), movement of secretory granules and neurosecretory vesicles, beating of cilia and flagella, and phagocytosis/lysosomal function.
4. The **microtubular organizing center (MTOC)** of the cell for the assembly of microtubules is called the **centrosome.** At the center of the centrosome are two **centrioles** that are oriented perpendicular to each other. During mitosis, each centriole duplicates by tubulin polymerization and the parent and daughter centrioles move to opposite poles of the cell.
5. **Clinical considerations**
   a. **Chédiak-Higashi syndrome** is a genetic disease characterized by neutropenia and impaired phagocytosis of bacteria resulting from a defect in microtubule polymerization that impairs lysosomal function of leukocytes. Large abnormal lysosomes can be observed in the cytoplasm of leukocytes in people with this syndrome.
   b. **Colchicine** is a M phase specific drug (anti-mitotic) that inhibits microtubule assembly (i.e., polymerization). It is used in the treatment of acute and chronic gout by reducing the motility, phagocytosis, and secretion in inflammatory leukocytes (i.e., anti-inflammatory effect).
   c. **Vinblastine (Velban) and vincristine (Oncovin)** are M-phase–specific drugs (anti-mitotic) that bind tubulin and inhibit microtubule assembly (i.e., polymerization).
   d. **Paclitaxel (Taxol)** is an M-phase–specific drug (anti-mitotic) that binds tubulin and inhibits microtubule disassembly (i.e., depolymerization).

XI Cell Inclusions

   A. **LIPOFUSCIN** is a **yellow-brown "wear and tear"** pigment found predominantly in residual bodies, which are the end point of lysosomal digestion. Lipofuscin is composed of **phospholipids complexed with proteins,** suggesting that it is derived from the lysosomal digestion of cellular membranes. Lipofuscin is a telltale sign of **free radical damage** and is found prominently within hepatocytes, skeletal muscle cells, and nerve cells of elderly people or patients with severe malnutrition.

B. HEMOSIDERIN is a **golden brown hemoglobin-derived** pigment consisting of iron. Iron is absorbed mainly by surface absorptive cells within the duodenum, transported in the plasma by a protein called **transferrin** and is normally stored in cells as **ferritin,** which is a protein–iron complex. Small amounts of ferritin normally circulate in the plasma, making plasma ferritin a good indicator of the adequacy of body iron stores. In iron deficiency, serum ferritin is <12 mg/L. In iron overload, serum ferritin approaches 5,000 mg/L. Also during iron overload, intracellular ferritin undergoes lysosomal degradation, in which the ferritin protein is degraded and the iron aggregates within the cell as hemosiderin in a condition called **hemosiderosis.** The more extreme accumulation of iron is called **hemochromatosis,** which is associated with liver and pancreas damage. Hemosiderosis can be observed in patients with **increased absorption of dietary iron, impaired utilization of iron, hemolytic anemias, and blood transfusions.**

C. GLYCOGEN is the **storage form of glucose** and is composed of glucose units linked by **1,4 glycosidic bonds.** Glycogen synthesis is catalyzed by **glycogen synthase.** Glycogen degradation is catalyzed by **glycogen phosphorylase.** Liver hepatocytes and skeletal muscle cells contain the largest glycogen stores, but the function of glycogen differs widely.

1. **Liver glycogen** functions in the **maintenance of blood glucose levels.** Liver glycogen is synthesized (using glycogen synthase) during a high-carbohydrate meal because of **hyperglycemia** and an **increase in the insulin:glucagon ratio.** Liver glycogen is degraded (using liver glycogen phosphorylase isoenzyme) during **hypoglycemia** (e.g., fasting), **exercise,** or other **stressful situations** because of a **decrease in the insulin:glucagon ratio** and the **secretion of epinephrine** from the adrenal medulla, which binds to a- and b-adrenergic receptors on the hepatocyte. Liver glycogen is degraded to **glucose-6-phosphate,** which is catalyzed to free glucose by the enzyme glucose-6-phosphatase. **Glucose-6-phosphate** is found only in the liver and kidney.

2. **Skeletal muscle glycogen** functions in the **formation of ATP** through glycolysis. Skeletal muscle glycogen is synthesized (using glycogen synthase) during a high-carbohydrate meal because of **hyperglycemia** and an **increase in the insulin:glucagon ratio.** Skeletal muscle glycogen is degraded (using muscle glycogen phosphorylase isoenzyme) during **exercise** or **stressful situations** because of a decrease in ATP, **calcium released during contraction,** and **secretion of epinephrine** from the adrenal medulla, which binds to a- and b-adrenergic receptors on the skeletal muscle cell. Skeletal muscle glycogen is degraded to **glucose-6-phosphate,** which enters glycolysis to produce ATP. The **absence of glucose-6-phosphatase** enzyme in skeletal muscle prevents the degradation of glycogen to free glucose.

3. **Glycogen storage diseases** are genetic diseases that involve mutations in one of the enzymes of glycogen synthesis or degradation.
   a. **Von Gierke disease (type 1 glycogenosis)** results from a deficiency in the enzyme glucose-6-phosphatase, causing an enlarged liver and severe hypoglycemia.
   b. **McArdle disease (type V glycogenosis)** results from a deficiency in the enzyme muscle glycogen phosphorylase, causing exercise-induced muscle pain and cramps.

XII Selected Photomicrographs

A. Electron micrographs of cytoplasmic organelles (Figure 2-3).

B. Electron micrographs of the cytoskeleton and light micrograph of cytokeratin immunocytochemical localization (Figure 2-4).

C. Electron micrographs of cell inclusions (Figure 2-5)

D. Electron micrographs of a protein-secreting cell and steroid-secreting cell (Figure 2-6).

● **Figure 2-3 Cytoplasmic organelles. (A)** Polyribosomes or polysomes are arranged in a spiral or rosette pattern. **(B)** Rough endoplasmic reticulum (rER) shows membranous cisterna covered with ribosomes (*arrows*). **(C)** Golgi complex (gol) shows *cis*-face and *trans*-face. Note the clathrin-coated vesicles budding from the *trans*-face (*arrows*). Sg = secretory granules. **(D)** Smooth endoplasmic reticulum (sER) shows membranous cisternae with no ribosomes. **(E)** Mitochondria and cristae (*arrows*). **(F)** Lysosome (Lys) and peroxisome (Per). **(G)** Residual body (RB).

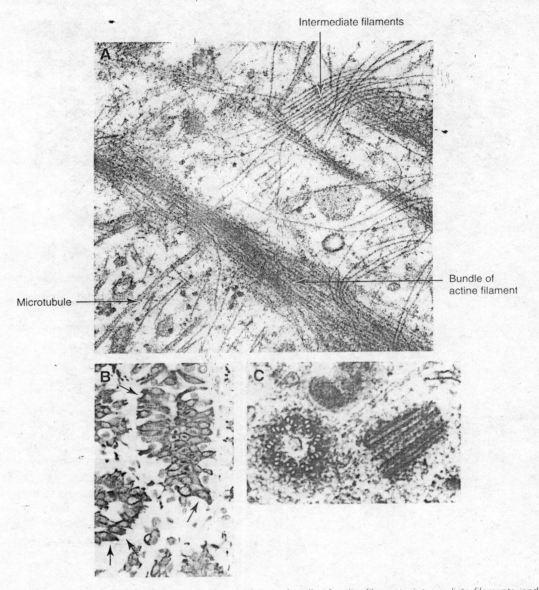

Intermediate filaments

Microtubule

Bundle of
actine filament

● **Figure 2-4 Cytoskeleton. (A)** Electron micrograph shows a bundle of actine filaments, intermediate filaments, and microtubules of a negatively stained actin filament. Note the plus end and the minus end. **(B)** Immunocytochemical staining for the intermediate filament (cytokeratin) in breast carcinoma. Note the localization of cytokeratin within the cytoplasm of the malignant epithelial cells *(arrows)*. **(C)** Electron micrograph of two centrioles, which are composed of microtubules. One centriole is cut in cross-section and the other cut in longitundinal section.

● **Figure 2-5 Cell inclusions. (A)** Electron micrograph of lipofuscin pigment, which is the "wear and tear" pigment generally found in residual bodies. **(B)** Light micrograph of hemosiderin within cardiac myocytes (hemosiderosis). The cardiac myocytes were stained with Prussian Blue, which is specific for iron. **(C)** Electron micrograph of glycogen particles within a hepatocyte *(arrow)*.

● **Figure 2-6 Protein versus steroid-secreting cell. (A)** Electron micrograph demonstrates the hallmarks of a protein-secreting cell. rER *(arrows)*, Gogli (gol), and secretory granules (sg). **(B)** Electron micrograph demonstrates the hallmarks of a steroid-secreting cell: sER, mitochondria with tubular cristae (m), and lipid droplets (lp). N = nucleus *Inset*: High magnification of a mitochondria with tubular cristae.

Case Study

A 25-year-old man comes to your office complaining that "I feel weak when I do my exercise routine in the morning. I like to work-out hard like a Navy Seal." He also tells you that "sometimes my urine is red and it scares me." After some discussion, he informs you that he takes a rest period when the weakness occurs and the symptoms resolve. But the symptoms reappear when he resumes exercise. The man is obviously frustrated and says, "Doc, I can't stay in shape if this keeps happening." What is the most likely diagnosis?

Differentials

- Anemia, muscular dystrophy, myasthenia gravis, polymyositis

Relevant Physical Exam Findings

- Burning pain, cramping, and exhaustion in legs and arms during strenuous exercise
- Normal muscle tone and strength bilaterally
- No enlargement of the liver or spleen

Relevant Lab Findings

- Blood chemistry: CPK = 100 U/L (High); Hct = 45% (Normal); Hgb = 15.2 g/dL (Normal); BUN = 15 mg/dL (Normal)
- Urinalysis: RBCs = 20–30 (High); Glucose = High
- Diagnostic anaerobic exercise test showed muscle pain, cramping, and exhaustion; CPK increase; blood lactate = no increase
- Muscle biopsy showed elevated glycogen content and low phosphorylase activity

Diagnosis

McArdle disease. McArdle disease (Type V glycogenosis) is an autosomal recessive disease and results from a deficiency in muscle glycogen phosphorylase, causing exercise-induced muscle pain and cramping. Myoglobulinuria results from a breakdown of muscle protein in an attempt to liberate amino acids for conversion to glucose. Other glycogen storage diseases: Cori disease (Type III glycogenosis) results from a deficiency in the enzyme, amylo-α-1,6 glucosidase. Von Gierke disease (Type I glycogensis) results from a deficiency in the enzyme, glucose-6-phosphatase. Duchenne muscular dystrophy (DMD) is a genetic disease that shows X-linked recessive inheritance. The DMD gene is located on the short (p) arm of chromosome X in band 21 (i.e., Xp21) and encodes for the dystrophin protein. Dystrophin anchors within skeletal muscle fibers to the extracellular matrix, thereby stabilizing the cell membrane. A mutation of the DMD gene alters the normal function of dystrophin, leading to progressive muscle weakness and wasting. The muscle weakness begins as early as 1 year of age. Myasthenia gravis is an autoimmune disease characterized by circulating antibodies against the nACh receptor (nicotinic acetylcholine receptor; anti-nAChR) and decreased number of nACh receptors. Clinical findings of myasthenia gravis include: muscle weakness that fluctuates daily or even within hours; extraocular muscle involvement with ptosis and diplopia being the first disability. Polymyositis is a connective tissue disease. Clinical findings of polymyositis include: progressive, bilateral weakness of the proximal muscles.

The Cell Membrane: Eicosanoids and Receptors/Signal Transduction

I ## The Lipid Component of the Cell Membrane (Figure 3-1)

A. The lipid component consists of four phospholipids: **phosphatidylcholine, sphingomyelin, phosphatidylethanolamine,** and **phosphatidylserine.** The lipid component exhibits **asymmetry** in which phosphatidylcholine and sphingomyelin are located in the **outer leaflet** (extracellular side); phosphatidylethanolamine and phosphatidylserine are located in the **inner leaflet** (cytoplasmic side). The asymmetry is maintained by **flippase,** which is a member of the ABC transporter superfamily. Flippase removes phosphatidylethanolamine and phosphatidylserine from the outer leaflet of the cell membrane and uses the energy from ATP hydrolysis to flip (or transport) them into the inner leaflet.

B. The four phospholipids are **amphiphilic;** i.e., they have a **hydrophilic (polar) head** and a **hydrophobic (nonpolar) tail.**

C. The lipid component exhibits **fluidity,** which means that the phospholipids diffuse laterally within the lipid bilayer. Fluidity is enhanced by **increased temperature** and a **high degree of unsaturation of fatty acid tails.** Fluidity is diminished by a **high cholesterol content.**

D. CHOLESTEROL is a component of the cell membrane and is thought to be distributed in both the outer and inner leaflets.

E. GLYCOLIPIDS are sugar-containing sphingolipids and are confined exclusively to the outer leaflet. The types of glycolipids include:
1. **Cerebrosides,** which contain a single sugar moiety (e.g., galactose).
2. **Other neutral glycolipids** (e.g., red blood cell group antigens A, B, and O), which contain many sugar moieties (e.g., glucose, galactose, N-acetyl-D-galactosamine, fucose).
3. **Gangliosides** (e.g., ganglioside GM_1), which contain many sugar moieties and negatively charged N-acetylneuraminic acid (or sialic acid).

F. PRODUCTION OF EICOSANOIDS. The lipid component produces **arachidonic acid,** which leads to the formation of **eicosanoids** through the following process:
1. In response to physical injury or inflammatory response, **phospholipase A_2 or C** catalyzes the breakdown of membrane lipids to **arachidonic acid.**
2. Arachidonic acid may be converted to straight-chain eicosanoids called **leukotrienes (LTB$_4$, LTC$_4$, LTD$_4$)** by **lipoxygenase.**

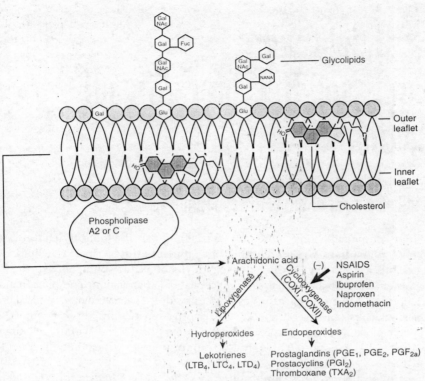

Eicosonoid	Function
LTB$_4$	Stimulates leukocyte chemotaxis.
LTC$_4$	Potent bronchoconstrictor. Component of slow-reacting substance of anaphylaxis (SRS-A)
LTD$_4$	Potent bronchoconstrictor. Component of slow-reacting substance of anaphylaxis (SRS-A)
PGE$_1$	Potent vasodilator (used to maintain patency of ductus arteriosus). Misoprostol (a PGE1 analogue) is used with mifepristone (RU-486; a progesterone receptor blocker) to induce therapeutic abortion. Inhibits gastric HCL secretion. Stimulates gastric secretion of bicarbonate and mucus (misbprostol is used to treat peptic ulcers).
PGE$_2$	Causes contraction of uterine smooth muscle at parturition (induces labor or therapeutic abortion in 2nd trimester). Potent vasodilator. Potent bronchodilator. Inhibits platelet aggregation. Inhibits mast cell secretion. Potentiates the inflammatory response.
PGF$_{2a}$	Causes contraction of uterine smooth muscle at parturition (induces labor or therapeutic abortion in 2nd trimester).
PGI$_2$	Potent vasodilator. Inhibits platelet aggregation. Potentiates the inflammatory response.
TXA$_2$	Potent vasodilator. Stimulates platelet aggregation.

● **Figure 3-1 Diagram of the lipid component of the cell membrane and its biological actions.** Note that two molecules of cholesterol are shown in the outer and inner leaflets. COX = cyclooxygenase; Gal = galactose; Glu = glucose; GalNAc = N-acetyl-D-galactosamine; Fuc = fucose; NANA = N-acetylneuraminic acid (or sialic acid).

3. Arachidonic acid may be converted to cyclical eicosanoids called **prostaglandins (PGE$_1$, PGE$_2$ and PGF$_{2a}$), prostacyclin (PGI$_2$), and thromboxane (TXA$_2$)** by **cyclo-oxygenase (COX I and COX II)**. COX I produces eicosanoids used in many normal physiologic processes, hence it is sometimes referred to as "good COX." COX II produces eicosanoids used in the inflammatory response, hence it is sometimes referred to as "bad COX."

4. **Pharmacology. Aspirin (acetylsalicylic acid, Bayer, Bufferin)** is a non-steroidal anti-inflammatory drug (NSAID) that irreversibly inhibits cyclo-oxygenase and is used clinically to ameliorate effects of myocardial infarction, inhibit platelet aggregation, reduce pain, reduce fever, and as a general anti-inflammatory agent. **Ibuprofen (Advil, Motrin, Nuprin) and Naproxen (Aleve)** are NSAIDs (a propionic acid derivatives) that reversibly inhibit cyclo-oxygenase and are used clinically to reduce pain, treat rheumatoid arthritis, and treat osteoarthritis. **Indomethacin** is an NSAID (an acetic acid derivative) that reversibly inhibits cyclo-oxygenase and is used clinically to treat acute gout, treat ankylosing spondylitis, and promote closure of the ductus arteriosus.

II The Protein Component of the Cell Membrane

(Figure 3-2). The protein component exhibits **patching or capping**, which means that proteins diffuse laterally within the lipid bilayer. The protein component consists of **peripheral and integral proteins. Peripheral proteins** can be easily disassociated from the lipid bilayer by changes in ionic strength of pH. **Integral proteins** are difficult to disassociate from the lipid bilayer unless detergents [e.g., sodium dodecyl sulfate or Triton X-100] are used. **Transmembrane proteins** are integral proteins that span the lipid bilayer, exposing the protein to both the extracellular space and the cytoplasm.

● **Figure 3-2 Diagram of the protein component of the cell membrane.** PL$_C$ = phospholipase C; AC = adenylate cyclase; LDL = low density lipoprotein.

III Membrane Transport Proteins

allow for the passage of polar molecules (e.g., ions, sugars, amino acids, nucleotides, and metabolites) across a membrane. There are two main classes of transport proteins: carrier proteins and ion channel proteins.

A. **CARRIER PROTEINS (TRANSPORTERS).** Carrier proteins or transporters bind a specific molecule and undergo **conformational changes** in order to transport the molecule across the membrane. Carrier proteins that transport a single molecule are called **uniporters.** Other carrier proteins function as **coupled transporters** in which the transport of one molecule depends on the simultaneous transport of another molecule either in the same direction **(symporters)** or in the opposite direction **(antiporters).**

Carrier proteins participate predominantly in **active transport** whereby molecules are transported **"uphill"** of the concentration and membrane potential, i.e., electrochemical gradient. Some important carrier proteins include the following:

1. **Ca^{2+} ATPase** is a uniporter carrier protein most commonly found in the sarcoplasmic reticulum (SR) of skeletal muscle that pumps Ca^{2+} from the cytoplasm back into the SR.

2. **H^+ ATPase** is a uniporter carrier protein most commonly found in lysosomes/endosomes that pumps H^+ into lysosomes/endosomes to create an acid pH that activates lysosomal enzymes.

3. **Na^+-K^+ ATPase** is an antiporter carrier protein found in almost all cells that pump Na^+ out of the cell and K^+ into the cell to maintain a low intracellular $[Na^+]$. **Quabain** is a specific inhibitor that competes for the K^+-binding site. **Cardiac glycosides (digoxin and digitoxin)** are Na^+-K^+ ATPase blockers that elevate intracellular Na^+ levels within cardiac myocytes. The elevated Na^+ overwhelms the Na^+-Ca^{2+} exchanger so that more Ca^{2+} can be reaccumulated by the sarcoplasmic reticulum. During the next contraction, more Ca^{2+} is released from the sarcoplasmic reticulum, which increased the force of the contraction. Cardiac glycosides are used in congestive heart failure to increase the force of contraction.

4. **H^+-K^+ ATPase** is an antiporter carrier protein most commonly found in the parietal cells of the stomach mucosa that pumps H^+ into the lumen of the stomach to form HCl gastric acid.

5. **Na^+-glucose cotransporter** is a symporter carrier protein most commonly found in surface absorptive cells of the small intestine mucosa and the simple columnar epithelim of the proximal convoluted tubule of the kidney that transports Na^+ across the luminal membrane into the cytoplasm by contransport with glucose.

6. **Na^+-amino acid cotransporter** is a symporter carrier protein found in surface absorptive cells of the small intestine mucosa that transports Na^+ across the luminal membrane into the cytoplasm by cotransport with amino acids. There are four separate cotransporters for neutral, basic, acidic, and imino amino acids.

7. **Fatty acid transporter (FAT)** is a uniporter carrier protein found in surface absorptive cells of the small intestine mucosa that transports long chain fatty acids (>12 carbons), monacylglycerols, cholesterol, and fat-soluble vitamins (A, D, E, and K), which are packaged as micelles across the luminal membrane into the cytoplasm.

8. **The ABC transporter superfamily.** This is a family of transport ATPases in which each member of the family contains two highly conserved **ATP-binding cassettes** (hence the name). ABC transporters use ATP binding and ATP hydrolysis to transport substrates across the cell membrane. The variety of substrates transported by this superfamily is diverse. In addition, members of this superfamily are involved in flipping of lipids between the outer and inner leaflets of the cell membrane. Members of this superfamily include:

   a. **Multidrug resistance (MDR) proteins.**
      (1) **MDR1** is a uniporter carrier protein found in hepatocytes of the liver that transports cholesterol into the bile canaciculus.
      (2) **MDR2** is a uniporter carrier protein found in hepatocytes of the liver that transports phospholipids (mainly lecithin) into the bile canaliculus.
      (3) **MDR1 and MDR2** are expressed by human cancer cells and unfortunately confer resistance to cancer chemotherapeutic drugs by transporting the hydrophobic drugs out of the cancer cell.

   b. **Chloroquine transporter** is expressed by *Plasmodium falciparum* (which causes malaria) and confers resistance to the antimalarial drug choloroquine by transporting the drug out of *P. falciparum*.

    c.   **Cystic fibrosis (CF) transporter.** CF is a disease caused by a mutation in the CF gene, which is located on the long arm of chromosome 7(7q). The CF gene encodes for a protein called CF transporter that transports Cl^- out of the cell.

    d.   **Multispecific organ anion transporter (MOAT)** is a uniporter carrier protein found in hepatocytes of the liver that transports bilirubin glucoronide (bile pigment) and glutathione into the bile canaliculus.

    e.   **Biliary acid transporter (BAT)** is a uniporter carrier protein found in hepatocytes of the liver that transports bile salts (cholic acid and chenodeoxycholic acid) into the bile canaliculus.

    f.   **Flippase** removes phosphatidylethanolamine and phosphatidylserine from the outer leaflet of the cell membrane and uses the energy from ATP hydrolysis to flip them into the inner leaflet.

9. **The glucose transporter family (GLUTI-5).** The initial event in the cellular metabolism of glucose is its transport across the cell membrane into the cytoplasm of the cell. This step is performed by the glucose transporter family. Members of this family include:

    a.   **GLUT-1** is a uniporter carrier protein found in **red blood cells** and **neurons** where it functions in the basal transport of glucose into the cell.

    b.   **GLUT-2** is a uniporter carrier protein found in: **hepatocytes** where it functions in bidirectional glucose transport (e.g., after a meal, glucose transport into hepatocytes is increased; during fasting, glucose transport out of hepatocytes is increased); **kidney cells** where it functions in glucose transport out of the cell (e.g., during fasting, glucose transport out of kidney cells is increased); **surface absorptive cells** of the small intestine mucosa where it functions in glucose, galactose, and fructose transport out of the cell across the basolateral membrane into the portal blood; pancreatic beta cells where it functions as a glucose sensor for the secretion of insulin.

    c.   **GLUT-3** is a uniporter carrier protein found in **neurons** where it functions in the basal transport of glucose into the cell.

    d.   **GULT-4** is a uniporter carrier protein found in **adipocytes, skeletal muscle cells,** and **cardiac myocytes** where it functions in the insulin-stimulated transport of glucose into the cell.

    e.   **GLUT-5** is a uniporter carrier protein found in **surface absorptive cells** of the small intestine mucosa where it functions in the transport of fructose into the cell.

10. **Urea transporter** is a uniporter carrier protein found in the inner medullary collecting ducts of the kidney that transports urea across the luminal and basolateral membranes.

11. **Na^+-dicarboxylate/tricarboxylate cotransporter** is a symporter carrier protein found in proximal convoluted tubule of the kidney that transports Na^+ across the basolateral membrane into the cytoplasm by cotransport with dicarboxylates or tricarboxylates into the cytoplasm.

12. **Organic anion-dicarboxylate/tricarboxylate exchanger** is an antiporter carrier protein found in the proximal convoluted tubule of the kidney that transports organic anions across the basolateral membrane into the cytoplasm by countertransport with dicarboxylates or tricarboxylates into the interstitial fluid.

13. **Organic anion-X^- exchanger** is an antiporter carrier protein found in the proximal convoluted tubule of the kidney that transports organic anions across the luminal membrane into the tubular fluid by countertransport with any of a large number of other organic anions into the cytoplasm.

14. **Organic cation-X^+ exchanger** is an antiporter carrier protein found in the proximal convoluted tubule of the kidney that transports organic cations across the

luminal membrane into the tubular fluid by countertransport with any of a large number of other organic cations into the cytoplasm.

15. **Na⁺-H⁺ exchanger** is an antiporter carrier protein found in the proximal convoluted tubule of the kidney that transports Na^+ across the luminal membrane into the cytoplasm by countertransport with H^+ into tubular fluid. The H^+ are supplied by the reaction $H_2CO_3 \rightarrow H^+ + HCO_3^-$, which is catalyzed by **carbonic anhydrase.**

16. **Na⁺ - HCO₃⁻ cotransporter** is a symporter carrier protein that transports HCO_3^- across the basolateral membrane into the interstitial fluid by cotrasport with Na^+ into the interstitial fluid that accounts for 80% of HCO_3^- reabsorption. **Acetazolamide (Diamox)** inhibits carbonic anhydrase by acting primarily on the early PCT resulting in decreased reabsorption of HCO_3^-. It is used clinically to treat glaucoma and altitude sickness.

17. **Na⁺-K⁺-2Cl⁻ cotransporter** is a symporter carrier protein that transports Na^+ across the luminal membrane into the cytoplasm by cotransport with K^+ and Cl^- into the cytoplasm that occurs because cytoplasmic $[Na^+]$ is kept low by Na^+-K^+ ATPase. **Furosemide (Lasix; last 6 hours), bumetanide (Bumex), and torsemide (Demadix)** inhibit the Na^+-K^+-$2Cl^-$ cotransporter by acting primarily on the **DST of the loop of Henle ("loop diuretics").** Loop diuretics are the most efficacious diuretics available and are sometimes called **"high ceiling diuretics."** They are used clinically to treat edema associated with congestive heart failure, pulmonary edema, and hypertension.

18. **Na⁺-Cl⁻ cotransporter** is a symporter carrier protein that transports Na^+ across the luminal membrane into the cytoplasm by cotransport with Cl^- into the cytoplasm that occurs because cytoplasmic $[Na^+]$ is kept low by Na^+-K^+ ATPase. **Hydrochlorothiazide (HydroDIURIL), chlorthalidone (Hygroton), indapamide (Lozol), and metolazone (Mykrox)** inhibit the Na^+-Cl^- cotransporter by acting primarily on the **DCT** resulting in decreased Na^+ reabsorption **("thiazide diuretics").** They are used clinically to treat edema associated with congestive heart failure and hypertension.

19. **Cl⁻ -base exchanger** is an antiporter carrier protein found in the proximal convoluted tubule of the kidney that transports Cl^- across the luminal membrane into the cytoplasm by countertransport with an organic base (e.g., formate, oxalate) into the tubular fluid.

20. **K⁺-Cl⁻ cotransporter** is a symporter carrier protein found in the proximal convoluted tubule of the kidney that transports Cl^- across the basolateral membrane into the interstitial fluid by cotransport with K^+ into the interstitial fluid.

21. **Cl⁻-HCO₃⁻ exchanger** is an antiporter carrier protein found in the collecting duct of the kidney that transports Cl^- across the luminal membrane into the cytoplasm by countertransport with HCO_3^- into the tubular fluid. The HCO_3^- is supplied by the reaction $H_2CO_3 \rightarrow H^+ + HCO_3^-$, which is catalyzed by **carbonic anhydrase.** In the red blood cell, **Band 3 protein** is a Cl^--HCO_3^- exchanger that transports Cl^- across the RBC membrane into the cytoplasm by countertransport with HCO_3^- into the plasma (called the **chloride shift**).

22. **Na⁺-Ca²⁺ exchanger** is an antiporter carrier protein found in the distal convoluted tubule of the kidney that transports Na^+ across the basolateral membrane into the cytoplasm by countertransport with Ca^{2+} into the interstitial fluid.

23. **Na⁺-PO₄²⁺ cotransporter** is a symporter carrier protein found in the proximal convoluted tubule of the kidney that transports PO_4^{2-} across the luminal membrane into the cytoplasm by cotransport with Na^+ into the cytoplasm.

24. **PO₄²⁺ - Anion exchanger** is an antiporter carrier found in the proximal convoluted tubule of the kidney that transports PO_4^{2-} across the basolateral membrane

into the interstitial fluid by countertransport with a non-specific anion into the cytoplasm.

25. **Na$^+$-NH$_4^+$ exchanger** is an antiporter carrier protein found in the proximal convoluted tubule of the kidney that transports Na$^+$ across the luminal membrane into the cytoplasm by countertransport with NH$_4^+$ into tubular fluid. The NH$_4^+$ is supplied by the reaction 1 glutamine $\rightarrow$ 2 NH$_4^+$ + 2HCO$_3^-$.

B. **ION CHANNEL PROTEINS.** Ion channel proteins form **hydrophilic pores** in order to transport **inorganic ions** across the membrane and generally called **ion channels.** Ion channels participate only in **passive transport (facilitated diffusion)** whereby molecules are transported **"downhill"** of the concentration and membrane potential, i.e., electrochemical gradient. Ion channels are **ion selective** and **gated** (i.e., open briefly and then close). Stimuli that open gates include: mechanical stress (**mechanical-gated ion channels**), changes in voltage across the cell membrane (**voltage-gated ion channels**), and ligand binding (**ligand-gated ion channels**). One of the more important types of ligand-gated ion channels are the **transmitter-gated ion channels** that bind neurotransmitters and mediate ion movement. Depending on the type of ion involved, transmitter-gated ion channels may have an excitatory or inhibitory effect. Some important ion channel proteins include the following:

1. **Voltage-gated ion channels**
   a. **L-type Ca^{2+} channel protein (dihydropyridine receptor;** L = long-lasting) is an important determinant of vascular tone and cardiac contractility.
      (1) **In skeletal muscle cells,** the L-type Ca^{2+} channel protein is found on the T-tubular and changes its conformation in response to the depolarization of an action potential and induces the action of the fast Ca^{2+} release channel protein (ryanodine receptor). Skeletal muscle depends mainly on intracellular pools of Ca^{2+} from the sarcoplasmic reticulum for contraction and does not require much transmembrane Ca^{2+} influx through the L-type Ca^{2+} channel protein. Therefore, skeletal muscle is not significantly affected by Ca^{2+} channel blockers.
      (2) **In vascular smooth muscle cells,** the L-type Ca^{2+} channel protein is found on the cell membrane and changes its conformation in response to the depolarization of an action potential to allow transmembrane Ca^{2+} influx into the cytoplasm and also induces more Ca^{2+} release from the sarcoplasmic reticulum via the fast Ca^{2+} release channel protein. The Ca^{2+} binds to calmodulin and the Ca^{2+}-calmodulin complex that activates myosin kinase which in turn phosphorylates the myosin crossbridge– ADP–PO$_4^{2-}$ complex. ADP + PO$_4^{2-}$ is released, leaving the phosphorylated myosin crossbridge bound to actin, which initiates vascular smooth muscle contraction.
      (3) **In the heart,** L-type Ca^{2+} channel protein is found in the SA nodal cells, AV nodal cells, and ventricular myocytes. In the SA and AV nodes, phase 0 of the slow action potential is caused by Ca^{2+} influx into nodal cells through the L-type Ca^{2+} channel protein. In ventricular myocytes, phase 2 of the fast action potential is caused by Ca^{2+} influx into ventricular myocytes through the L-type Ca^{2+} channel protein. This transmembrane Ca^{2+} influx is called **"trigger Ca^{2+}"** and is involved in myocyte contraction.
      (4) **Ca^{2+} channel antagonists (blockers).** All Ca^{2+} channel antagonists in current use act by blocking Ca^{2+} influx through the L-type Ca^{2+} channel protein. **Nifedipine** and **amlodipine** (representatives of the dihydropyridine class of Ca^{2+} channel blockers) predominantly block Ca^{2+} influx in vascular smooth muscle cells (i.e., cause arterial vasodilation). **Diltiazem**

(a representative of the benzothiazepine class of Ca^{2+} channel blockers) and **verapamil** (a representative of the phenylalkylamine class of Ca^{2+} channel blockers) act preferentially on the SA and AV nodal cells because these pacemaker areas depend on Ca^{2+} currents for phase 0 of the action potential. Diltiazem and verapamil have two major actions: slow the rise of phase 0 of the action potential, which leads to a slowed conduction velocity through the AV node; prolong the repolarization of the AV node, which increases the effective refractory period of the AV node. Both of these actions are very effective in treating re-entrant arrhythmias.

b.   Fast Ca^{2+} release channel protein (ryanodine receptor)

(1) In skeletal muscle cells, the fast Ca^{2+} release channel protein is found on the sarcoplasmic reticulum and changes its conformation in response to its interaction with the L-type Ca^{2+} channel protein to allow transmembrane Ca^{2+} influx into the cytoplasm. The Ca^{2+} binds to troponin C, which allows the myosin crossbridge–ADP–PO_4^{2-} complex to bind actin. ADP + PO_4^{2-} is released leaving the myosin crossbridge bound to actin which initiates skeletal muscle contraction.

(2) In smooth muscle cells, the fast Ca^{2+} release channel protein is found on the sarcoplasmic reticulum and changes its conformation in response to its interaction with the L-type Ca^{2+} channel protein to allow transmembrane Ca^{2+} influx into the cytoplasm. The Ca^{2+} binds to calmodulin and the Ca^{2+}-calmodulin complex that activates myosin kinase which in turn phosphorylates the myosin crossbridge–ADP–PO_4^{2-} complex. ADP + PO_4^{2-} is released, leaving the phosphorylated myosin crossbridge bound to actin, which initiates vascular smooth muscle contraction.

(3) In the heart, the fast Ca^{2+} release channel protein is found on the sarcoplasmic reticulum of cardiac myocytes. "Trigger Ca^{2+}" stimulates the release of a large pool of Ca^{2+} stored in the sarcoplasmic reticulum through the fast Ca^{2+} release channel protein into the cytoplasm. The Ca^{2+} binds to troponin C, which allows the myosin crossbridge–ADP–PO_4^{2-} complex to bind actin. ADP + PO_4^{2-} is released leaving the myosin crossbridge bound to actin which initiates cardiac myocyte contraction.

c.   T-type Ca^{2+} channel protein (T = transient)

(1) In the heart, the T-type Ca^{2+} channel protein is found on SA and AV nodal cells and plays a role in phase 4 of the action potential. Phase 4 is caused by Ca^{2+} influx into nodal cells through the T-type Ca^{2+} channel protein and Na^+ influx into nodal cells through slow (funny) Na^+ channels.

(2) In the brain, the T-type Ca^{2+} channel protein is found a relay neurons connecting the thalamus to the cortex. In the awake state, these neurons faithfully transmit sensory signals to the cortex and the T-type Ca^{2+} channel protein is depolarized and inactive. In the sleep state, the transient, bursting activity of the T-type Ca^{2+} channel protein alters incoming signals so that output to the cortex have an oscillatory firing rate that has a characteristic "spike and wave" readout on an EEG. For reasons not yet understood, absence seizures (petit mal seizure) are associated with paroxysmal hyperpolarization and activation of the T-type Ca^{2+} channel protein in the awake state. Patients experiencing absence seizures have EEG readings somewhat similar to patterns generated in slow-wave (stage 3) sleep. **Ethosuximide** is a specific T-type Ca^{2+} channel protein antagonist and is the first-line therapy for uncomplicated absence seizures.

d. K$^+$ channel protein. These are the most abundant class of ion channel proteins whereby at least 16 types and many more subtypes have been described but their physiologic functions are far from being fully understood. There are voltage-gated K$^+$ channel proteins that include the: **delayed rectifier (K$_V$), inward rectifier (K$_{IR}$),** and **transient outward rectifier (K$_A$).** There are also Ca^{2+}-activated K$^+$ channel proteins that include the: **large conductance channel (BK$_{Ca}$), intermediate conductance channel (IK$_{Ca}$),** and **small conductance channel (SK$_{Ca}$).** There are also metabolically gated K$^+$ channel proteins which include the: **ATP-sensitive K$^+$ channel (K$_{ATP}$), arachidonic acid modulated K$^+$ channel (K$_{AA}$),** and **acetylcholine-activated K$^+$ channel (K$_{ACh}$).** In the heart, the K$^+$ channel protein is found on SA and AV nodal cells and cardiac myocytes.

(1) In SA and AV nodal cells. Adenosine stimulates P$_1$ purinergic receptors which causes the opening of a G protein-linked K$^+$ channel (possibly K$_{IR}$ or K$_{ATP}$) so that K$^+$ moves from the cytoplasm (intracellular) into the extracellular space resulting in a hyperpolarization. This inhibits the SA nodal, atrial, and AV nodal conduction. The AV node is more sensitive to adenosine than the SA node. Adenosine has a half-life of 10 seconds and is often used as a first-line therapy for converting narrow-complex paroxysmal supraventricular tachycardia to a normal sinus rhythm.

(2) In cardiac myocytes. Phase 2 (plateau phase) of the action potential in cardiac myocytes is determined by the depolarizing Ca^{2+} influx through the L-type Ca^{2+} channel protein and the hyperpolarizing K$^+$ efflux through the K$^+$ ion channel protein. Larger hyperpolarizing K$^+$ currents shorten the phase 2 plateau duration causing the membrane potential to return to its resting value more rapidly. Shorter hyperpolarizing K$^+$ currents lengthen the phase 2 pleateau duration causing the membrane potential to return to its resting value more slowly. When K$^+$ channel proteins are blocked, a smaller hyperpolarizing K$^+$ current is generated and therefore cause a longer phase 2 (plateau phase) and prolonged repolarization. On the beneficial side, a longer phase 2 (plateau phase) increases the effective refractory period and decreases the incidence of re-entry. On the toxic side, a longer phase 2 (plateau phase) increases the likelihood of early afterdepolaizations and *torsades de pointes*. **Ibutilide** is a Class III antiarrhythmic K$^+$ channel protein antagonist (blocker) that also enhances a slow Na$^+$ influx that further prolongs repolarization. **Sotalol** is a mixed Class II (nonselectively antagonizes ß-adrenergic receptors) and a Class III antiarrhythmic K$^+$ channel protein antagonist (blocker). **Bretylium** is an antihypertensive agent (performs a "chemical sympathetectomy" by inhibiting the release of norepinephrine) and a Class III antiarrhythmic K$^+$ channel protein antagonist (blocker). **Amiodarone** is mainly a Class III antiarrhythmic K$^+$ channel protein antagonist (blocker). Amiodarone is also a Class I (blocks Na$^+$ channels and therefore decreases the rate of firing of SA and AV nodal cells), Class II (noncompetitive antagonist of α- and- β-adrenergic receptors), and Class IV (L-type Ca^{2+} channel protein antagonist) antiarrhythmic.

e. Slow (funny) Na$^+$ channel protein. The slow (funny) Na$^+$ channel protein is found on SA and AV nodal cells in the heart and causes a slow, inward current of Na$^+$. Phase 4 of the slow action potential observed in SA and AV nodal cells is caused by Ca^{2+} influx into nodal cells through T-type Ca^{2+} channel proteins and Na$^+$ influx into nodal cells through slow (funny) Na$^+$ channel proteins.

f. Fast Na$^+$ channel protein. The fast Na$^+$ channel protein is found on cardiac myocytes and causes a fast, inward current of Na$^+$. Phase 0 of the fast action potential observed in cardiac myocytes is caused by Na$^+$ influx into cardiac myocytes through fast Na$^+$ channel proteins. Na$^+$ channel protein antagonists (blockers) decrease the upstroke velocity of phase 0 and thereby decrease the conduction velocity through cardiac tissue. Class IA Na$^+$ channel protein antagonists prolong repolarization and thereby increase the effective refractory period. In addition, Na$^+$ channel protein antagonists decrease the slope of phase 4 depolarization and increase the threshold potential in SA and AV nodal cells and thereby decrease the automaticity in SA nodal cells. **Quinidine, procainamide, disopyramide** are Class IA antiarrhythmic Na$^+$ channel protein antagonists (blockers) that bind preferentially to **open** Na$^+$ channel proteins. **Lidocaine, tocainide, and mexiletine** are Class IB antiarrhythmic Na$^+$ channel protein antagonists (blockers) that bind preferentially to **open and inactivated** Na$^+$ channel proteins. A major distinguishing characteristic of Class IB antiarrhythmics is their **fast dissociation** from Na$^+$ channel proteins. **Flecainide, propaferone, moricizine, and encainide** are Class IC antiarrhythmic Na$^+$ channel protein antagonists (blockers), which are the most potent Na$^+$ channel protein blockers.

2. Transmitter-gated ion channels

a. Nicotinic acetylcholine (nACh) receptor. The nACh receptor is composed of two α, one ß, one δ, and either one ϵ or one γ subunit (i.e., five subunits). The a_2ßde nACh receptor is found at the neuromuscular junction of mature skeletal muscle and the a_2ßdy nACh receptor is found at the neuromuscular junction of embryonic skeletal muscle. The α **subunits** are responsible for binding acetylcholine (ACh) which is the structural basis for the binding of **two ACh molecules per receptor.** When two molecules of ACh bind to the nACh receptor during a discrete, brief pulse, the gate is opened and the influx of Na$^+$ and Ca^{2+} and efflux of K$^+$ occurs. The gate remains open for only about 1 msec when it is non-selectively permeable to all cations (but excludes anions). The **influx of Na$^+$** (~30,000 Na$^+$/nACh receptor/msec) is primarily responsible for the depolarization of the postsynaptic membrane and mediates the excitatory postsynaptic potential (EPSP). During a continuous exposure of nACh receptor to ACh, the nACh receptor undergoes a change to a desensitized conformation whereby the channel is locked closed. nACh Receptors are also found in the CNS, autonomic ganglia, and the adrenal medulla where they are termed **N$_2$ or N$_N$.** nAChRs found in skeletal muscle are termed **N$_1$ or N$_M$.** **Succinylcholine (Anectine, Quelicin, Sucostrin)** is an nACh receptor agonist that competes with ACh for the nACh receptor. Succinylcholine maintains an open Na$^+$ channel eventually causing skeletal muscle relaxation and paralysis. Succinylcholine is used to induce paralysis during surgery by means of a **depolarizing blockade.** Succinylcholine may cause malignant hyperthermia which is a major cause of anesthesia related deaths. Malignant hyperthermia results from an excessive release of Ca^{2+} from the sarcoplasmic reticulum and presents as hyperthermia, metabolic acidosis, tachycardia, and accelerated muscle contractions. Treatment includes: rapid cooling, 100% oxygen, control of acidosis, and administration of **Dantrolene,** which blocks release of Ca^{2+} from the sarcoplasmic reticulum. **Nicotine** is considered a nACh receptor agonist because it binds to ACh-binding sites and activates the nACh receptor. Nicotine may be responsible for the psychophysical effects of smoking addiction by its interaction with N$_2$ or N$_N$ nACh receptors in the CNS. **Tubocurarine, pancuronium, vecuronium, rocuronium** are nACh receptor antagonists (blockers) that block endogenous ACh binding. These blockers are used to induce paralysis during surgery by means of a **non-depolarizing blockade.** Since nACh receptors (i.e., N_2 or N_N) are found on autonomic ganglia, these blockers often have side effects associated with **ganglionic blockade** that can be reversed by acetylcholinesterase inhibitors (e.g., neostigmine).

b. Glutamate receptors. Glutamate is the **major excitatory neurotransmitter in the CNS** and elicits its action by binding to glutamate receptors. There are two main classes of glutamate receptors: transmitter-gated-ion channel proteins (discussed here) and G protein-linked receptors (sometimes called metabotropic receptors will be discussed later). The glutamate-gated ion channel proteins include the following:

- **(1) N-methyl-D-aspartate (NMDA) receptor.** The NMDA receptor is found throughout the CNS (e.g., hippocampus, cerebral cortex, and spinal cord). When **glutamate** and the cofactor **glycine** bind to the NMDA receptor, the gate is opened and the influx of Na^+ and Ca^{2+} and efflux of K^+ occurs. In addition, a **voltage-dependent membrane depolarization** is required to open the gate because the NMDA receptor is "plugged" by extracellular Mg^{2+} at resting membrane potential. **Amantadine** is a non-competitive NMDA receptor antagonist (blocker). **Memantine** is a non-competitive, use-dependent NMDA receptor antagonist. **Ketamine** (Ketalar; Special K; K) is an NMDA receptor antagonist that acts as a CNS depressant and a dissociative anesthetic. Ketamine has sedative, analgesic, and hallucinogenic effect and is used as a "date rape" drug. **Phencyclidine (PCP; angel dust)** and **dizocilpine (MK-801)** are NMDA receptor antagonists that cause hallucinogenic behavior and require the NMDA receptor to be open in order to gain access to their binding sites (i.e., open channel blockers).

- **(2) Kainate receptor.** The kainate receptor is found throughout the CNS (e.g., hippocampus, cerebellum). When glutamate binds to the kainite receptor, the gate is opened and the influx of Na^+ and the efflux of K^+ occurs.

- **(3) a-amino-3-hydroxy-5-methyl-4-isoxazole proprionic acid (AMPA) receptor.** The AMPA receptor is found throughout the CNS (e.g., hippocampus, cerebral cortex). When glutamate binds to the AMPA receptor, the gate is opened and the influx of Na^+ and Ca^{2+} and the efflux of K^+ occurs. Ca^{2+} influx through AMPA receptors may play a role in neuronal cell death. **Excitotoxicity** refers to neuronal cell death caused by a toxic level of glutamatergic neurotransmission that increases neuronal Ca^{2+} levels. Some diseases associated with excitotoxicity include: CNS ischemia, physical trauma, epilepsy, Parkinson disease, amyotrophic lateral sclerosis (ALS), and Alzheimer's disease.

c. 5-Hydroxytryptamine$_3$ (5-HT$_3$) serotonin receptor. When serotonin binds to the 5-HT$_3$ receptor, the gate is opened and the influx and Na^+ and efflux of K^+ occurs. The 5-HT$_3$ receptor belongs to a family of 5-HT receptors whose other members are G protein-linked receptors that will be discussed later.

d. Purinergic$_{2X}$ (P$_{2X}$) receptor. Adenosine and **ATP** are neurotransmitters that elicit their action by binding to purinergic receptors. The P_{2X} receptor found on peripheral terminals of nociceptive neurons is involved in the sensation of acute pain caused by tissue damage and inflammation (i.e., nociception). When adenosine or ATP binds to the P_{2X} receptor, the gate is opened and the influx and Na^+ and Ca^{2+} and efflux of K^+ occurs. The P_{2X} receptor belongs to a family of purinergic receptors whose other members are G protein-linked receptors that will be discussed later.

e. **Gamma-aminobutyric acid$_A$ (GABA$_A$) receptors.** GABA is the **major inhibitory neurotransmitter in the CNS** and elicits its action by binding to GABA receptors. There are two main classes of GABA receptors: transmitter-gated ion channel proteins (**GABA$_A$ receptor** discussed here) and G protein–linked receptors (**GABA$_B$ receptor,** sometimes called metabotropic receptors is discussed later). The GABA$_A$ receptor is found in most areas of the CNS and generates a **fast inhibitory postsynaptic potentials (IPSPs).** The GABA$_A$ receptor is composed of two α subunits and three ß or γ subunits (i.e., five subunits). The α subunits are responsible for binding GABA, which is the structural basis for the binding of **two GABA molecules per receptor.** When two molecules of GABA bind to the GABA$_A$ receptor, the gate is opened and the influx of Cl$^-$ occurs (causes **hyperpolarization** of the cell). **Muscimol** is a GABA$_A$ receptor agonist. **Bicuculline** is a GABA$_A$ receptor competitive antagonist. **Picrotoxin** is a GABA$_A$ receptor non-competitive antagonist. The drugs used in clinical practice (i.e., barbiturates and benzodiazepines) to effect the GABA$_A$ receptor fall into the category of **GABA$_A$ receptor modulators.**

   (1) **Barbiturates. Thiopental, methohexital, pentobarbital, secobarbital, amobarbital,** and **phenobarbital** are GABA$_A$ receptor modulators that enhance the **efficacy** of GABA by increasing the **duration of Cl$^-$ channel opening** leading to membrane hyperpolarization and decreased neuronal excitability.

   (2) **Benzodiazepines. Midazolam, clorazepate, alprazolam, lorzepam, chlordiazepoxide, clonazepam, diazepam, triazolam, estazolam, temazepam, flurazepam,** and **quazepam** are GABA$_A$ receptor modulators that enhance the **potency** of GABA by increasing the **frequency of Cl$^-$ channel opening** leading to membrane hyperpolarization and decreased neuronal excitability. **Flunitrazepam (Rohypnol; "roofies"; Forget Me Pill)** is a fast-acting benzodiazepine that causes amnesia and is used as a "date rape" drug.

f. **Glycine receptor.** The amino acid glycine is the **major inhibitory neurotransmitter in the spinal cord** and elicits its action by binding to glycine receptors. The glycine receptor is composed of α subunits and ß subunits. When glycine binds to the glycine receptor, the gate is opened and the influx of Cl$^-$ occurs (causes **hyperpolarization** of the cell).

Ⅳ G Protein–linked Receptors (Figure 3-3).

G protein-linked receptors are proteins that span the cell membrane seven times (**seven pass receptor**) and are linked to **trimeric GTP-binding proteins (called G proteins)** composed of an **α-chain, ß-chain,** and **γ-chain.** These receptors activate a chain of cellular events either through the **adenylate cyclase (AC) pathway** (by increasing or decreasing cAMP levels) or the **phospholipase C (PL$_C$) pathway.**

A. **AC PATHWAY (↑ CAMP LEVELS).** When norepinephrine (NE) binds to the ß$_1$, ß$_2$, or ß$_3$ receptor, **inactive G$_S$ protein** (which exists as a trimer with GDP bound to the α$_S$ chain) exchanges its GDP for GTP to become **active G$_S$ protein.** This allows the α$_S$ chain to disassociate from the β$_S$ chain and γ$_S$ chain and **stimulate adenylate cyclase** to **increases cAMP levels.** Active G$_S$ protein is short-lived since the α$_S$ chain has **GTPase activity** which quickly hydrolyzes GTP to GDP to form inactive G$_S$ protein. cAMP activates the enzyme **cAMP-dependent protein kinase (or protein kinase A; PKA),** which catalyzes the **covalent phosphorylation** of serine and threonine within certain intracellular proteins to increase their activity. The enzyme **serine/threonine**

● **Figure 3-3 Diagram of G protein-linked receptor action. (A)** Adenylate cyclase pathway (increase cAMP levels).
(B) Adenylate cyclase pathway (decrease cAMP levels).

● Figure 3-3 (Continued) (C) Phospholipase C pathway.
NE = norepinephrine; ACh = acetylcholine, AC = adenylate cyclase; SER = smooth endoplasmic reticulum; PL_C = phospholipase C; CaM = Ca^{2+}/calmodulin-dependent protein kinase; IP_3 = inositol triphosphate; DAG = diacylglycerol; PIP_2 = phosphatidylinositol biphospate.

protein phosphatase reverses the effects of protein kinase A by dephosphoylating serine and threonine. **Cholera toxin** (an enzyme that catalyzes **ADP ribosylation of the** α_S **chain**) blocks α_S chain GTPase activity so that the effects of active G_S protein continue indefinitely. Within intestinal epithelium, this causes Na^+ ion and water movement into the gut lumen resulting in severe **diarrhea.**

B. AC PATHWAY ($\downarrow$ cAMP LEVELS). When norepinephrine (NE) binds to the α_2 adrenergic receptor, **inactive G_i protein** (which exists as a trimer with GDP bound to the α_i chain) exchanges its GDP for GTP to become **active G_i protein.** This allows the α_i chain to disassociate from the β_i chain and γ_i chain and **inhibit adenylate cyclase** to **decrease cAMP levels.** The β_i and γ_i complex stimulates a K^+ channel protein (probably K_{IR}) so that the channel opens and K^+ flows out of the cell causing a hyperpolarization of the cell (probably the main effect). **Pertussis toxin** (an enzyme that catalyzes **ADP ribosylation of the α_i chain**) blocks the dissociation of the α_i chain from the β_i chain and γ_i chain so that adenylate cyclase is not inhibited.

C. PL_C PATHWAY. When acetylcholine (ACh) binds to the M_3 muscarinic acetylcholine receptor, **inactive G_q protein** (which exists as a trimer with GDP bound to the α chain) exchanges its GDP for GTP to become **active G_q protein.** Active G_q protein activates **phospholipase C,** which cleaves **phosphatidylinositol biphosphate (PIP_2)** into **inositol triphosphate (IP_3)** and **diacylglycerol (DAG).** IP_3 causes the **release of Ca^{2+} from the endoplasmic reticulum,** which activates the enzyme Ca^{2+}/calmodulin-dependent protein kinase (or CaM-kinase), which catalyzes the **covalent phosphorylation** of serine and threonine within certain intracellular proteins to increase their activity. DAG activates the enzyme **protein kinase C (PKC),** which catalyzes the covalent phosphorylation of serine and threonine within certain intracellular proteins to increase their activity.

Ⓥ Types of G Protein—linked Receptors

A. MUSCARINIC ACETYLCHOLINE (mACh) RECEPTORS (M_1, M_2, M_3, M_4, M_5). The **M_1 receptor** is found in the CNS and autonomic ganglia (mediates the slow excitatory postsynaptic potential), where it elicits its action through the PL_C pathway ($\uparrow IP_3$ + DAG). The **M_2 receptor** is found in the heart (SA and AV nodes, atrial and ventricular cardiac myocytes), where it elicits its action through the AC pathway ($\downarrow$ cAMP levels + opens a K^+ channel protein so that K^+ flows out of the cell causing a hyperpolarization). The **M_3 receptor** is found in smooth muscle and secretory glands, where it elicits its action through the PL_C pathway ($\uparrow IP_3$ + DAG). The **M_4 receptor** in found in the CNS, where it elicits its action through the AC pathway ($\downarrow$ cAMP levels + opens a K^+ channel protein so that K^+ flows out of the cell causing a hyperpolarization. The **M_5 receptor** is found in the CNS, where it elicits its action through the PL_C pathway ($\uparrow IP_3$ + DAG). **Methacholine, carbachol, bethanechol,** and **pilocarpine** (an alkaloid) are mACh receptor agonists. Methacholine is used only in the diagnosis of asthma. Carbachol is used topically (cannot be used systemically) as a miotic agent in the treatment of glaucoma. Bethanechol is used to promote gastrointestinal and urinary tract motility. Pilocarpine is used as a miotic agent and sialogogue (saliva-producing agent) in the treatment of xerostomia. **Atropine, scopolamine, pirenzepine,** and **ipratropium** (a synthetic quaternary ammonium compound) are mACh receptor antagonists. Atropine is used to induce mydriasis (pupil dilation) for ophthalmic examination, to reverse sinus bradycardia caused by excessive vagal tone in the setting of acute myocardial infarction or asystole, to inhibit excessive salivation and mucus secretion during surgery, prevent vagal reflexes induced by surgical trauma of visceral organs, and counteract the effects of muscarine poisoning from certain mushrooms. Scopolamine is used to prevent motion sickness. Pirenzepine is used in the treatment of peptic ulcers. Ipratropium is used in the treatment of chronic pulmonary obstructive disease.

B. ADRENERGIC RECEPTORS (α_1, α_2, β_1, β_2, β_3). The adrenergic receptors bind **epinephrine** and **norepinephrine.** The **α_1 receptor** is found in the dilator pupillae muscle, arteriolar smooth muscle, GI and GU sphincters, arrector pili muscle, genitourinary smooth muscle, and liver where it elicits its action through the PL_C pathway ($\uparrow IP_3$ + DAG). The **α_2 receptor** is found in pancreatic ß cells, platelets, and autonomic ganglia (mediates the slow inhibitory postsynaptic potential) where it elicits its action through the AC pathway ($\downarrow$ cAMP + opens a K^+ channel protein so that K^+ flows out of the cell causing hyperpolarization). The **β_1 receptor** is found in the heart and juxtaglomerular cells, where it elicits its action through the AC pathway ($\downarrow$ cAMP). The **β_2 receptor** is found in vascular smooth muscle (within skeletal muscle), bronchiolar smooth muscle, GI and urinary bladder smooth muscle, uterine smooth muscle, skeletal muscle, and liver, where it elicits its action through the AC pathway ($\uparrow$ cAMP). The **β_3 receptor** is found in adipose tissue, where it elicits its action through the AC pathway ($\uparrow$ cAMP).

1. **α-Agonists.** Phenylephrine, oxymetazoline, and tetrahydrozoline are α_1-agonists and are used in the non-prescription remedies Afrin and Visine to constrict vascular smooth muscle for the treatment of nasal congestion or ophthalmic hyperemia. Clonidine and methyldopa (a prodrug metabolized to methylepinephrine) are α_2-agonists. **Clonidine** and **methyldopa** are used to treat hypertension by activating α_2 receptors in cardiovascular control centers of the CNS and thereby inhibiting sympathetic stimulation of the heart and vasculature.

2. **α-Antagonists. Phenoxybenzamine** and **phentolamine** are non-selective α_1 and α_2 antagonists used in the preoperative treatment of a pheochromocytoma. **Prazosin, terazosin,** and **doxazosin** are α_1 antagonists that decrease peripheral vascular resistance and venous return to the heart and are used to treat hypertension and congestive heart failure. **Tamsulosin** is an α_1A antagonist (the α_{1A} receptor is preferentially expressed in genitourinary smooth muscle) that relaxes genitourinary smooth muscle and is used to treat benign prostatic hyperplasia. **Yohimbine** is an α_2 antagonist that acts at the level of the autonomic ganglia and leads to the increase in epinephrine release.

3. **ß-Agonists. Isoproterenol** is a non-selective β_1 and β_2 agonist that increases the heart rate (positive chronotropism; β_1 effect), increases cardiac contractility (positive inotropism; β_1 effect), and relaxes bronchiolar smooth muscle (β_2 effect). **Dobutamine** is a β_1 agonist that increases the heart rate (positive chronotropism) and increases cardiac contractility (positive inotropism) and is used to treat decompensated heart failure. **Metaproterenol, terbutaline, albuterol,** and **salmeterol** (long-acting) are β_2 agonists that relax bronchiolar smooth muscle and are used to treat obstructive airway disease and bronchospasm.

4. **ß-Antagonists. Propanolol, nadolol,** and **timolol** are β_1 and β_2 antagonists that decrease the heart rate (positive chronotropism; β_1 effect), cardiac contractility (positive inotropism; $\beta 1$ effect), and peripheral vascular resistance (β_2 effect) and are used to treat hypertension, angina, and glaucoma. **Labetalol** and **carvedilol** are α_1, β_1, and β_2 antagonists that are used to treat hypertension. **Pindolol** is a partial β_1 and β_2 agonist that is used to treat hypertension. **Acebutolol** is a partial β_1 agonist that is used to treat hypertension. **Esmolol, metoprolol,** and **atenolol** are β_1 antagonists that decrease the heart rate (positive chronotropism; β_1 effect) and decrease cardiac contractility (positive inotropism; β_1 effect) and are used to treat hypertension, myocardial infarction, and mild congestive heart failure.

C. **METABOTROPIC GLUTAMATE RECEPTOR (mGLuR).** Glutamate is the main excitatory neurotransmitter in the CNS. **Group I receptors (mGluR1 and mGluR5)** are found in the CNS and elicit their action through the AC pathway ($\uparrow$ cAMP) and PL$_C$ pathway ($\uparrow$ IP$_3$ + DAG). **Group II receptors (mGluR2 and mGluR3)** are found in the CNS and elicit their action through the AC pathway ($\downarrow$ cAMP). **Group III receptors (mGluR4, mGluR6, mGluR7, and mGluR8)** are found in the CNS and elicit their action though the AC pathway ($\downarrow$ cAMP).

D. **5-HYDROXYTRYPTAMINE$_{1,2,4,6,7}$ (5-HT$_{1,2,4,6,7}$) SEROTONIN RECEPTOR.** The **5-HT$_1$** serotonin receptor is found in the CNS and elicits its action through the AC pathway ($\downarrow$ cAMP). The **5-HT$_2$** serotonin receptor is found in the CNS and elicits its action through the PL$_C$ pathway ($\uparrow$ IP$_3$ + DAG). The **5-HT$_{4,6,7}$** serotonin receptor is found in the CNS and elicits its action through the AC pathway ($\uparrow$ cAMP).

E. **PURINERGIC$_{1,2Y}$ (P$_1$ AND P$_{2Y}$) RECEPTORS.** Adenosine and ATP are neurotransmitters that elicit their action by binding to purinergic receptors. The **P$_1$ receptor** is found in the CNS and elicits its action through the AC pathway ($\downarrow$ cAMP). The **P$_{2Y}$ receptor** is found in the CNS and peripheral terminals of nociceptive neurons and elicits its action through the PL$_C$ pathway ($\uparrow$ IP$_3$ + DAG). The P$_{2Y}$ receptor is involved in the sensation of acute pain caused by tissue damage and inflammation (i.e., nociception).

F. **GAMMA-AMINOBUTYRIC ACID$_B$ (GABA$_B$) RECEPTOR.** GABA is the main inhibitory neurotransmitter of the CNS. The GABA$_B$ receptor is found in the CNS and mediates slow inhibitory postsynaptic potentials (IPSPs). The $GABA_B$ receptor elicits its action through the AC pathway ($\downarrow$ cAMP levels + opens a K^+ channel protein so that K^+ flows out of the cell causing a hyperpolarization + closes a Ca^{2+} channel).

G. **DOPAMINE 1,2 (D1 AND D2) RECEPTOR.** The **D1 receptor family (D_1 and D_5)** is found in the CNS (i.e., striatum, nucleus accumbens, amygdale, olfactory tubercle, hippocampus, and neocortex) and elicits its excitatory action through the AC pathway ($\uparrow$ cAMP) and PL_C pathway ($\uparrow IP_3$ + DAG). The **D2 receptor family (D_2, D_3, D_4)** is found in the CNS (i.e., striatum, nucleus accumbens, amygdale, olfactory tubercle, hippocampus, neocortex, hypothalamus, ventral tegmental area, substantia nigra, and anterior pituitary) and elicits its inhibitory action through the AC pathway ($\downarrow$ cAMP + opens a K^+ channel protein so that K^+ flows out of the cell causing a hyperpolarization). These receptors play an important role in schizophrenia and Parkinson disease. **Bromocriptine** (D_2 agonist; ergot derivative), **pergolide** (D_1 and D_2 agonist; ergot derivative), **pramipexole** ($D_3 > D_2$ agonist), and **ropinirole** ($D_3 > D_2$ agonist) are dopamine receptor agonists.

H. **HISTAMINE$_{1,2}$ (H_1 AND H_2) RECEPTOR.** The **H_1 receptor** is found in the CNS, hypothalamus, vascular endothelial cells, and smooth muscle cells and elicits its action through the PL_C pathway ($\uparrow IP_3$ + DAG). The H_1 receptor is involved in inflammation and allergic reactions (IgE-mediated hypersensitivity reaction) causing edema, bronchoconstriction, and sensitization of sensory neurons. The **H_2 receptor** is found in the CNS, parietal cells of the stomach that produce HCl, cardiac myocytes, and mast cells and elicits its action through the AC pathway ($\uparrow$ cAMP). **Diphenhydramine, doxylamine,** and **chlorpheniramine** are first generation H_1 antagonists. **Loratadine** is a second-generation H_1 antagonist. **Cimetidine, ranitidine, famotidine,** and **nizatidine** are H_2 antagonists used to treat heartburn and peptic ulcer disease.

I. **THYROID STIMULATING HORMONE (TSH) RECEPTOR.** The TSH receptor is found on thyroid follicular cells and elicits its action through the AC pathway ($\uparrow$ cAMP). When TSH binds to the TSH rerceptor, virtually every step in T_3 and T_4 biosynthesis and secretion is stimulated.

K. **LUTEINIZING HORMONE (LH) RECEPTOR.** The LH receptor is found on Leydig cells (in the male) and theca interna cells of secondary and Graafian follicles (in the female) and elicits its action through the AC pathway ($\uparrow$ cAMP). When LH binds to the LH receptor in the male, testosterone biosynthesis is stimulated in Leydig cells. When LH binds to the LH receptor in the female, androgen biosynthesis is stimulated in theca interna cells.

L. **FOLLICLE-STIMULATING HORMONE (FSH) RECEPTOR.** The FSH receptor is found on Sertoli cells (in the male) and granulose cells of secondary and Graafian follicles (in the female) and elicits its action through the AC pathway ($\uparrow$ cAMP). When FSH binds to the FSH receptor in the male, androgen-binding protein (ABP) biosynthesis is stimulated in Sertoli cells. When FSH binds to the FSH receptor in the female, aromatase activity is increased which converts androgens to estrogens in granulosa cells.

M. **ADRENOCORTICOTROPIN HORMONE (ACTH) RECEPTOR.** The ACTH receptor is found on zona fasciculata and zona reticularis cells of the adrenal cortex and elicits its action through the AC pathway ($\uparrow$ cAMP). When ACTH binds to the ACTH receptor, cortisol, androstenedione, and dehydroepiandrosterone (DHEA) biosynthesis, and secretion are stimulated.

N. GLUCAGON RECEPTOR. The glucagons receptor is found on hepatocytes and adipocytes and elicits its action through the AC pathway ($\uparrow$ cAMP). When glucagons binds to the glucagons receptor, glycogen degradation and gluconeogenesis are increased in hepatocytes and lipolysis and β-oxidation of free fatty acids is increased in adipocytes.

O. SOMATOSTATIN RECEPTOR. The somatostatin receptor is found in the CNS and the delta cells of the pancreatic islets and elicits its inhibitory action through the AC pathway ($\downarrow$ cAMP levels + opens a K^+ channel protein so that K^+ flows out of the cell causing hyperpolarization).

P. PARATHYROID HORMONE (PTH) RECEPTOR. The PTH receptor is found on renal tubular cells of the kidney (i.e., proximal convoluted tubule, distal convoluted tubule, and collecting duct) and osteoblasts and elicits its action through the AC pathway ($\uparrow$ cAMP). When PTH binds to the PTH receptor, kidney reabsorption of Ca^{2+} from the tubular fluid $\rightarrow$ plasma is increased, 1a-hydroxylase synthesis is increased, and osteoblasts are stimulated to secrete macrophage colony-stimulating factor (M-CSF) and express RANKL.

Q. NEUROPEPTIDE RECEPTORS.

1. **Vasopressin$_{1,2}$ receptors (V$_1$ and V$_2$).** Antidiuretic hormone (ADH; or vasopressin) binds to V$_1$ and V$_2$ receptors. The **V$_1$ receptor** is found on arterioles and elicits its action of vasoconstriction through the PL$_C$ pathway ($\uparrow$ IP$_3$ + DAG). The **V$_2$ receptor** is found on principal cells of the cortical and medullary collecting ducts in the kidney and elicits its action of increasing the expression of aquaporin water channels through the AC pathway ($\uparrow$ cAMP).

2. **Oxytocin receptor.** The **oxytocin receptor** is found on myoepithelial cells in the mammary gland and smooth muscles cells of the myometrium in the uterus and elicits its action of milk ejection and uterine contraction through the PL$_C$ pathway ($\uparrow$ IP$_3$ + DAG).

3. **Angiotensin (AT$_1$) receptor.** The **AT$_1$ receptor** is found on vascular smooth muscle cells (including the afferent and efferent arterioles), CNS, zona glomerulosa cells of adrenal cortex, and renal tubular cells of the proximal convoluted tubule and elicits its action of increased arteriolar constriction, increased sensation of thirst, increased ADH secretion, increased aldosterone secretion, and increased Na^+ reabsorption through the PL$_C$ pathway ($\uparrow$ IP$_3$ + DAG).

4. **Opiate receptors (μ, δ, κ, σ).** The μ, δ, κ, σ **receptors** are found throughout the CNS and spinal cord. The μ **receptor** elicits its action through the PL$_C$ pathway ($\uparrow$ IP$_3$ + DAG and close voltage-gated Ca^{2+} channels when acting presynaptically) and the AC pathway ($\downarrow$ cAMP levels + opens a K^+ channel protein so that K^+ flows out of the cell causing a hyperpolarization when acting postsynaptically). ß-endorphin, enkephalins, and dynorphins are naturally occurring opioids that bind to the μ,δ,κ,σ receptors. **Morphine (Roxanol, MS Contin), meperidine (Demerol), methadone (Dolophine), fentanyl (Sublimaze, Duragesic), alfentanil, sufentanil, remifentanil, hydromorphone (Dilaudid), and heroin** are μ receptor agonists and are used to treat severe pain. **Hydrocodone (Hycodan), oxycodone (Roxicodone, Supeudol), codeine, propoxyphene (Darvon)** are μ receptor agonists and are used to treat moderate to mild pain. **Butorphanol** and **buprenorphine** are partial μ receptor agonists. **Nalbuphine** is a mixed agonist with κ agonist activity and μ-antagonist activity. **Naloxone (Narcan)** and **naltrexone (Trexan)** are μ-receptor antagonists and are used to treat opioid toxicity, respiratory depression, and opioid addiction.

5. **Bradykinin$_{1,2}$ (B$_1$ and B$_2$) receptors.** The **B$_1$ receptor** is found on peripheral terminals of nociceptive neurons (its expression is induced by inflammatory cytokines and bacterial lipopolyusaccharide) and elicits its action through the PL$_C$ pathway ($\uparrow$ IP$_3$ + DAG). The **B$_2$ receptor** is found on peripheral terminals of nociceptive neurons and elicits its action of forming prostaglandins PGE$_2$ and PGI$_2$ through the PL$_C$ pathway ($\uparrow$ IP$_3$ + DAG). **Kinin peptides** are produced from kininogens by serine protease kallikreins in the setting of tissue damage and inflammation and bind to B$_1$ and B$_2$ receptors. The B$_1$ and B$_2$ receptors are involved in the sensation of acute pain caused by tissue damage and inflammation (i.e., nociception).

6. **Neurotensin receptor**
7. **Neuropeptide Y receptor**
8. **Vasoactive intestinal polypeptide (VIP) receptor**
9. **Cholecystokinin (CCK) receptor**

VI **Enzyme-Linked Receptors.** All enzyme-linked receptors are composed structurally of single or multiple polypeptides that span the cell membrane once (**one-pass transmembrane receptors**). These receptors are unique in that their cytoplasmic domain has **intrinsic enzyme activity** or **associates directly with an enzyme.** The various types of enzyme-linked receptors include:

A. **Receptor guanylate cyclase.** When the appropriate signal binds to receptor guanylate cyclase, its intrinsic enzyme guanylate cyclase activity produces cGMP. cGMP activates **cGMP-dependent protein kinase (protein kinase G; PKG),** which catalyzes the **covalent phosphorylation** of serine and threonine within certain intracellular proteins to increase their activity. An example of a receptor guanylate cyclase is **atrial natriuretic peptide (ANP) receptor.**

B. **Receptor tyrosine phosphatase.** When the appropriate signal binds to a receptor tyrosine phosphatase, its intrinsic tyrosine phosphatase will catalyze the **dephosphorylation** of tyrosine within certain intracellular proteins to increase their activity. An example of a receptor tyrosine phosphatase is **CD45.**

C. **Receptor serine/threonine kinase.** When the appropriate signal binds to a receptor serine/threonine kinase, its intrinsic serine/threonine kinase activity catalyzes the **covalent phosphorylation** of serine and threonine within certain intracellular proteins to increase their activity. An example of a receptor serine/threonine kinase is **transforming growth factor ß (TGFß) receptor.**

D. **Tyrosine kinase-associated receptor.** When the appropriate signal binds to a tyrosin kinase-associated receptor, the tyrosine kinase that is associated with the receptor will catalyze the **covalent phosphorylation** of tyrosine within certain intracellular proteins to increase their activity. One important tyrosine kinase that is associated with the receptor is the Src protein. Src protein is a tyrosine kinase that is the gene product of the **src proto-oncogene.** Examples of tyrosine kinase-associated receptors include **cytokine receptors, growth hormone receptor, prolactin hormone receptor, antigen-specific receptors on B and T lymphocytes, interleukin-2 (IL-2) receptor, and the erythropoietin receptor.**

E. **Receptor tyrosine kinase** (Figure 3-4). When the appropriate signal binds to a receptor tyrosine kinase, its intrinsic tyrosine kinase activity catalyzes the **autophosphorylation** of tyrosine (producing **phosphotyrosine**) within the receptor. There is a vast array of intracellular proteins that bind to the phosphotyrosine residues all of which share a sequence homology (called SH$_2$ domain) and are called **SH$_2$-domain proteins.** The SH$_2$-domain protein interacts with **Sos protein (son-of-sevenless).** The Sos protein activates **Ras protein** by causing Ras protein to bind GTP. Ras protein is a monomeric G protein that is the gene product of the **ras proto-oncogene.** The activated Ras protein activates **Raf protein kinase.** The activated Raf protein kinase activates **mitogen-activated protein kinase (MAP kinase)** by covalent phosphorylation of tyrosine and threonine. The activated MAP kinases leaves the cytoplasm and enters the nucleus, where it phosphorylates gene regulatory proteins that then causes **gene transcription.** Examples of receptor tyrosine kinases include: **epidermal growth factor (EGF) receptor, platelet-derived growth factor (PDGF) receptor, fibroblast growth factor (FGF) receptor, nerve growth factor (NGF) receptor, vascular endothelial growth factor (VEGF) receptor,** and the **insulin receptor.**

VII **Low Density Lipoprotein (LDL) Receptor.** The LDL receptor has an extracellular portion that consists of a one domain with seven cysteine-rich areas called the **LDL-binding region;** a second domain with EGF homology; and a third domain with serine and threonine-rich areas linked to oligosaccharides. When LDL (the principal carrier of serum cholesterol) binds to the LDL receptor, **receptor-mediated endocytosis** forms in the following steps:

A. Receptor-mediated endocytosis forms **clathrin-coated vesicles** that fuse with an **endosome** or **compartment for uncoupling of receptor and ligand (called the CURL)** where the LDL and LDL receptor are disassociated from each other because of the low pH. The LDL receptor is recycled back to the cell membrane.

B. **ENDOLYSOSOMES** fuse with the endosome and LDL is lysosomally degraded to **cholesterol,** which is released into the cytoplasm.

C. The cholesterol inhibits the enzyme **3-hydroxy-3-methylglutaryl-CoA (HNG-CoA) reductase,** which catalyzes the committed step in cholesterol biosynthesis and thereby suppresses *de novo* cholesterol biosynthesis. This process contributes to keeping serum cholesterol levels in the normal range.

D. Receptor-mediated endocytosis is clinically relevant in a condition called **familial hypercholesteremia (FH).**
   1. FH is a genetic disease (autosomal dominant) involving mutations in the gene (located on chromosome 19p13.1–13.3) for the LDL receptor.
   2. The mutations can result in two scenarios: the LDL receptor fails to bind LDL; or the LDL receptor binds LDL, but fails to undergo receptor-mediated endocytosis.
   3. In FH, HMG-CoA reductase activity and *de novo* cholesterol biosynthesis are unchecked.
   4. Clinical findings in FH include: premature coronary artery disease; myocardial infarcts in third decade; Achilles tendon xanthomas; yellow patches on eyelids (xanthelasmas); lipid deposits in the eye in front of the iris (arcus senilis); **Type IIa:** ↑LDL (>260 mg/dL), ↑cholesterol, normal triglycerides; **Type IIb:** ↑LDL, ↑LDL, ↑cholesterol, ↑triglycerides.

● **Figure 3-4 Signal transduction of a receptor tyrosine kinase.** EGF = epidermal growth factor; Sos = son-of-sevenless; Ras = rat sarcoma; MAP = mitogen-activated protein; SH_2 = sequence homology; DNA = deoxyribonucleic acid.

VIII Summary Table (Table 3-1)

TABLE 3-1

Carrier Proteins (transporters)	Ion Channel Proteins	G Protein-Linked Receptors	Enzyme-Linked Receptors
Ca^{2+} ATPase H$^+$ ATPase Na$^+$-K$^+$ ATPase H$^+$-K$^+$ ATPase Na$^+$-glucose cotransporter Na$^+$-amino acid cotransporter FAT	**Voltage-gated** L-type Ca^{2+} channel protein (dihydropyridine receptor) Fast Ca^{2+} release channel protein (ryanodine receptor) T-type Ca^{2+} channel protein K$^+$ channel protein Slow (funny) Na$^+$ channel protein Fast Na$^+$ channel protein	**mACh receptors** M$_1$ ($\uparrow$IP3 + DAG) M$_2$ ($\downarrow$cAMP + open K$^+$ channel) M$_3$ ($\uparrow$IP3 + DAG) M$_4$ ($\downarrow$cAMP + open K$^+$ channel) M$_5$ ($\uparrow$IP$_3$ +DAG)	**Receptor guanylate cyclase** ANP receptor **Receptor tyrosine phosphatase** CD45
ABC transporter superfamily MDR1 MDR2 Chloroquine transporter CF transporter MOAT BAT Flippase		**Adrenergic Receptors** a$_1$ ($\uparrow$IP$_3$ + DAG) a$_2$ ($\downarrow$cAMP + open K$^+$ channel) ß$_1$ ($\uparrow$cAMP) ß$_2$ ($\uparrow$cAMP) ß$_3$ ($\uparrow$cAMP)	**Receptor serine/threonine kinase** TGFß
	Transmitter-gated nACh receptor	mGluR1,5 ($\uparrow$cAMP and $\uparrow$IP$_3$ + DAG) mGluR2,3 ($\downarrow$cAMP) mGluR4,6,7,8 ($\downarrow$cAMP)	**Tyrosine kinase-associated receptors** Cytokine receptors Growth hormone receptor Prolactin receptor
Glucose transporter family GLUT 1 GLUT 2 GLUT 3 GLUT 4 GLUT 5	**Glutamate receptors** NMDA receptor Kainate receptor AMPA receptor 5-HT$_3$ receptor P$_{2x}$ receptors GABA$_A$ receptor Glycine receptor	5-HT$_1$ ($\downarrow$cAMP) 5-HT$_2$ ($\uparrow$IP$_3$ + DAG) 5-HT$_{4,6,7}$ ($\uparrow$cAMP) P$_1$ receptor ($\downarrow$cAMP) P$_{2Y}$ receptor ($\uparrow$IP$_3$ + DAG) GABA$_B$ receptor ($\downarrow$cAMP + open K$^+$ channel)	Antigen-specific receptors IL-2 receptor Erythropoietin receptor
Urea transporter Na$^+$-dicarboxylate/ tricarboxylate cotransporter Organic anion-dicarboxylate/ tricarboxylate cotransporter Organic anion- X$^-$ exchanger Organic cation-X$^+$ exchanger Na$^+$-H$^+$ exchanger Na$^+$-HCO$_3^-$ cotransporter Na$^+$-K$^+$-2C1$^-$ cotransporter		D1 receptor ($\uparrow$cAMP and $\uparrow$IP$_3$ + DAG) D2 receptor ($\downarrow$cAMP + open K$^+$ channel) H$_1$ receptor ($\uparrow$IP$_3$ + DAG) H$_2$ receptor ($\uparrow$cAMP) TSH receptor ($\uparrow$cAMP) LH receptor ($\uparrow$cAMP) FSH receptor ($\uparrow$cAMP) ACTH receptor ($\uparrow$cAMP) Glucagon receptor ($\uparrow$cAMP) Somatostatin receptor ($\downarrow$cAMP + open K$^+$ channel) PTH receptor ($\uparrow$cAMP)	**Receptor tyrosine kinase** EGF receptor PDGF receptor FGF receptor NGF receptor VEGF receptor Insulin receptor

TABLE 3.1		*(Continued)*	
Carrier Proteins (Transporters)	**Ion Channel Proteins**	**G Protein-Linked Receptors**	**Enzyme-Linked Receptors**
Na^+-Cl^- cotransporter		**Neuropeptide receptors**	
Cl^--Base exchanger		V_1 receptor ($\uparrow IP_3$ + DAG)	
K^+-Cl^- cotransporter		V_2 receptor ($\uparrow$ cAMP)	
Cl^--HCO_3^- exchanger		Oxytocin receptor ($\uparrow IP_3$ + DAG)	
Na^+-Ca^{2+} exchanger		AT_1 receptor ($\uparrow IP_3$ + DAG)	
Na^+-PO_4^{2-} cotransporter		μ,δ,κ,σ, Opiate receptors	
PO_4^{2-}-anion exchanger		μ receptor ($\uparrow IP_3$ + DAG and close Ca^{2+} channel) or ($\downarrow$ cAMP + open K^+ channel)	
Na^+-NH_4^+ exchanger		B_1 and B_2 receptors ($\uparrow IP_3$ + DAG)	
		Neurotensin receptor	
		Neuropeptide Y receptor	
		VIP receptor	
		CCK receptor	

mGluR = metabotropic glutamate receptor; 5-HT = 5-hydroxytryptamine serotonin receptor; P = purinergic; GABA = gamma-aminobutyric acid; D = dopamine; H = histamine; TSH = thyroid stimulating hormone; LH = luteinizing hormone; ACTH = adrenocorticotrophin hormone; PTH = parathyroid hormone; V = vasopressin; VIP = vasoactive intestinal polypeptide; CCK = cholecystokinin; mACh = muscarinic acetylcholine; FAT-fatty acid transporter; MDR = multidrug resistance; CF = cystic fibrosis; MOAT = multispecific organ anion transporter; BAT = biliary acid transporter; GLUT = glucose transporter; FSH = follicle stimulating hormone; AT = angiotensin; B = bradykinin; ANP = atrial natriuretic peptide; TGF = transforming growth factor; IL = interleukin; EGF = epidermal growth factor; PDGF = platelet derived growth factor; FGF = fibroblast growth factor; NGF = nerve growth factor; VEGF = vascular endothelial growth factor.

From Dudek RW: *High Yield Cell and Molecular Biology; 2nd ed.* Philadelphia: Lippincott Williams & Wilkins, 2000.

Chapter 4

Epithelium

I   **Introduction.** Epithelium is a tissue that **covers the body surface, lines body cavities** (e.g., peritoneal, pleural), **lines tubules** (e.g., gastrointestinal tract, blood vessels, kidney tubules), and **forms glands** (e.g., exocrine, endocrine). Epithelium is **avascular** and has a **high regeneration capacity** ranging from a **few days** (e.g., epithelium lining small intestine) to **1 month** (e.g., epidermis of the skin).

II   **Classification** (Table 4-1)

III   **Polarity** of an epithelial cell is made evident by specializations that are found in various regions of the cell (Figure 4-1).

A. THE APICAL REGION

1. **Microvilli** contain a core of **actin** filaments that are anchored to the **terminal web.** The actin filaments are cross-linked by villin. Microvilli of intestinal epithelium are

TABLE 4-1	CLASSIFICATION OF EPITHELIUM
Type of Epithelium	**Location in Body**
Simple squamous	**Type I pneumocytes** of alveoli, parietal layer of Bowman's capsule, **endothelium** of blood and lymph vessels, **mesothelium** of body cavities, **corneal endothelium**
Simple cuboidal	Lining of respiratory bronchioles, thyroid **follicular cells, germinal epithelium** of ovary, lens of eye, **pigment epithelium** of retina, **ependymal cells** of choroid plexus
Simple columnar	Lining of pulmonary bronchioles, lining of gastrointestinal tract, lining of anal canal **above anal valves,** lining of uterus and uterine tubes, lining of large excretory ducts of glands, lining of efferent ductules
Stratified squamous	**Epidermis** of skin, lining of oral cavity and esophagus, lining of anal canal **below anal valves,** lining of vagina, **corneal epithelium,** lining of female urethra, lining of **fossa navicularis** of the penile urethra
Stratified columnar	Lining of membranous and penile urethra up to fossa navicularis
Pseudostratified columnar	Lining of trachea and primary bronchi, lining of epididymis, ductus deferens, ejaculatory duct
Transitional	Lining of renal calyces, renal pelvis, ureters, urinary bladder, prostatic urethra

Reprinted with permission from Dudek RW. *High-Yield Histology,* 2nd ed. P 20, table 2-1. Philadelphia: Lippincott Williams & Wilkins, 2000.

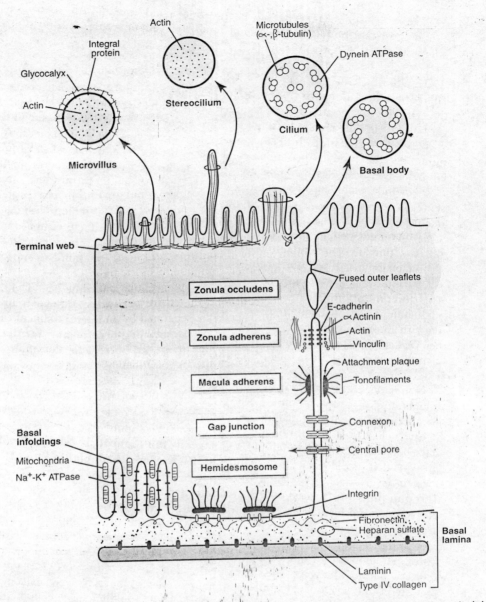

Actin

Integral protein

Glycocalyx

Actin

Microvillus

Actin

Stereocilium

Microtubules (∝-, β-tubulin)

Dynein ATPase

Cilium

Basal body

Terminal web

Fused outer leaflets

| Zonula occludens |

E-cadherin
∝Actinin
Actin
Vinculin

| Zonula adherens |

| Macula adherens |

Attachment plaque
Tonofilaments

Basal infoldings

Mitochondria

Na⁺-K⁺ ATPase

| Gap junction |

Connexon

Central pore

| Hemidesmosome |

Integrin

Fibronectin
Heparan sulfate

Basal lamina

Laminin

Type IV collagen

● Figure 4-1 Diagram of a hypothetical epithelial cell demonstrating the specializations in the apical, lateral, and basal regions.

coated with a **glycocalyx** that consists of **terminal oligosaccharides of integral membrane proteins.** The glycocalyx has enzymatic activity involved in carbohydrate digestion.

2. **Stereocilia** are long microvilli found on epididymal epithelium and hair cells of the inner ear.

3. **Cilia** are motile cell processes that contain a core of microtubules (α- and β-tubulin) called the **axoneme.** The axoneme consists of nine doublet microtubules uniformly spaced around two central microtubules (**9 + 2 arrangement**). **Nexin** connects the nine doublet microtubules. Each doublet has **short arms** that consist of **dynein**

ATPase, which splits ATP to provide energy for cilia movement. At the base of each cilium is a **basal body** that consists of nine triplet microtubules and no central microtubules (**9 + 0 arrangement**).

B. THE LATERAL REGION

1. **The zonula occludens (or tight junction)** extends around the **entire perimeter** of the cell. The outer leaflets of the cell membrane of the two adjoining cells **fuse** at various points. The zonula occludens is the gatekeeper of the **paracellular pathway,** thereby regulating the passage of fluid, electrolytes, macromolecules, and immune cells through the intercellular space between epithelial cells. Various epithelia have been classified either as "tight" or "leaky" based on the permeability of the zonula occludens. The zonula occludens can be rapidly formed and disassembled (e.g., during leukocyte migration across endothelium). The protein **occludin** (~65 kDa; the first tight junction protein identified) interacts with many structural and signaling molecules and participates in the regulation of tight junction function. The protein family of **claudins** (~23 kDa; >20 family members) are the major structural and functional components of the tight junction and are considered the major players in regulating the paracellular pathway.

2. **The zonula adherens** extends around the **entire perimeter** of the cell. The cell membranes of the two adjoining cells are separated by an intercellular space filled with an amorphous material. There is a dense area on the cytoplasmic side of each cell that consists of **actin** filaments, which are linked by **α-actinin** and **vinculin** to a transmembrane protein called **E-cadherin** (or adherens cell adhesion molecule [A-CAM]).

3. **The macula adherens (desmosome)** occurs at **small discrete sites.** The cell membranes of the two adjoining cells are separated by an intercellular space filled with a **thin dense line** of material. An **attachment plaque** on the cytoplasmic side of each cell anchors **tonofilaments.** Several protein components of the desmosome have been identified: **desmoglein I** and **desmocollin I and II** are calcium-binding proteins that mediate calcium-dependent cell adhesion; **desmoplakin I and II** are located in the attachment plaque.

4. **The gap junction (nexus)** occurs at **small discrete sites** for the **metabolic and electrical coupling** of cells. The cell membranes of the two adjoining cells are separated by an intercellular space that is bridged by **connexons.** Connexons consist of a transmembrane protein (**connexin**) complex. Connexons contain central pores that allow passage of ions, cAMP, amino acids, steroids, and small molecules (<1,200 daltons) between cells. The opening and closing of the pores is regulated by intracellular levels of calcium. Gap junctions are also found between osteocytes, astrocytes, cardiac muscle cells, smooth muscle cells, and endocrine cells. Cancer cells generally do not have gap junctions, so the cancer cells cannot communicate their mitotic activity to each other, which may explain their uncontrolled growth.

C. THE BASAL REGION

1. **Basal infoldings** are invaginations of the cell membrane that contain **ion pumps** (Na^+-K^+ **ATPase**) found in close association with **mitochondria,** which provide the substrate ATP. Basal infoldings are found in the proximal and distal convoluted tubules of the kidney and in ducts of salivary glands.

2. **Hemidesmosomes** are junctions that anchor epithelial cells to the underlying basal lamina via a transmembrane protein called **integrin.** As a result, hemidesmosomes provide a connection between the **cytoskeleton** of the epithelial cell and the **extracellular matrix.**

3. **Basal lamina.** The principal constituents are **fibronectin** (binds to integrin of the hemidesmosome), **heparan sulfate, laminin,** and **type IV collagen.** Functions of the basal lamina include:
   a. **Forming a barrier** between epithelium and connective tissue. **In normal conditions,** lymphocytes may pass the basal lamina during immune surveillance. **In cancerous conditions,** neoplastic cells may pass the basal lamina during malignant invasion.
   b. **Serving as a filter** (e.g., renal glomerulus)
   c. **Playing a role in regeneration** (epithelial, nerve, or muscle cells use the basal lamina as a scaffolding during regeneration or wound healing)

IV Clinical Considerations

A. **IMMOTILE CILIA SYNDROME (KARTAGENER SYNDROME)** is a genetic disease involving mutations in genes that code for ciliary proteins (e.g., tubulin, dynein). This results in **situs inversus** (organ reversal as a result of failure of cells to migrate properly during embryogenesis), **recurrent sinus and pulmonary infections** (inability to move mucus), and **sterility in males** (retarded sperm movement).

B. **BULLOUS PEMPHIGOID** is an autoimmune disease in which antibodies against desmosomal proteins are formed. This results in widespread skin and mucous membrane blistering as desmosomes fall apart.

C. **CARCINOMA** is a malignant neoplasm derived from epithelium.

D. **ADENOCARCINOMA** is a malignant neoplasm derived from glandular epithelium.

V Selected Photomicrographs (Figure 4-2).

● **Figure 4-2 Epithelial components. (A)** EM of a junctional complex that exists between adjoining epithelial cells. Note the zonula occludens (*ZO*), zonula adherens (*ZA*), and macula adherens or desmosome (*D*). Note the actin core of the microvilli (*MV*) extending into the terminal web (*arrows*) within the cytoplasm. **(B)** A freeze-fracture replica of a zonula occludens or tight junction. A beltlike band of anastomosing strands (*ZO*) can be observed. The strands are seen as ridges of intramembranous particles on the P-face or complementary grooves on the E-face. Microvilli (*MV*) are apparent. **(C)** EM of a gap junction (*GJ;* or nexus) between adjoining cells. **(D)** A freeze-fracture replica of a gap junction or nexus shows a cluster of intramembranous particles (*arrow*) on the P-face. Each intramembranous particle corresponds to a connexon. Gap junctions are constructed from transmembrane proteins (called connexins) that form structures called connexons. Two connexons bridge across the intercellular space to form a channel (or pore) connecting two cells. **(E)** EM of microvilli in cross-section demonstrating the actin core (*arrow* 1) and the fuzzy glycocalyx (*arrow* 2). **(F)** EM of cilia. Note the microtubule core (*arrow*) extending into the basal body within the cytoplasm. **(G)** EM of cilia in cross-section. Note the arrangement of microtubules in a 9 + 2 arrangement and the dynein arm (*arrow*).

Connective Tissue

① Introduction. Types of connective tissue include loose connective tissue (e.g., fascia, lamina propria), dense connective tissue (e.g., tendons), adipose tissue, cartilage, and bone. The common features of all connective tissues are the **ground substance, fibers, and cells,** as described below.

② Ground Substance contains the following components:

A. Proteoglycans consist of a **core protein,** which binds many side chains of **glycosaminoglycans (GAGs),** and a **link protein,** which binds hyaluronic acid. GAGs are highly sulfated (SO_4^{2-}) and consist of **repeating disaccharide units** of a **hexosamine** (e.g., N-acetylglucosamine, N-acetylgalactosamine) and a **uronic acid** (e.g., glucuronic acid). Specific GAGs include the following:

1. **Hyaluronic acid** is found in most connective tissues and binds to the link protein of a large number of proteoglycans to form a proteoglycan aggregate.
2. **Chondroitin sulfate** is found in cartilage and bone.
3. **Keratan sulfate** is found in cartilage and bone, cornea, and intervertebral disk.
4. **Dermatan sulfate** is found in dermis of skin, blood vessels, and heart valves.
5. **Heparan sulfate** is found in the basal lamina, lung, and liver.

B. GLYCOPROTEINS
1. **Fibronectin** is a component of the basal lamina.
2. **Laminin** is a component of the basal lamina.
3. **Chondronectin** is found in cartilage.
4. **Osteocalcin, osteopontin, and bone sialoprotein** are found in bone.

C. THE MINERAL (INORGANIC) COMPONENT varies depending on the type of connective tissue.

D. WATER (TISSUE FLUID). The high concentration of negative charges as a result of sulfation (SO_4^{2-}) and carboxylation (COO–) of GAGs attracts water into the ground substance.

③ Fibers

A. COLLAGEN contains two characteristic amino acids, **hydroxyproline** and **hydroxylysine.**
1. **Synthesis of collagen** involves intracellular and extracellular events.
   a. **Intracellular events** include:

(1) **Synthesis of preprocollagen** within rER
(2) **Hydroxylation of proline and lysine** within rER catalyzed by **peptidyl proline hydroxylase** and **peptidyl lysine hydroxylase** Vitamin C is essential in this step. When vitamin C deficiency (i.e., scurvy) occurs, wounds fail to heal, bone formation is impaired, and teeth become loose.
(3) **Glycosylation of hydroxylysine** within rER
(4) **Formation of triple helix procollagen** within rER (involves registration peptides)
(5) **Addition of carbohydrates** within Golgi complex
(6) **Secretion of procollagen**

  b.   **Extracellular events** include:
(1) **Cleavage of procollagen** to form **tropocollagen** by extracellular peptidases
(2) **Self-assembly of tropocollagen** into fibrils **(67 nm periodicity)**
(3) **Cross-linking of adjacent** tropocollagen molecules catalyzed by lysyl oxidase

2. **Types of collagen** (Table 5-1)

B. **ELASTIC FIBERS** consist of an amorphous core of the **elastin** protein surrounded by microfibrils of the **fibrillin** protein. Elastic fibers contain two unique amino acids called **desmosine** and **isodesmosine,** which are involved in cross-linking.

TABLE 5-1	DISTRIBUTION OF COLLAGEN TYPES IN THE BODY
Type	**Location in Body**
I	Fibrocartilage, bone, dermis of skin, tendons, cornea, fascia In **wound healing,** type 1 replaces the initial type III collagen Most ubiquitous type of collagen Involved in Ehlers-Danlos syndrome and osteogenesis imperfecta
I;	Hyaline cartilage, elastic cartilage, nucleus pulposus, vitreous body
III	Liver, spleen, tunica media of blood vessels, muscularis externa of gastrointestinal tract In **wound healing,** type III is laid down first In **keloid formation,** increased amounts of type III are laid down Traditionally called **reticular fibers** Involved in Ehlers-Danlos syndrome
IV	Basal lamina Involved in Alport syndrome (hereditary nephritis)

Reprinted with permission from Dudek RW. *High-Yield Histology,* 2nd ed. p 26, table 3-1. Philadelphia: Lippincott Williams & Wilkins, 2000.

 Cells

A. **RESIDENT OR FIXED CELLS** are a stable population of cells that remain in the connective tissue. These include the following types of cells:

1. **Fibroblasts and fibrocytes** are fixed cells that are involved in the synthesis and secretion of collagen, elastic fibers, and ground substance.

2. **Macrophages (histiocytes)**
  a.   Macrophages arise from **monocytes** within the circulating blood and bone marrow.

b. They have a **phagocytic function.**

    (1) F_c **antibody receptors** on the macrophage cell membrane bind antibody-coated foreign material and subsequently phagocytose the material for lysosomal digestion.

    (2) **C3 (a component of complement) receptors** on the macrophage cell membrane bind bacteria and subsequently phagocytose the bacteria (called opsonization) for lysosomal digestion.

    (3) Certain phagocytosed material (e.g., bacilli of tuberculosis and leprosy, *Trypanosoma cruzi, Toxoplasma, Leishmania,* asbestos) cannot undergo lysosomal digestion, so macrophages will fuse to form **foreign body giant cells.**

    (4) In sites of chronic inflammation, macrophages may assemble into epithelial-like sheets called **epithelioid cells of granulomas.**

c. Macrophages have an **antigen-presenting function.**

    (1) **Exogenous antigens** circulating in the bloodstream are phagocytosed by macrophages and undergo degradation in endosomal acid vesicles.

    (2) Antigen proteins are degraded into **antigen peptide fragments,** which are presented on the macrophage cell surface in conjunction with class II major histocompatibility complex (MHC).

    (3) **CD4+ helper T cells** with antigen-specific T cell receptor (TcR) on its cell surface recognize the antigen peptide fragment.

d. Macrophages are activated by **lipopolysaccharides** (a surface component of Gram-negative bacteria) and **γ-interferon.**

e. They secrete **interleukin 1** (IL-1; stimulates mitosis of T cells), **interleukin 6** (IL-6; stimulates differentiation of B cells into plasma cells), **pyrogens** (mediate fever), **tumor necrosis factor-α (TNF-α),** and **granulocyte-macrophage colony-stimulating factor (GM-CSF).**

f. Macrophages have granules that are endolysosomes, which contain **acid hydrolases, aryl sulfatase, acid phosphatases, and peroxidase.**

g. Macrophages impart natural (innate) immunity along with neutrophils and NK cells.

3. **Mast cells**

a. Mast cells arise from stem cells in the bone marrow.

b. They have a function in **type I anaphylactic reactions, inflammation, and allergic reactions.**

c. They have **IgE antibody receptors** on their cell membranes that **bind IgE** produced by plasma cells on **first exposure** to an allergen (e.g., plant pollen, snake venom, foreign serum), which sensitizes the mast cells.

d. Mast cells secrete the following substances on **second exposure** to the same allergen, causing the classic **wheal-and-flare reaction** in the skin:

    (1) **Heparin,** an anticoagulant and cofactor for lipoprotein lipase (LPL)

    (2) **Histamine** (produced by decarboxylation of histidine), which increases vascular permeability, causes vasodilation, causes smooth muscle contraction of bronchi, and stimulates HCl secretion from parietal cells in the stomach

    (3) **Leukotriene C_4 and D_4** (are eicosanoids and components of slow-reacting substance of anaphylaxis [SRS-A]), which increase vascular permeability, cause vasodilation, and cause smooth muscle contraction of bronchi

    (4) **Eosinophil chemotactic factor (ECF-A),** which attracts eosinophils to the inflammation site

4. **Adipocytes**

   a. Adipocytes in **multilocular (brown) adipose tissue** contain numerous fat droplets and **numerous mitochondria that lack elementary particles** on the inner membrane. The energy produced by these mitochondria is dissipated as heat instead of being stored as ATP. Brown adipose tissue is present in **human infants after birth** to assist in **regulation of body temperature** but disappears within a few years. Multilocular adipose tissue has a brown color as a result of the numerous mitochondria that contain **cytochromes,** which have a color similar to hemoglobin.

   b. Adipocytes in **unilocular (white) adipose tissue** contain a large, single fat droplet surrounded by a thin rim of cytoplasm. This tissue accounts for all of the stored fat in humans and has a yellow color as a result of the presence of carotene.

      (1) In general, adipocytes synthesize and store **triacylglycerols** (also called triglycerides, fats, or neutral fats), which are composed of **three fatty acids in ester linkage with glycerol.**

      (2) **In the fed state,** an increased insulin:glucagon ratio stimulates adipocytes to produce the following reactions:

         (a) **Lipoprotein lipase (LPL)** attached to endothelial cells of capillaries within white adipose tissue catalyzes the digestion of triacylglycerols (carried by VLDL and chylomicrons) into fatty acids and glycerol. The fatty acids enter the adipocyte to be stored as triacylglycerols. The glycerol travels to the liver.

         (b) Adipocytes **take up and metabolize glucose** and use it for energy (via glycolysis) and as a source of the glycerol moiety of the stored triacylglycerols.

      (3) **In the fasted state,** a decreased insulin:glucagon ratio and epinephrine stimulate adipocytes to **begin lipolysis** as a result of increased levels of cAMP, which activate hormone-sensitive lipase. **Hormone-sensitive lipase** catalyzes the cleavage of fatty acids from triacylglycerol. The fatty acids become the major fuel of the body because they are used by muscle and kidney for production of energy (i.e., ATP) and converted in the liver to ketone bodies. The glycerol is used as a source of carbon by the liver for gluconeogenesis.

      (4) Adipocytes secrete a hormone called **leptin** that has an anorexic action in that leptin **decreases appetite** and **decreases body weight** (caused exclusively by a reduction of fat stores). The action of leptin is mediated through satiety centers in the **hypothalamus** (i.e., **paraventricular and arcuate nuclei**) where **leptin receptors** are found. The gene for leptin has been cloned and is called the *LEP* gene in humans.

5. **Chondroblasts and chondrocytes** are discussed in Chapter 6.

6. **Osteoblasts and osteocytes** are discussed in Chapter 7.

B. **TRANSIENT OR FREE CELLS** enter connective tissue from blood, usually during inflammation. These cells include neutrophils, eosinophils, basophils, monocytes, B cells, plasma cells, and T cells, which are discussed in Chapter 11.

Ⓥ Clinical Considerations

A. **EHLERS-DANLOS SYNDROME** is a genetic defect involving **peptidyl lysine hydroxylase** that affects **type I and type III** collagen synthesis, resulting in hypermobile joints, excessive stretchability of the skin, and rupture of large bowel and large arteries.

B. MARFAN SYNDROME is a genetic defect involving **fibrillin** (a component of elastic fibers), resulting in weakened tunica media of aorta (aortic dissection) and ectopia lentis.

C. HOMOCYSTINURIA is a genetic defect involving the enzyme cystathionine synthetase, resulting in abnormal cross-linking of collagen.

D. OSTEOGENESIS IMPERFECTA is a genetic defect involving **type I collagen**, resulting in spontaneous fractures of bone and blue sclera of the eye.

E. ALPORT SYNDROME (HEREDITARY NEPHRITIS) is a genetic defect involving **type IV collagen**, resulting in renal failure and deafness.

F. KELOID FORMATION is a deviation in normal wound healing whereby an excessive accumulation of collagen occurs, resulting in a raised, tumorous scar.

G. AMYLOIDOSIS is a group of diseases that have in common the **deposition of amyloid** (a proteinaceous substance) in the intercellular space of various organs.
1. By light microscopy, amyloid is an eosinophilic, amorphous substance. By electron microscopy, amyloid is composed of **nonbranching fibrillar proteins** (95%) and a glycoprotein called **P component**, which is pentagonal in shape (5%).
2. A number of different nonbranching fibrillar proteins have been identified, which include:
   a. **Amyloid light chain,** an immunoglobulin protein secreted by plasma cells
   b. **Amyloid-associated protein,** synthesized by the liver
   c. **β_2-microglobulin,** a component of the major histocompatibility complex class I proteins
   d. **β_2-amyloid,** a 4,000-dalton peptide
   e. **Islet amyloid polypeptide (amylin),** which is increased within pancreatic islets of Langerhans in patients with type 2 diabetes
3. **Types of amyloidosis** include the following:
   a. **Immunocyte dyscrasias with amyloidosis (primary amyloidosis)** are the most common form of amyloidosis and are associated with the amyloid light chain protein. Some patients with **multiple myeloma** (a plasma cell neoplasia) demonstrate amyloidosis along with the presence of light chains (**Bence Jones proteins**) in the serum and urine.
   b. **Reactive systemic amyloidosis (secondary amyloidosis)** occurs as a secondary complication to **chronic inflammation** (e.g., rheumatoid arthritis, regional enteritis, ulcerative colitis) and is associated with the amyloid-associated protein.
   c. **Hemodialysis-associated amyloidosis** occurs in patients on **long-term hemodialysis** and is associated with the β_2-microglobulin protein.
   d. **Senile cerebral amyloidosis** occurs in patients with **Alzheimer disease** and is associated with β_2-amyloid protein deposition in cerebral plaques.
   e. **Endocrine amyloid** occurs in patients with **type 2 diabetes** and is associated with islet amyloid polypeptide deposition in the pancreatic islets.

VI SELECTED PHOTOMICROGRAPHS (Figure 5-1).

● **Figure 5-1 Connective tissue. (A1)** A group of collagen fibers. Note the 67 nm periodicity of collagen (*arrows*). **(A2)** Ehlers-Danlos syndrome. Note the extremely stretchable skin at the elbow. **(B1)** EM of an elastic fiber consisting of an amorphous core (*CR*) of elastin protein and microfibrils (*arrows*) of the fibrillin protein. **(B2)** Marfan syndrome. Note the tall stature, exceptionally long limbs, and arachnodactyly (elongated hands and feet with very slender digits). **(C)** EM of a fibroblast. Fibroblasts (*F*) have a centrally located, cigar-shaped nucleus (*N*). A well-developed rER, mitochondria (M), Golgi (*G*), and secretory vesicles reflecting active collagen (*Col*) synthesis characterize the cytoplasm. **(D)** EM of a macrophage. Macrophages have an ovoid nucleus that is frequently indented on one side to become bean-shaped. The cell surface is uneven, varying from short projections to long, thin fingerlike projections. The cytoplasm is characterized by phagolysosomes (*arrowhead*) and phagocytic vacuoles (*arrows*) reflecting their phagocytic activity. **(E)** EM of a mast cell. Mast cells have a centrally located, ovoid-shaped nucleus. The cytoplasm is characterized by numerous secretory granules (Gr) that display variations in morphology even within the same cell. **(F)** EM of an adipocyte. Adipocytes have an eccentrically located nucleus (*N*) and a thin rim of cytoplasm giving the "signet ring" appearance. A small Golgi, few mitochondria, sparse rER, abundant free ribosomes, and a large lipid droplet (*lp*) that is not membrane bound characterize the cytoplasm.

Chapter 6

Cartilage

① Introduction. Cartilage is a type of connective tissue that includes the bluish-white and translucent **hyaline cartilage** (e.g., articular ends of long bones), yellowish **elastic cartilage** (e.g., pinna of ear), and **fibrocartilage** (e.g., annulus fibrosus of the intervertebral disk and meniscus of the knee joint). Cartilage has all the common features of connective tissue, which include ground substance, fibers, and cells, as indicated below.

② Ground Substance consists of:

    A. PROTEOGLYCANS, containing side chains of glycosaminoglycans (GAGs), specifically **chondroitin sulfate** and **keratan sulfate**

    B. GLYCOPROTEINS, including **chondronectin** and **chondrocalcin** (a Ca^{2+}-binding protein)

    C. NO MINERAL (INORGANIC) COMPONENT, because cartilage is not mineralized

    D. WATER (TISSUE FLUID)—high degree of hydration (75%)

③ Fibers

    A. TYPE I COLLAGEN is found in fibrocartilage.

    B. TYPE II COLLAGEN is found in hyaline and elastic cartilage.

④ Cells

    A. CHONDROGENIC CELLS are found in the perichondrium, where they undergo mitosis and differentiate into chondroblasts.

    B. CHONDROBLASTS arise from chondrogenic cells and may undergo mitosis.

    C. CHONDROCYTES reside in lacunae. They form **isogenous groups** that are surrounded by a **territorial matrix** that stains basophilic because of the higher local concentration of chondroitin sulfate. Chondrocytes may undergo mitosis.

⑤ Blood Vessels and Nerves are absent. Like epithelium, cartilage is avascular. It receives its nutrients by diffusion through the ground substance.

VI **Chondrogenesis** occurs in the embryo when mesodermal cells withdraw their processes and condense into aggregations called **centers of chondrification.** Cartilage may then grow in the following ways:

A. **INTERSTITIAL GROWTH** occurs by mitosis of preexisting chondrocytes.

B. **APPOSITIONAL GROWTH** occurs by differentiation of chondrogenic cells in the perichondrium into chondroblasts.

VII **Hormonal Influence**

A. **PROTEIN HORMONES. GROWTH HORMONE (GH)** is converted by the liver to **somatomedin C,** which stimulates cartilage growth.

B. **STEROID HORMONES.**
   1. Triiodothyronine (T_3), thyroxine (T_4), and **testosterone** stimulate cartilage growth.
   2. Estradiol, **cortisone,** and **hydrocortisone** inhibit cartilage growth.

VIII **Repair.** In the adult, damaged cartilage shows limited repair (regeneration) and may form scar tissue instead of cartilage. In young children, damaged cartilage shows a greater capacity for repair.

Chapter 7

Bone

I **Introduction.** Bone is a type of connective tissue that has a **supportive and protective function** and also serves as a **reservoir for Ca^{2+} and PO$_4^{2-}$**. Bone has all the common features of connective tissue, which include ground substance, fibers, and cells, as indicated below.

II **Ground Substance** consists of:

    A. PROTEOGLYCANS containing a side chain of glycosaminoglycans (GAGs), specifically **chondroitin sulfate** and **keratan sulfate**

    B. GLYCOPROTEINS, such as **osteonectin, osteocalcin** (a Ca^{2+}-binding protein), and **osteopontin**

    C. A MINERAL (INORGANIC) COMPONENT that includes: **Ca$_{10}$(PO$_4$)$_6$OH$_2$ (hydroxyapatite crystals), C$_6$H$_5$O$_7^{3-}$ (citrate ions), and CO$_3^{2-}$ (carbonate ions).** The mineral component comprises approximately 75% of the bone mass and contributes to the **hardness and rigidity** of bone. A dilute acid or chelating agent, such as ethylenediaminetetraacetic acid (EDTA), demineralizes bone.

    D. WATER (TISSUE FLUID), which contributes to a low degree of hydration (7%)

III **Fibers** consist of **type I collagen** that provides **tensile strength** to bone.

IV **Cells**

    A. OSTEOPROGENITOR CELLS differentiate into osteoblasts during osteogenesis and bone repair and may undergo mitosis.

    B. OSTEOBLASTS
      1. Osteoblasts are derived from osteoprogenitor cells.
      2. Osteoblasts secrete **osteoid,** which is unmineralized bone matrix consisting of proteoglycans, glycoproteins, and type I collagen.
        a. For mineralization to occur, osteoblasts secrete **osteocalcin** and **alkaline phosphatase,** which hydrolyzes PO$_4^{2-}$-containing substrates as well as Ca^{2+} β-glycerophosphate to release Ca^{2+} and PO$_4^{2-}$.
        b. In addition, osteoblasts release **matrix vesicles** (membrane-bound vesicles), which concentrate Ca^{2+} and PO$_4^{2-}$ and are the most important factor for mineralization to occur.

   c.   Clinical markers for osteogenesis or bone repair: **serum alkaline phosphatase** and **serum osteocalcin**
3. Osteoblasts secrete **interleukin 1 (IL-1)**, which is a potent stimulator of osteoclast activity.
4. Osteoblasts possess the **parathyroid hormone (PTH) receptor** (a G protein–linked receptor) and the **1,25-(OH)$_2$vitamin D receptor** (a steroid hormone receptor).
5. Osteoblasts do not undergo mitosis.

C. OSTEOCYTES
1. Osteocytes and their cytoplasmic processes are surrounded by bone matrix as they reside in spaces called **lacunae** and **canaliculi**, respectively. Cytoplasmic processes of neighboring osteocytes communicate via **gap junctions**.
2. Osteocytes do not undergo mitosis.

D. OSTEOCLASTS
1. Osteoclasts are derived from **granulocyte-monocyte progenitor cells** within the bone marrow.
2. Osteoclasts are multinucleated cells that reside in shallow depressions of the bone called **Howship's lacunae.**
3. Osteoclasts function in **bone resorption** in the following ways:
   a.   Secrete **lysosomal enzymes** (e.g., β-glucuronidase, aryl sulfatase) to digest the proteoglycans of the bone matrix
   b.   Secrete **collagenase** to digest type I collagen of the bone matrix
4. Osteoclasts have a ruffled border (infoldings of the cell membrane) closest to the bone that contains **H$^+$ ATPase** and **carbonic anhydrase**, which produces H$^+$ ions that create an acidic environment to digest the mineral component of the bone matrix.
5. Clinical markers for bone resorption: **urine hydroxyproline** (amino acid unique to collagen), **urine pyridinoline cross-links**, and **serum N-telopeptides.**
6. Osteoclasts possess the **calcitonin receptor** (a G protein–linked receptor).
7. Osteoclasts do not undergo mitosis.

V **Blood Vessels and Nerves** are present in Haversian canals and Volkmann's canals. However, they are absent in lacunae and canaliculi.

VI **Osteogenesis** always occurs by replacing preexisting connective tissue. In the embryo, two types of osteogenesis occur:

A. **INTRAMEMBRANOUS OSSIFICATION** occurs in the embryo when mesoderm condenses into sheets of highly vascular connective tissue, which then forms a primary ossification center. Bones that form via intramembranous ossification include **flat bones of the skull.**

B. **ENDOCHONDRAL OSSIFICATION** occurs in the embryo when mesoderm initially forms a hyaline cartilage model, which then develops a primary ossification center at the diaphysis. Later, secondary ossification centers form at the epiphysis at each end of the bone. Bones that form via endochondral ossification include the **humerus, femur, tibia, and other long bones.**
1. **Growth in length of long bones** occurs at the **epiphyseal plate,** which includes a number of zones as indicated below.
   a.   **Zone of reserve** contains resting chondrocytes.

b. **Zone of proliferation** contains chondrocytes undergoing mitosis and forming isogenous groups.

c. **Zone of hypertrophy** contains hypertrophied chondrocytes, which secrete alkaline phosphatase to increase Ca^{2+} and PO_4^{2-} levels.

d. **Zone of calcification** contains dead chondrocytes and calcified cartilage matrix called spicules.

e. **Zone of ossification** contains osteoprogenitor cells that congregate on spicules and differentiate into osteoblasts. Osteoblasts deposit bone on the surface of a spicule to form a **mixed spicule**, which consists of calcified cartilage matrix and bone.

2. **Growth in diameter of long bones** occurs at the **diaphysis** by deposition of bone at the periphery (**appositional growth**) as osteoprogenitor cells within the **periosteum** differentiate into osteoblasts.

VII **Bone Repair.** In the adult, bone shows a high capacity for repair through the proliferation of osteoprogenitor cells. After a bone fracture, the following actions take place:

A. Ruptured blood vessels form a **hematoma,** which bridges the fracture gap and provides a meshwork for the influx of inflammatory cells that secrete products (e.g., transforming growth factor β [TGF-β]; fibroblast growth factor [FGF]) to activate osteoprogenitor cells to form osteoblasts.

B. After 1 week, the hematoma is organized into a **soft tissue callus (procallus)** that anchors the ends of the fracture but provides no rigidity for weight bearing.

C. Osteoblasts begin to deposit **immature woven bone.** Woven bone is formed whenever osteoblasts produce osteoid rapidly and is characterized by an irregular arrangement of collagen.

D. Mesenchymal cells in the procallus form **hyaline cartilage** at the periphery that envelops the fracture site. The hyaline cartilage undergoes endochondral ossification.

E. The collection of bone at the fracture is now called a **bony callus.** As the bony callus mineralizes, controlled weight bearing can be tolerated.

F. Eventually all the woven bone of the bony callus is remodeled into **mature lamellar bone.** Lamellar bone is characterized by a regular layered arrangement of collagen.

VIII **Hormonal Influence**

A. **PROTEIN HORMONES**

1. **Growth hormone (GH)** stimulates hepatocytes in the liver to produce **somatomedin C (or insulin-like growth factor; IGF-1)**, which promotes skeletal growth and bone remodeling.

2. **PTH** acts directly on osteoblasts to secrete **macrophage colony-stimulating factor (M-CSF)** and expression of a cell surface protein called **RANKL.** M-CSF stimulates monocytes to differentiate into macrophages and express a cell surface receptor called **RANK.** RANKL (on the osteoblast) and RANK (on the macrophage) interact and cause the differentiation of macrophages into osteoclasts. Osteoclasts increase bone resorption, thereby elevating blood Ca^{2+} levels.

3. **Calcitonin** acts directly on osteoclasts to decrease bone resorption, thereby lowering blood Ca^{2+} levels.

B. **STEROID HORMONES**
  1. **T$_3$ and T$_4$** stimulate endochondral ossification and linear growth of bone.
  2. **Androgens** and **estrogens.** The closure of the epiphyseal plate is closely related to the development of the ovaries and testes. In **precocious sexual development,** skeletal growth is stunted because of premature closure of the epiphyseal plate. In **gonadal hypoplasia,** closure of the epiphyseal plate is delayed, and arms or legs become disproportionately long.
  3. **Cortisol** inhibits bone formation
  4. **1,25-(OH)$_2$ vitamin D** acts directly on osteoblasts to secrete IL-1, which stimulates osteoclasts to increase bone resorption, thereby elevating blood Ca^{2+} levels.

IX Cartilage and Bone Comparison (Table 7-1).

TABLE 7-1	CARTILAGE AND BONE COMPARISON	
Characteristic	**Cartilage**	**Bone**
Ground substance	Chondroitin sulfate, keratan sulfate Chondronectin, chondrocalcin No mineralization High degree of hydration (75%)	Chondroitin sulfate, keratan sulfate Osteonectin, osteocalcin, osteoporin Hydroxyapatite, citrate, bicarbonate Low degree of hydration (7%)
Fibers	Type I collagen (fibrocartilage) Type II collagen (hyaline and elastic)	Type I collagen (provides tensile strength)
Vascularity	Avascular; nutrients received via diffusion	Highly vascular
Nerves	Absent	Present
Growth	Interstitial and appositional	Appositional only
Repair	Low	High
Mitosis	Chondrogenic—yes Chondroblasts—yes Chondrocytes—yes	Osteoprogenitor—yes Osteoblasts—no Osteocytes—no Osteoclasts—no
Communication	No junctions	Gap junctions between osteocytes
Hormonal influence	Protein hormone: GH Steroids: T$_3$, T$_4$, testosterone, estradiol, cortisone, hydrocortisone	Protein hormone: GH, PTH, calcitonin Steroids: T$_3$, T$_4$, androgens, estrogens, cortisol, 1,25-(OH)$_2$ vitamin D
Vitamin influence	N/A	Vitamin D (deficiency = osteomalacia or rickets) Vitamin C (deficiency = scurvy) Vitamin A

Reprinted with permission from Dudek RW. *High-Yield Histology,* 2nd ed. p 37, table 5-1. Philadelphia: Lippincott Williams & Wilkins, 2000.
T$_3$ = triiodothyronine; T$_4$ = thyroxine; GH = growth hormone; PTH = parathyroid hormone; 1,25-(OH)$_2$ vitamin D = 1,25-dihydroxyvitamin D$_3$.

X   Clinical Considerations of Bone

A.   PRIMARY OSTEOPOROSIS (SENILE OR POSTMENOPAUSAL) is a critical loss of bone mass associated with a deficiency of either **GH (senile)** or **estrogen (post-menopausal)**. Decreased estrogen levels result in increased secretion of IL-1 (a potent stimulator of osteoclasts) from monocytes. Osteoporosis is widely recognized as a serious consequence of chronic glucocorticoid use to manage diseases including rheumatoid arthritis, inflammatory bowel diseases (e.g., Crohn's disease), asthma, emphysema, and rejection of organ transplant. Clinical findings include being asymptomatic in early stages, then presentation of vertebral compression fractures, femoral head fracture, or slow healing of fractured bones; severity is assessed by bone densitometry.

B.   OSTEOSARCOMA is a malignant tumor in which the tumor cells characteristically **produce bone.** This tumor is usually found in patients between **10 and 20 years of age** and most often around the **knee. Retinoblastoma** and mutations in the *p53* **gene (Li-Fraumeni syndrome)** have been implicated in increased risk for osteosarcomas.

C.   PAGET DISEASE is characterized by **uncontrolled osteoclast activity,** causing widespread bone resorption followed by intense osteoblast activity, producing woven bone that fills in the erosion. The net effect is paradoxically an increase in bone mass that is architecturally unsound because the woven bone persists.

D.   OSTEOMALACIA (in adults) and **rickets** (in children) are characterized by **lack of minerals within osteoid,** which occurs as a result of **vitamin D deficiency.**
   1.   To understand osteomalacia and rickets, normal **vitamin D metabolism** must be explained as indicated below:
      a.   Vitamin D sources include dietary intake and production by skin keratinocytes stimulated by ultraviolet light.
      b.   Vitamin D is hydroxylated by liver hepatocytes to **25-(OH) vitamin D.**
      c.   25-(OH) vitamin D is hydroxylated in the kidney to **1,25-(OH)$_2$ vitamin D,** the active metabolite that functions similar to a steroid hormone.
      d.   1,25-(OH)$_2$ vitamin D **stimulates absorption of Ca^{2+} and PO$_4$$^{2-}$ ions** from the intestinal lumen into the blood, thereby **elevating blood Ca^{2+} and PO$_4$$^{2-}$ levels. Ca^{2+} and PO$_4$$^{2-}$** are used in the normal mineralization of osteoid.
   2.   Physical signs of osteomalacia in adults include bowed legs, increased tendency to fracture, and scoliotic deformity of the vertebral column. Physical signs of rickets in nonambulatory children include craniotabes (elastic recoil of the skull on compression), "rachitic rosary" (excess osteoid at the costochondral junction), and "pigeon-breast deformity" (anterior protrusion of sternum).

E.   ACROMEGALY is characterized by thick bones as a result of excess GH.

F.   SCURVY is characterized by **lack of collagen** within osteoid, which occurs as a result of **vitamin C deficiency.** Vitamin C is necessary for the hydroxylation of proline and lysine amino acids during collagen synthesis. Physical signs of scurvy include poor bone growth and poor fracture repair as a result of lack of collagen within osteoid, as well as hemorrhages in the skin (purpura), gingival mucosa, and joints as a result of a weakened tunica media of blood vessels.

G.   VITAMIN A. An excess of vitamin A causes a premature closure of the epiphyseal plate, resulting in a person of small stature.

XI Clinical Considerations of Joints

A. DEGENERATIVE JOINT DISEASE (OSTEOARTHRITIS; OA) is characterized by progressive erosion or "wear and tear" of articular cartilage without a prominent inflammatory reaction (which seems to be a secondary event). Chondrocytes produce **IL-1**, which initiates matrix breakdown and **TNF-α and TNF-β** that stimulate release of lytic enzymes from chondrocytes and inhibit matrix synthesis. OA is considered a disease of the cartilage.

B. RHEUMATOID ARTHRITIS (RA) is characterized by erosion of articular cartilage and ankylosis of the joint as a result of a chronic proliferative synovitis (i.e., inflammatory reaction of the synovium). RA is an autoimmune disease that may affect many different tissues but typically begins in the proximal interphalangeal (PIP) and metacarpophalangeal (MP) joints of the hand and then spreads to other joints. Women are affected 3 to 5 times more often than men.

XII Selected Photomicrographs

A. Spongy bone, compact bone, and osteoclast (Figure 7-1)

B. Epiphyseal growth plate (Figure 7-2)

C. Osteoporosis, Paget disease (Figure 7-3)

D. Degenerative joint disease (osteoarthritis) and rheumatoid arthritis (Figure 7-4)

● **Figure 7-1 Spongy bone, compact bone, and the osteoclast. (A)** Coronal section through the epiphysis of an adult tibia. In terms of gross anatomy, two different types of bone can be described: spongy bone (*S*), arranged as trabeculae that are adapted to mechanical forces, and compact bone (*C*), forming a rigid outer shell. The *dotted line* is the site of the former epiphyseal plate. **(B)** LM of spongy bone (H&E-stained section). Trabeculae of spongy bone are shown with a lamellar (layered linearly) arrangement of osteocytes (*arrows*) and bone matrix. Osteoblasts (*arrowheads*) can be observed on the surface of the trabeculae. The interstices between the trabeculae are filled with bone marrow (*BM*). **(C)** LM of compact bone (ground bone section). An osteon or Haversian system of compact bone is shown with a lamellar (layered concentrically) arrangement of osteocytes within lacunae (*arrowheads*) and bone matrix. Osteocytes have many cytoplasmic processes within canaliculi (*arrows*) that extend throughout the bone matrix and communicate with other osteocytes. Within the center of an osteon is a Haversian canal (*HC*) that contains blood vessels and nerves. **(D)** LM of an osteoclast. Note the multinucleated osteoclast attached to the resorbing bone (*B*). The ruffled border (*RF*) is clearly shown at the resorbing surface (*arrows*). **(E)** EM of an osteoclast. The ruffled border (*RF*) adjacent to the resorbing bone (*B*) is shown.

● **Figure 7-2　LM of endochondral ossification at the epiphyseal plate. (A)** Zone of reserve consists of hyaline cartilage and chondrocytes (*arrows*). **(B)** Zone of proliferation consists of hyaline cartilage and chondrocytes undergoing mitosis, forming stacks of chondrocytes (*bracket*). **(C)** Zone of hypertrophy consists of hyaline cartilage and hypertrophied chondrocytes (*arrows*) that are secreting alkaline phosphatase to increase Ca^{2+} and PO_4^{2-} levels in the ground substance. **(D)** Zone of calcification consists of dead chondrocytes and calcified cartilage matrix called spicules (*asterisks*). **(E)** Zone of ossification consists of osteoprogenitor cells in the marrow cavity that differentiate into osteoblasts (*arrows*). Osteoblasts deposit bone (*black areas*) on the surface of a spicule to form a mixed spicule (*asterisks*).

Region	BMD	T score	Z score
Neck	0.52		
Troch	0.44		
Inter	0.90		
TOTAL	0.62	−3.0	−2.5

Inter = intertrochanteric line; Troch = trochanter

● **Figure 7-3 Osteoporosis and Paget disease. (A)** Scanning electron micrograph (SEM) of normal bone biopsy from a normal individual. **(B)** SEM of bone biopsy from female patient with osteoporosis. Compare A and B. **(C)** Table of the results after measurement of bone mass using DEXA (dual-energy x-ray absorptiometry) scan of the hip. All bone densitometry techniques measure the amount of Ca^{2+} present in the bone. BMD is the bone mass density expressed as grams per square centimeter. The T score compares the patient's bone density with a young, normal reference population. A T score greater than −1.0 is defined as normal bone. A T score less than −2.5 is defined as osteoporosis. The Z score compares the patient's bone density with an age-matched reference population. A Z score greater than −2.0 is defined as bone density appropriate for the patient's age. A Z score less than −2.0 is defined as bone density inappropriate for the patient's age, indicating a medical or lifestyle condition that has hastened bone loss. **(D)** LM of bone biopsy from patient with Paget disease. Note the bone spicules surrounded by an increased number of osteoclasts (*arrows*), causing widespread bone resorption.

● **Figure 7-4 Osteoarthritis and rheumatoid arthritis. (A, B, C)** Degenerative joint disease (osteoarthritis; OA). **(A)** Diagram shows the hallmarks of OA, which include articular cartilage erosion, osteophyte formation, cartilage and bone fragments ("joint mice"), and osteosclerosis. **(B)** Articular cartilage (*AC*) erosion produces cartilage fragments (*arrows*) that float within the joint space (joint mice). Fibrillations (microscopic vertical splits) of the articular cartilage (*asterisks*) are also seen. *B* = bone. **(C)** As the fibrillations become progressively deeper, synovial fluid may accumulate in the subchondral bone and form cysts (*CY*). **(D, E)** Rheumatoid arthritis (RA). **(D)** Diagram shows the hallmarks of RA, which include synovial villus protrusion with inflammation, pannus, destruction of articular cartilage, and osteoporosis. **(E)** Synovial villous protrusions (*VP*) are shown which are hyperemic (i.e., increased vascularity; *arrows*) and filled with an inflammatory infiltrate. These protrusions creep over the articular cartilage, forming a pannus that eventually erodes all the articular cartilage. In time, the pannus bridges the opposing bones (fibrous ankylosis), which eventually ossify, result-ing in bony ankylosis (fusion of the joint).

Chapter 8

Muscle

Skeletal Muscle. The terms muscle fiber and muscle cell are synonymous.

A. **MUSCLE FIBER TYPES** (Figure 8-1). Skeletal muscle fibers can be classified mainly into **red fibers (type I)** and **white (type II) fibers** that have quite different characteristics based on their function.
   1. **Red fibers (type I)** are **slow-twitch fibers** and are largely present, for example, in the long muscles of the back (antigravity muscles).
   2. **White fibers (type II)** are **fast-twitch fibers** and are largely present, for example, in the extraocular muscles of the eye.
   3. **Intermediate fibers** have characteristics intermediate between red and white fibers.

B. **CROSS-STRIATIONS** (Figure 8-1)
   1. The **A band** contains both thin and thick myofilaments and is the **dark band** seen when using an electron microscope.
   2. The **I band** contains only thin myofilaments and is the **light band** seen when using an electron microscope.
   3. The **H band** bisects the A band and contains only thick myofilaments.
   4. The **Z disk** bisects the I band. The distance between two Z disks delimits a sarcomere, which is the basic unit of contraction for the myofibril. The Z disk contains **α-actinin,** which anchors thin filaments to the Z disk.

C. **THIN MYOFILAMENTS**
   1. **F-actin** has an active site that interacts with the cross-bridges of myosin.
   2. **Tropomyosin** blocks the active site on F-actin during relaxation.
   3. **Troponin C** is a Ca^{2+}-binding protein.

D. **THICK MYOFILAMENTS**
   1. **Myosin** can be cleaved by trypsin into **light meromyosin** and **heavy meromyosin,** which contains myosin heads. The cross-bridges have **actin-binding sites** and **ATPase activity.**
   2. **Titin** anchors myosin to the Z disks and helps the muscle to accommodate extreme stretching.

E. **CHANGES IN CONTRACTED AND STRETCHED MUSCLE** (Figure 8-1). The cross-striational pattern of skeletal muscle changes when it is contracted or stretched. These changes are caused by the degree of interdigitation of the thin and thick myofilaments.

A

Characteristic	Red Fiber Type I	White Fiber Type II
Speed of contraction	Slow twitch	Fast twitch
Myoglobin content*	High	Low
Generation of ATP	Aerobic glycolysis† Oxidative phosphorylation	Anaerobic glycolysis‡
Number of mitochondria	Many	Few
Glycogen content	Low	High
Succinate dehydrogenase NADH dehydrogenase	High	Low
Glycolytic enzymes	Low	High

B

C

Band	Contracted	Relaxed	Stretched
A band	No change		No change
I band	Shortens		Lengthens
H band	Shortens		Lengthens
Z disks	Move closer together		Move farther apart

● **Figure 8-1 Skeletal muscle. (A)** Characteristics of muscle fiber types. LM of skeletal muscle stained for ATPase, which specifically identifies red, type I, slow-twitch fibers (R) and white, type II, fast-twitch fibers (W). *Myoglobin is an oxygen-binding protein similar to hemoglobin and accounts for the reddish appearance of red (type I) fibers. †Aerobic glycolysis (conversion of glucose to carbon dioxide and water) is a relatively slow process so that it can meet the demands of red fibers, but it yields 36 to 38 moles of ATP per mole of glucose. ‡Anaerobic glycolysis (conversion of glucose to lactate) is a relatively fast process so that it can meet the demands of white fibers, but it yields only 2 moles of ATP per mole of glucose. *NADH* = reduced nicotinamide adenine dinucleotide. **(B)** Organization of thin and thick myofilaments in skeletal muscle. **(C)** Changes in contracted and stretched muscle compared with relaxed muscle.

F. **THE TRIAD.** A triad consists of one **transverse tubule (T tubule)** located at the A–I junction flanked on either side by two **terminal cisternae (TC).**

   1. T tubules are invaginations of the cell membrane and transmit an action potential to the depths of a muscle fiber. T tubules contain a voltage-sensitive protein called the **L-type Ca^{2+} channel protein (dihydropyridine receptor).**

   2. TC are dilated sacs of sarcoplasmic reticulum (SR) that store, release, and reaccumulate Ca^{2+} critical for muscle contraction. TC and SR contain a **fast Ca^{2+}-release channel protein (ryanodine receptor)** that releases Ca^{2+} from the TC and SR into the cytoplasm and a **Ca^{2+} ATPase** that pumps Ca^{2+} from the cytoplasm into the TC and SR.

G. **CONTRACTION OF SKELETAL MUSCLE (FIGURE 8-2)**

H. **NEUROMUSCULAR JUNCTION** (also called **myoneural junction** or **motor endplate**)

   1. Synaptic terminals of **α-motorneurons** contain synaptic vesicles, which store **acetylcholine (ACh).** ACh is synthesized by the condensation of **acetyl CoA** and **choline,** which is catalyzed by **choline-O-acetyltransferase.** Choline is obtained by active uptake from the extracellular fluid.

   2. The cell membrane of the synaptic terminal is called the **presynaptic membrane** and is where exocytotic release of ACh occurs. The cell membrane of the muscle fiber is called the **postsynaptic membrane,** and it contains the **nicotinic acetylcholine receptor (nAChR).**

   3. The space between the presynaptic and postsynaptic membrane is called the **synaptic cleft,** and it contains the basal lamina associated with the enzyme **acetylcholinesterase (AChE),** which hydrolyzes ACh (ACh $\rightarrow$ acetate + choline).

   4. nAChR is a **transmitter-gated ion channel** such that when nAChR binds ACh, the "gate" is opened and allows Na^+ influx. Na^+ influx causes depolarization of the postsynaptic membrane called the **endplate potential.**

   5. Endplate potentials spread to areas of the cell membrane and T tubule by **electrotonic conduction** until a threshold is reached and an action potential is generated. (Note: An action potential is not generated per se at the neuromuscular junction.)

I. **PHARMACOLOGY**

   1. **Tubocurarine, pancuronium, vecuronium,** and **atracurium** are nondepolarizing drugs that competitively block nAChR (i.e., an **nAChR antagonist**). Anticholinesterase drugs that increase the amount of ACh within the synaptic cleft can reverse the effect of these drugs. Tubocurarine may cause histamine release, resulting in bronchospasm, skin wheals, and hypotension.

   2. **Succinylcholine (Anectine, Quelicin, Sucostrin)** is a depolarizing drug that competes with ACh for the nAChR (i.e., an **nAChR agonist**). Succinylcholine maintains an open Na^+ channel, eventually causing skeletal muscle relaxation and paralysis. Anticholinesterase drugs cannot reverse the effect of succinylcholine. Succinylcholine may cause **malignant hyperthermia,** which is a major cause of anesthesia-related deaths. Malignant hyperthermia results from an excessive release of Ca^{2+} from the SR and presents as hyperthermia, metabolic acidosis, tachycardia, and accelerated muscle contractions. Treatment includes rapid cooling, 100% oxygen, control of acidosis, and administration of **dantrolene,** which blocks release of Ca^{2+} from the SR.

   3. **Botulinus toxin** is a potent toxin produced by *Clostridium botulinus* bacteria that inhibits the release of ACh.

J. **INNERVATION.** A single axon of an α-motorneuron may innervate one to five muscle fibers (forming a small motor unit), or the axon may branch and innervate more than

● **Figure 8-2 Events in skeletal muscle contraction.** An action potential is generated, which releases stored Ca^{2+} from the terminal cisternae/sarcoplasmic reticulum (*TC/SR*) via **fast Ca^{2+}-release channel proteins (ryanodine receptors)** into the cytoplasm. Note that there is no entry of extracellular Ca^{2+}. **Dantrolene** interferes with the release of Ca^{2+} and thereby reduces skeletal muscle contractions. Dantrolene is used in treatment of cerebral palsy, multiple sclerosis, and malignant hyperthermia. Ca^{2+} binds to troponin C, which allows the **myosin head–ADP–PO_4^{2-} complex** to bind actin. $ADP+PO_4^{2-}$ is released, leaving the myosin head bound to actin. Thick and thin filaments slide past each other (i.e., power stroke). Repetitive action potentials may produce saturating levels of Ca^{2+} for troponin C and thereby cause **tetany.** The myosin head detaches from actin because of ATP binding. If ATP is not available, the myosin head will not detach from actin and **rigor mortis** results. ATP hydrolysis by **myosin ATPase** occurs, and the products ($ADP+PO_4^{2-}$) remain bound to the myosin head, thereby reforming the **myosin head–ADP–PO_4^{2-} complex.** Ca^{2+} is pumped from the cytoplasm back into the TC/SR by **Ca^{2+}ATPase,** causing muscle relaxation. Note the points at which tetany and rigor mortis occur.

150 muscle fibers (forming a large motor unit). **A motor unit is the functional contractile unit of a muscle** (not a muscle fiber).

K. DENERVATION. If a nerve to a muscle is severed, **fasciculations** (small irregular contractions) occur caused by release of ACh from the degenerating axon. Several days after denervation, **fibrillations** (spontaneous repetitive contractions) occur caused by a supersensitivity of the muscle to ACh as nAChRs spread out over the entire cell membrane of the muscle fiber.

L. SKELETAL MUSCLE REPAIR (regeneration) is limited. Skeletal muscle fibers develop embryologically from **rhabdomyoblasts.** After injury or extensive exercise, **satellite cells** present in the adult proliferate and fuse to form new skeletal muscle fibers. Adult skeletal muscle fibers do not undergo mitosis.

M. STRETCH (SENSORY) RECEPTORS
   1. **Muscle spindles** activate the **myotatic (stretch) reflex** and consist of **nuclear bag fibers** or **nuclear chain fibers.**
        a. **Nuclear bag fibers** contain nuclei that are bunched together centrally and that transmit sensory information to group **Ia afferent neurons.**
        b. **Nuclear chain fibers** contain nuclei that are linearly arranged and that transmit sensory information (muscle length and rate of change in muscle length) to group **Ia and group II afferent neurons.**
        c. Nuclear bag fibers and nuclear chain fibers are innervated by **γ-motorneurons** that set the sensitivity of the muscle spindle. The activity of γ-motorneurons is controlled by descending pathways of higher brain centers (upper motorneurons) such that after spinal cord transection, hyperactivity of γ-motorneurons plays a role in **spasticity** and **hypertonia.**
   2. **Golgi tendon organs** activate the **inverse myotatic (stretch) reflex** and consist of a bundle of collagen fibers within the tendon that transmit sensory information (force on the muscle) to group **Ib afferent neurons.**

N. CLINICAL CONSIDERATIONS
   1. **Duchenne muscular dystrophy (DMD)** is a genetic disease that shows X-linked recessive inheritance. The DMD gene is located on the short (p) arm of chromosome X in band 21 (i.e., Xp21) and encodes for the **dystrophin** protein. Dystrophin anchors within skeletal muscle fibers to the extracellular matrix, thereby stabilizing the cell membrane. A mutation of the DMD gene alters the normal function of dystrophin, leading to progressive muscle weakness and wasting.
   2. **Myasthenia gravis** is an autoimmune disease characterized by circulating antibodies against the nAChR (anti-nAChR) and decreased number of nAChRs. It is characterized by muscle weakness that is made worse with exercise and improved by rest. Muscle weakness fluctuates daily or even within hours. The extraocular muscles are generally involved, with ptosis and diplopia being the first disability.

Ⅱ Cardiac Muscle will be discussed in Chapter 10.

Ⅲ Smooth Muscle (Figure 8-3)

A. TYPES OF SMOOTH MUSCLE
   1. **Single-unit smooth muscle (SU).** SU is found in the **respiratory system, genitourinary system, and gastrointestinal tract.** SU demonstrates spontaneous oscillating

● **Figure 8-3 Extension smooth muscle contraction. (A)** Organization of the cytoskeleton and actin and myosin filaments. Intermediate filaments connect dense bodies in the cytoplasm and dense plaques beneath the cell membrane. Movement of actin and myosin filaments during contraction transmits the force throughout the smooth muscle cell. **(B)** Characteristics of single-unit and multiunit types of smooth muscle. Single-unit smooth muscle has characteristics that include: gap junctions, autonomic nerves synapsing en passant and diffusing neurotransmitter to numerous cells, hormonal control, and action potentials (*AP*) superimposed on slow waves. Multiunit smooth muscle has characteristics that include: no gap junctions, autonomic nerves synapsing en passant and diffusing neurotransmitter to an individual cell; action potential (*AP*) is spiked. **(C)** Events in smooth muscle contraction. An action potential is generated which either (*a*) causes extracellular Ca^{2+} to enter through L-type Ca^{2+} channel proteins and induces more Ca^{2+} release from sarcoplasmic reticulum (*SR*; neural control) or (*b*) intracellular Ca^{2+} stored in the SR is released through inositol triphosphate (*IP_3*)-gated Ca^{2+} channels (hormonal control). Ca^{2+} binds to calmodulin, which activates **myosin kinase.** Myosin kinase phosphorylates the myosin head–ADP–PO_4^{2-} complex. ADP+PO_4^{2-} is released, leaving the phosphorylated myosin head bound to actin. Thin and thick filaments slide past each other (i.e., power stroke). The phosphorylated myosin head detaches from actin as a result of ATP binding. ATP hydrolysis by myosin ATPase occurs, and the products (ADP+PO_4^{2-}) remain bound to the phosphorylated myosin head. **Myosin phosphatase** dephosphorylates the myosin head, causing relaxation.

membrane potentials called **slow waves**, which determine the pattern of action potentials. Action potentials, which produce contraction, are superimposed on a background of slow waves. SU has **gap junctions**, which permit coordinated contraction. SU activity is modulated by:

    a. **Postganglionic parasympathetic neurons** that release ACh, which binds to M_3 muscarinic ACh receptor (mAChR).

    b. **Postganglionic sympathetic neurons** that release norepinephrine (NE), which binds to α_1- and β_1-adrenergic receptors.

    c. **Hormones (oxytocin, epinephrine, cholecystokinin [CCK]).** For example, oxytocin binds to the oxytocin receptor, a G protein–linked receptor that generates inositol triphosphate (IP_3). IP_3 opens IP_3-gated Ca^{2+} channels in the TC and SR.

  2. Multiunit smooth muscle (MU). MU is found in the **dilator and sphincter pupillae muscles of the iris and ciliary muscle of the lens.** MU behaves as individual motor units and is highly innervated. MU has no gap junctions. MU activity is generated by:

    a. **Postganglionic parasympathetic neurons** that release ACh, which binds to mAChR.

    b. **Postganglionic sympathetic neurons** that release NE, which binds to α_1- and β_2-adrenergic receptors.

  3. SU/MU smooth muscle has properties of both SU and MU smooth muscle and is found in the **tunica media of blood vessels.**

B. CONTRACTION OF SMOOTH MUSCLE (SEE FIGURE 8-3)

IV Comparisons and Contrasts of Skeletal, Cardiac, and Smooth Muscle (Table 8-1)

TABLE 8-1	COMPARISONS OF MUSCLE TYPES	
Skeletal Muscle	**Cardiac Muscle**	**Smooth Muscle**
Types: Red fibers (type I) White fibers (type II) Intermediate fibers	Types: Cardiac myocytes Purkinje myocytes Myocardial endocrine cells	Types: Single-unit Multiunit Single/Multiunit
Long parallel cylinders with multiple peripheral nuclei	Short branching cylinders with single central nucleus	Spindle-shaped, tapering ends with single central nucleus
A band, I band, H band, and Z disks are present	A band, I band, H band, and Z disks are present	Dense bodies and dense plaques connected by intermediate filaments; actin and myosin filaments
T tubules present at A–I junction and form triads with terminal cisternae	T tubules present at Z disks and form diads with a terminal cisterna	Caveolae present
Extensive sarcoplasmic reticulum	Intermediate sarcoplasmic reticulum	Limited sarcoplasmic reticulum
Cell junctions absent	Intercalated disks present (fascia adherens, desmosomes, gap junctions)	Gap junctions present in single unit Gap junctions absent in multiunit

(Continued)

TABLE 8-1   **COMPARISONS OF MUSCLE TYPES (Continued)**

Skeletal Muscle	Cardiac Muscle	Smooth Muscle
Muscle spindles present	Muscle spindles absent	Muscle spindles absent
Neuromuscular junction	Synapse en passant	Synapse en passant
Voluntary regulation of "all-or-none" contraction by α-motorneurons	Involuntary regulation of pacemaker-generated heart beat by autonomic nervous system	Involuntary regulation of contraction by autonomic nervous system and hormonal control
α-Motorneuron releases ACh at neuromuscular junction, which binds to nAChR	Postganglionic parasympathetic neuron releases ACh, which binds to M_2 mAChR. Postganglionic sympathetic neuron releases NE, which binds to β_1-adrenergic receptor	Postganglionic parasympathetic neuron releases ACh, which binds to M_3 mAChR. Postganglionic sympathetic neuron releases NE, which binds to α_1- and β_2-adrenergic receptors. Hormonal control: oxytocin, epinephrine, CCK
Troponin C is the Ca^{2+} binding protein	Troponin C is the Ca^{2+} binding protein	Calmodulin is the Ca^{2+} binding protein
Intracellular Ca^{2+} stored in the TC/SR is released for contraction	Extracellular Ca^{2+} enters ("trigger Ca^{2+}") and induces more Ca^{2+} release from TC/SR	Extracellular Ca^{2+} enters ("trigger Ca^{2+}") and induces more Ca^{2+} release from SR (neural control) or Intracellular Ca^{2+} stored in the SR is released (hormone control)
Growth by hypertrophy	Growth by hypertrophy	Growth by hypertrophy and hyperplasia
Regeneration limited Satellite cells give rise to myoblasts	No regeneration	Regeneration high Pericytes give rise to new cells
No mitosis	No mitosis	Mitosis

ACh = acetylcholine; NE = norepinephrine; CCK = cholecystokinin; TC/SR = terminal cisternae/sarcoplasmic reticulum; nAChR = nicotinic ACh receptor; mAChR = muscarinic ACh receptor.

 Selected Photomicrographs

A. Skeletal muscle (Figure 8-4)

B. Neuromuscular junction and muscle spindle (Figure 8-5)

C. Cardiac muscle and smooth muscle (Figure 8-6)

● **Figure 8-4 Skeletal muscle. (A)** LM of skeletal muscle cut longitudinally. Note the A band (dark) and I band (light). The I band is bisected by the Z disk. A sarcomere (Z disk to Z disk) is indicated by the *double-headed arrow*. **(B)** EM of skeletal muscle cut longitudinally. Note the A band (dark), I band (light), and H band. The M line is also indicated. The I band is bisected by the Z disk (Z). A sarcomere is indicated. **(C–E)** Schematics of skeletal muscle cut in cross section showing the characteristic arrangement of myofilaments in the H band, A band, and I band, respectively. The H band shows only thick myofilaments (*large black dots*). The A band shows both thick myofilaments (*large black dots*) surrounded by six thin myofilaments (*small black dots*). The I band shows only thin myofilaments (*small black dots*). **(F)** EM of the sarcoplasmic reticulum (*SR*), which is an extensive network of smooth endoplasmic reticulum that ends as dilated sacs called terminal cisternae (*TC*). A T tubule (*T*), which is an invagination of the cell membrane, is indicated. Two terminal cisternae are always found in close association with a T tubule, forming a triad.

● Figure 8-5 Neuromuscular junction and muscle spindle. (A) LM of a neuromuscular junction (*NMJ*) in whole mount. *M* = muscle; *N* = nerve. **(B)** EM of a neuromuscular junction. A myelinated axon (*N*) loses its myelin sheath (at the *arrow*) and ends in a synaptic terminal on the surface of a skeletal muscle fiber (*M*). At the junction of the nerve and muscle fiber, the cell membrane of the muscle fiber is thrown into junctional folds (*JF*; brackets). **(C)** High magnification of the neuromuscular junction (boxed area in B). A collection of synaptic vesicles (*SV*) that contain acetylcholine (*ACh*) is indicated along with the presynaptic membrane (*single arrow*) where ACh is released. The postsynaptic membrane (*double arrows*), which contains nicotinic ACh receptors (*nAChR*), is shown. The bracket indicates the postsynaptic membrane of the skeletal muscle fiber thrown into junctional folds (*JF*). The synaptic cleft (*large arrow*) containing the electron-dense basal lamina and acetylcholinesterase (*AChE*) is shown. Hemicholium blocks uptake of choline from the synaptic cleft into the synaptic terminal and thereby depletes ACh stores. Neostigmine (an AChE inhibitor) inhibits the degradation of ACh, which prolongs its action at the neuromuscular junction. **(D)** LM of a muscle spindle (*ms*) showing both the nuclear bag fibers and nuclear chain fibers. Note the surrounding muscle fibers (*M*).

● **Figure 8-6 Cardiac muscle and smooth muscle. (A)** LM of cardiac muscle in longitudinal section. Note the intercalated disks (*arrowheads*) and centrally located nucleus (*arrow*). The cytoplasm demonstrates a striated appearance, although less prominent than in skeletal muscle. **(B)** LM of cardiac muscle in cross section. Note the centrally located nucleus (*arrow*). **(C)** EM of cardiac muscle in longitudinal section. Note the centrally located nucleus (*arrow*), numerous mitochondria (mit), and striations (*). **(D)** EM of an intercalated disk in cardiac muscle. An intercalated disk is found at the junction of two cardiac myocytes and is typically arranged in a stairstep pattern. The intercalated disk consists of a fascia adherens (*fa*), desmosomes (*des*), and gap junction (*gap*). The gap junction is always oriented parallel to the myofilaments. **(E)** LM of smooth muscle in longitudinal section. Note the centrally located nuclei and lack of cytoplasmic striations. **(F)** LM of smooth muscle in cross section. Note the centrally located nucleus. **(G and H)** Viable smooth muscle cell in relaxed state **(G)** and contracted state **(H)**. **(I)** EM of smooth muscle in longitudinal section. Note the centrally located nucleus and lack of cytoplasmic striations. Note also the cytoplasmic dense bodies (*arrows*) and the dense plaques (*arrowheads*) located at the cell membrane. The dense bodies and dense plaques are connected by an array of intermediate filaments, which participate in contraction generated by actin and myosin interaction. **(J)** EM of smooth muscle in cross section. Note the dense plaques (*arrowheads*) located at the cell membrane. *N* = nucleus.

Chapter 9

Nervous Tissue

The Neuron is the structural and functional unit of the nervous system. The neuron consists of a **perikaryon (cell body)**, **dendrite**, and **axon**, each of which contains certain ultrastructural components (Table 9-1). The axon arises from an extension of the perikaryon called the **axon hillock.** The part of the axon between the axon hillock and the start of the myelin sheath is called the **initial segment** and is where the action potential is initiated.

TABLE 9-1	ULTRASTRUCTURAL COMPONENTS OF NEURON
Neuron Part	**Components**
Perikaryon	Nucleus with prominent nucleolus, rER and polyribosomes (Nissl substance), Golgi, some sER, mitochondria, lysosomes, microfilaments (actin), neurofilaments (intermediate), microtubules, and
	Pigments: **Lipofuscin granules** are pigmented residual bodies derived from lysosomal degradation that accumulate with age. **Melanin** is a black cytoplasmic pigment found in the substantia nigra and locus ceruleus. Melanin disappears from nigral neurons in Parkinson disease.
	Inclusion bodies: **Lewy bodies** are round, eosinophilic inclusions that are characteristic of Parkinson disease. **Negri bodies** are inclusions that are pathognomonic of rabies. **Hirano bodies** are rodlike, eosinophilic inclusions that are found in Alzheimer disease. **Neurofibrillary tangles** are degenerated neurofilaments that are found in Alzheimer disease. **Cowdry Type A** are intranuclear inclusions that are found in herpes simplex encephalitis.
Dendrite	Similar to the perikaryon
Axon	Some sER, mitochondria, neurofilaments (intermediate), microtubules, and neurosecretory vesicles *Absent: rER and polyribosomes (Nissl substance), Golgi, and lysosomes*

rER = rough endoplasmic reticulum; sER = smooth endoplasmic reticulum.

con-
truc-
axon
alled

A. AXONAL TRANSPORT

1. **Fast anterograde transport** is responsible for transporting **vesicles** (containing enzymes, proteins, phospholipids, and neurotransmitter) necessary for neuro-transmission. This transport occurs at the rate of 200–400 mm/day, is mediated by **microtubules**, and uses **kinesin**, which is a motor protein with **ATPase activity**.

2. **Slow anterograde transport** is responsible for transporting **cytosolic and cytoskeletal components (enzymes, actin, myosin, etc.)** from the perikaryon to the synaptic terminal. This transport occurs at the rate of 1 to 5 mm/day.

3. **Fast retrograde transport** is responsible for transporting **nerve growth factor, tetanus toxin, polio virus, rabies virus, and herpes simplex virus** from the synaptic terminal to the perikaryon. This transport occurs at the rate of 100 to 200 mm/day, is mediated by **microtubules**, and uses **dynein**, which is a motor protein with **ATPase activity**.

B. ACTION POTENTIAL AND SYNAPSE (Figure 9-1)

C. CONDUCTION VELOCITY of action potentials down an axon is influenced by **axon diameter** and **degree of myelination.** Large-diameter and highly myelinated axons have a high conduction velocity (fast). Small-diameter and unmyelinated axons have a low conduction velocity (slow) (Table 9-2).

D. NODE OF RANVIER is a segment of the axon exposed to the extracellular milieu because of gaps in the myelin sheath. It is the site where action potentials are regenerated as a result of the **presence of Na^+ channels (i.e., saltatory conduction).**

E. FUEL SOURCES. Glucose is the major fuel source for neurons. During starvation, **ketones** can be metabolized by neurons.

TABLE 9-2		CLASSIFICATION OF NERVE FIBERS	
Fiber	Diameter (μm)*	Conduction Velocity (m/sec)	Function
Sensory axons			
Ia (A-α)	12–20	70–120	Proprioception, muscle spindles
Ib (A-α)	12–20	70–120	Proprioception, Golgi tendon organs
II (A-β)	5–12	30–70	Touch, pressure, vibration, muscle spindles
III (A-δ)	2–5	12–30	Touch, pressure, fast pain, and temperature
IV (C)	0.5–1	0.5–2	Slow pain and temperature, unmyelinated fibers
Motor axons			
Alpha (A-α)	12–20	15–120	Alpha motor neurons of ventral horn (innervate extrafusal muscle fibers)
Gamma (A-γ)	2–10	10–45	Gamma motor neurons of ventral horn (innervate intrafusal muscle fibers)
Preganglionic autonomic fibers (B)	<3	3–15	Myelinated preganglionic autonomic fibers
Postganglionic autonomic fibers (C)	1	2	Unmyelinated postganglionic autonomic fibers

*Myelin sheath included if present.
Type A = high myelination
Type B = intermediate myelination
Type C = no myelination

● **Figure 9-1 Action potential and synapse. (A)** Diagram depicting the [Na⁺] and [K⁺] in the neuron and extracellular milieu. Within the neuronal cytoplasm, the [Na⁺] is low and the [K⁺] is high. Within the extracellular milieu, the [Na⁺] is high and the [K⁺] is low. **(B)** Diagram of an action potential. The influx of Na⁺ (*thick dashed line*) and efflux of K⁺ (*thin dashed line*) are indicated. Because of K⁺ leakage from the cytoplasm into the extracellular milieu and the Na⁺-K⁺ ATPase pump, a **resting membrane potential (–70 mV)** is established. When the membrane potential reaches **threshold (–55 mV),** an action potential occurs. At the peak of the action potential, the membrane potential reaches approximately **+50 mV** because of a depolarization as a result of an **influx of Na⁺.** At the nadir of the action potential, the membrane potential reaches approximately **–80 mV** because of a hyperpolarization caused by an **efflux of K⁺.** Tetrodotoxin (a poison found in puffer fish) and **saxitoxin** (a poison found in dinoflagellates ["red tides"]) are potent **Na⁺ channel blockers.** Tetraethylammonium (a poison) is a potent **K⁺ channel blocker. (C)** Axosomatic synapse and generation of action potential (*AP*). Synapses are areas of interaction between two neurons, for example, an axon and cell body, forming an axosomatic synapse. Binding of the neurotransmitter to receptor alters the conductance of the postsynaptic membrane to ions. Two synapses (*1* and *2*) are shown. Synapse 1 allows for the influx of Na⁺ (depolarization), causing an **excitatory postsynaptic potential** (*EPSP*). Synapse 2 allows for the influx of Cl⁻ (hyperpolarization), causing an **inhibitory postsynaptic potential** (*IPSP*). The EPSPs and IPSPs spread over the postsynaptic neuron by **electrotonic conductance** (*dotted lines*). If the momentary sum of the EPSPs and IPSPs reaches –55 mV (threshold), an AP is generated at the **initial segment of the axon.** The AP is conducted along the axon and propagated, which means "new" APs are regenerated at the nodes of Ranvier because of an influx of Na⁺. Note that an AP does not occur at the synapse. **(D)** Diagram of a neuron cut so as to sever the perikaryon from the axon. If an AP is experimentally induced at mid-axon, the AP will be propagated along the axon in both directions, that is, toward both the perikaryon and synaptic terminal.

Neurotransmitters are listed in Table 9-3.

TABLE 9-3	NEUROTRANSMITTERS
Neurotransmitter	**Characteristics**
Acetylcholine (ACh) $CH_3 - N - CH_2 - CH_2O - C - CH_3$ with CH_3 groups and O	Binds to nAChR, which is a **transmitter-gated ion channel** permeable to Na^+, K^+, and Ca^{2+} ions Binds to M_1, M_2, M_3 mAChRs, which are **G protein–linked receptors** Is the neurotransmitter of: Neuromuscular junction, preganglionic parasympathetic neurons, preganglionic sympathetic neurons (ACh + nAChR) Postganglionic parasympathetic neurons (ACh + M_2 or M_3 mAChR) Somatic and visceral motor nuclei in the brainstem, basal nucleus of Meynert, which degenerates in Alzheimer disease, and striatum (caudatoputamen), which degenerates in Huntington disease (ACh + M_1 mAChR) Postganglionic sympathetic neurons that innervate eccrine sweat glands for thermoregulation and some blood vessels in skeletal muscle for dilation (ACh + mAChR)
Catecholamines **Norepinephrine** (structure with OH, $CH - CH_2 - NH_2$, HO, HO)	Binds to α_1-, α_2-, β_1-, β_2-, or β_3-adrenergic receptors, which are **G protein–linked receptors** Is the neurotransmitter of postganglionic sympathetic neurons and locus ceruleus in pons and midbrain Is metabolized by MAO and COMT to form metabolites NMN, MOPEG, and VMA Plays a role in anxiety states, panic attacks, depression, and mania
Epinephrine (structure with OH, CH_3, $CH - CH_2 - NH$, HO, HO)	Binds to α_1-, α_2-, β_1-, β_2-, or β_3-adrenergic receptors, which are **G protein–linked receptors** Plays an insignificant role in the CNS Is secreted by chromaffin cells of the adrenal medulla
Dopamine (structure with $CH_2 - CH_2 - NH_2$, HO, HO)	Binds to D_1 and D_2 dopamine receptors, which are **G protein–linked receptors** Is the neurotransmitter of the arcuate nucleus in hypothalamus, ventral tegmental area, and substantia nigra Plays a role in Parkinson disease (dopamine decreased) and schizophrenia (dopamine increased)
Serotonin **(5-hydroxytryptamine;** **5-HT)** (structure with HO, $CH_2 - CH_2 - NH_2$, N)	Binds to $5\text{-HT}_{1A,B,C,D,E,F}$ receptors, which are **G protein–linked receptors** ($\downarrow$cAMP) found in the CNS (raphe nuclei of the brainstem and hippocampus) Binds to $5\text{-HT}_{2A,B,C}$ serotonin receptors, which are **G protein–linked receptors** ($\uparrow$IP$_3$ + DAG) found in the CNS Binds to the 5-HT_3 serotonin receptor, which is a **transmitter-gated ion channel** permeable to Na^+ and K^+ ions Binds to $5\text{-HT}_{4,6,7}$ serotonin receptors, which are G protein–linked receptors ($\uparrow$cAMP) found in the CNS
γ-Aminobutyric acid **(GABA)** NH_2 $H_2C - CH_2 - CH_2 - COOH$	Binds to GABA$_A$ receptor, which is a **transmitter-gated ion channel** permeable to Cl^- ions Binds to GABA$_B$ receptor, which is a **G protein–linked receptor** Is the **major inhibitory neurotransmitter of the CNS**

(Continued)

TABLE 9-3	NEUROTRANSMITTERS (*Continued*)

Neurotransmitter	Characteristics
Glycine $$H_3N - \overset{\text{COOH}}{\underset{\text{H}}{\overset{|}{C}}} - H$$	Binds to glycine receptor, which is a **transmitter-gated ion channel** permeable to Cl^- ions Is the **major inhibitory neurotransmitter of the spinal cord**
Glutamate $$COOH - \overset{H}{\underset{NH_2}{\overset{|}{C}}} - CH_2 - CH_2 - COOH$$	Binds to *N*-methyl-D-aspartate (NMDA), kainate, or quisqualate A receptors, which are **transmitter-gated ion channels** permeable to Na^+, K^+, and Ca^{2+} ions Is the **major excitatory neurotransmitter of the CNS**
Opioid peptides (β-endorphin, leu-enkephalin, met-enkephalin)	Bind to μ, δ, κ, and σ receptors, which are **G protein–linked receptors** Play a role in pain suppression
Neuropeptides	Use **G protein–linked receptors**

COMT = catechol *O*-methyltransferase; NMN = normetanephrine; MOPEG = 3-methoxy-4-hydroxyphenylglycol; VMA = vanillylmandelic acid.

 ## III Parasympathetic Pharmacology

A. CHOLINERGIC AGONISTS

1. **Carbachol, methacholine, bethanechol, pilocarpine,** and **nicotine** are cholinergic agonists that bind directly to muscarinic acetylcholine receptors (mAChR).
2. **Edrophonium, neostigmine,** and **physostigmine** are indirect cholinergic agonists that inhibit acetylcholinesterase.

B. CHOLINERGIC ANTAGONISTS (BLOCKERS)

1. **Atropine** is the classic cholinergic antagonist (mAChR blocker; muscarinic blocker; or antimuscarinic) that blocks mAChR. Atropine overdose is associated with dry mouth, dry skin, and inhibition of sweating ("dry as a bone"); red, flushed, hot skin ("red as a beet"); blurred vision ("blind as a bat"); and delirium and hallucinations ("mad as a hatter").
2. **Scopolamine, propantheline, methantheline, benztropine, cyclopentolate,** and **pirenzepine** are other cholinergic antagonists that block mAChR.

 ## IV Sympathetic Pharmacology

A. ADRENERGIC AGONISTS

1. **Phenylephrine, tetrahydrozoline, oxymetazoline, naphazoline, methoxamine,** and **clonidine** are α-adrenergic agonists that bind directly to α_1 and α_2 adrenergic receptors.
2. **Methyldopa** is a pro-drug to the α_2-adrenergic agonist **methylnorepinephrine**.
3. **Isoproterenol, dobutamine, metaproterenol, albuterol, tubertaline, salmeterol,** and **ritodrine** are β-adrenergic agonists that bind directly to β_1, β_2, and β_3 adrenergic receptors.
4. **Tyramine, amphetamine,** and **methamphetamine** are indirect adrenergic agonists that act either by increasing norepinephrine release or inhibiting norepinephrine reuptake.

5. **Ephedrine and phenylpropanolamine** are mixed adrenergic agonists that act either directly or indirectly.

B. **ADRENERGIC ANTAGONISTS ("BLOCKERS")**

1. **Prazosin (Minipress), terazosin, doxazosin, phenoxybenzamine, phentolamine, tamsulosin,** and **yohimbine** are α-adrenergic antagonists ("α-blockers") that block α_1 and α_2 adrenergic receptors.

2. **Metoprolol (Lopressor), propranolol (Inderal), atenolol, esmolol, acebutolol, pindolol, timolol, celiprolol,** and **nadolol** are β-adrenergic antagonists (β-blockers) that block β_1, β_2, and β_3 adrenergic receptors.

3. **Labetalol** and **Carvedilol** are α and β-adrenergic antagonists (α- and β-blocker) that block α_1, α_2, β_1, β_2 and β_3 -adrenergic receptors

Ⓥ CNS Pharmacology

A. **BENZODIAZEPINES (ANXIOLYTIC DRUGS)**

1. **Chlordiazepoxide (Librium), diazepam (Valium), flurazepam (Dalmane), alprazolam (Xanax), lorazepam (Ativan), temazepam (Restoril), clonazepam (Klonopin), oxazepam (Serax), midazolam (Versed),** and **triazolam (Halcion)** are γ-aminobutyric acid (GABA$_A$) receptor agonists that increase the frequency of Cl^- channel opening, leading to membrane hyperpolarization and decreased neuronal excitability. The GABA$_A$ receptor is an inhibitory transmitter-gated ion channel that is permeable to Cl^-. A classic side effect of these drugs is "rebound insomnia" as a withdrawal symptom.

2. **Flumazenil (Romazicon)** is a GABA$_A$ receptor antagonist that is used clinically in suspected acute benzodiazepine overdose.

B. **BARBITURATES (HYPNOTIC DRUGS).** Phenobarbital (Luminal), pentobarbital (Nembutal), secobarbital (Seconal), amobarbital (Amytal), thiopental (Pentothal), and methohexital (Brevital) are GABA$_A$ receptor agonists that prolong the duration of Cl^- channel opening, leading to membrane hyperpolarization and decreased neuronal excitability.

C. **ANTIDEPRESSANT DRUGS**

1. **Isocarboxazid (Marplan), phenelzine (Nardil),** and **tranylcypromine (Parnate)** are **monamine oxidase (MAO) inhibitors.** MAO is a mitochondrial enzyme that oxidatively deaminates catecholamines (i.e., epinephrine, norepinephrine, and serotonin). MAO inhibitors reversibly or irreversibly inhibit MAO, which results in the accumulation of catecholamines in the presynaptic neuron and synaptic cleft. A side effect of these drugs is a hypertensive crisis that can be eliminated by avoiding foods (e.g., cheese and wine) that contain tyramine.

2. **Imipramine (Tofranil), desipramine (Norpramin), amitriptyline (Elavil), nortriptyline (Aventyl),** and **clomipramine (Anafranil)** are tricyclic antidepressants (TCAs) that inhibit the reuptake of norepinephrine and serotonin at the presynaptic membrane.

3. **Fluoxetine (Prozac), sertraline (Zoloft), paroxetine (Paxil), trazodone (Desyrel),** and **bupropion (Wellbutrin)** are selective serotonin reuptake inhibitors (SSRIs).

D. **NEUROLEPTIC DRUGS** (e.g., schizophrenia, acute manic depression)

1. **Chlorpromazine (Thorazine), fluphenazine (Permitil), trifluoperazine (Stelazine), thioridazine (Mellaril), thiothixene (Navane), haloperidol (Haldol), clozapine (Clozaril),** and **risperidone (Risperdal)** are **D$_2$** dopamine

receptor antagonists. The extrapyramidal side effects of these drugs include parkinsonism (i.e., rigidity, tremor), akathisia (inability to remain in a seated position), and acute dystonic reactions.

2. **Lithium carbonate (Eskalith)** is an antimanic agent that decreases the levels of inositol triphosphate (IP_3) and diacylglycerol (DAG).

E. ANTIEPILEPTIC DRUGS

1. **Phenytoin (Dilatin), carbamazepine (Tegretol), lamotrigine, and primidone (Mysoline)** are drugs that prolong the inactivated state of Na^+ ion channels. They are used to treat partial seizures and tonic-clonic (grand mal) seizures.
2. **Ethosuximide (Zarontin)** inhibits Ca^{2+} influx by low threshold T-type calcium channels in thalamic neurons. It is used to treat absence ("petit mal") seizures.
3. **Valproic acid (Depakene)** inhibits Na^+ influx by Na^+ ion channels and inhibits Ca^{2+} influx by low threshold T-type calcium channels in thalamic neurons. It is used to treat absence (petit mal) seizures.

F. DRUGS FOR PAIN MANAGEMENT.
Endogenous-occuring opioids (e.g., β-endorphin, enkephalins, and dynorphins) impart their analgesic effect via the **μ, κ, δ, and σ receptors,** which are found on neurons throughout the CNS. Stimulation of opioid receptors suppress peripheral nociceptive pathways and pain-processing centers within the cerebral cortex.

1. **Morphine (Roxanol, MS Contin), levorphanol, meperidine (Demerol), methadone (Dolophine), hydromorphone (Dilaudid), fentanyl (Sublimaze, Duragesic), alfentanil, sufentanil, remifentanil, and heroin** are μ-opioid receptor agonists that are used to treat severe pain. Miosis (papillary constriction) is characteristic of all opioids, except meperidine (Demerol), which causes mydriasis (dilation of the pupil).
2. **Butorphanol and buprenorphine** are μ-opioid receptor partial agonists that are used to treat severe pain.
3. **Loperamide (Imodium)** acts on opioid receptors in the enteric nervous system to decrease intestinal motility. It is used to treat diarrhea (e.g., traveler's diarrhea).
4. **Dextromethorphan (Benylin)** is a derivative of morphine, which acts on cough center within the medulla to suppress the cough reflex (i.e., an antitussive). It does not have any activity at opioid receptors.
5. **Naloxone (Narcan) and naltrexone (Trexan)** are opioid receptor antagonists. They are used to treat opioid toxicity, respiratory depression, and opioid addiction.

G. CENTRAL NERVOUS SYSTEM (CNS) STIMULANTS

1. **Caffeine** is a purinergic receptor antagonist, which uses adenosine as a neurotransmitter.
2. **Nicotine** is an nAChR agonist initially; it eventually becomes an nAChR antagonist. At low doses, nicotine is an nAChR agonist. At high doses, nicotine is an mAChR agonist and elicits no response at nAChR (i.e., "nicotinic escape").
3. **Dextroamphetamine (Dexedrine), methamphetamine (Methedrine; "speed"), and methylphenidate (Ritalin)** stimulate the release of dopamine from neurons.
4. **Cocaine, "free base" cocaine (free alkaloid cocaine), and "crack" cocaine (cocaine salt combined with bicarbonate)** prevent dopamine, norepinephrine, and serotonin reuptake.

H. OTHER RECREATIONAL DRUGS

1. **Lysergic acid diethylamide (LSD), psilocybin, and mescaline** interact with 5-hydroxytryptamine (5-HT) receptors.

2. **Phencyclidine (PCP; "angel dust")** is an N-methyl-D-aspartate (NMDA) receptor antagonist.

3. **Ketamine (Ketalar; Special K; K)** is an NMDA receptor antagonist that acts as a CNS depressant and a dissociative anesthetic. It has sedative, analgesic, and hallucinogenic effects. It is also used as a "date rape" drug.

4. **Marijuana (Dronabinol)** contains the active compound δ-9 tetrahydrocannabinol (δ-9 THC) whose mechanism of action is unknown but probably acts through its own receptors.

5. **3,4-Methylenedioxymethamphetamine (MDMA; Ectasy; XTC)** causes damage to serotonin-containing neurons.

6. **γ-Hydroxybutyrate (GHB; G; Grievous Bodily Harm)** is a CNS depressant that has a sedative or euphoric effect. It is used by bodybuilders because it stimulates growth hormone release. It is also used as a "date rape" drug.

7. **Rohypnol (flunitrazepam; Roofies; Forget Me Pill)** and **clonazepam** are very similar to other benzodiazepine drugs. They have sedative or hypnotic, muscle relaxant, and amnesia effects. They are used as "date rape" drugs.

I. **PHARMACOLOGY OF MIGRAINE HEADACHES. Sumatriptan (Imitrex), rizatriptan, naratriptan, zolmitriptan, almotriptan, and eletriptan** are 5-HT_{1B} and 5-HT_{1D} serotonin receptor agonists that reduce: sensory activation in the periphery, nociceptive transmission in the brainstem trigeminal nucleus, and vasoconstriction of cerebral blood vessels opposing the vasodilation thought to be involved in migraine attacks.

VI **NEUROGLIAL CELLS** are the nonneural cells of the nervous system.

A. **OLIGODENDROCYTES** produce myelin in the CNS. One oligodendrocyte can myelinate several (up to 30) axons.

B. **ASTROCYTES** have the following characteristics and functions: project foot processes to capillaries that contribute to the blood-brain barrier, play a role in the metabolism of neurotransmitters (e.g., glutamate, GABA, serotonin), buffer the $[K^+]$ of the CNS extracellular space, form the external and internal glial-limiting membrane in the CNS, form glial scars in a damaged area of the CNS (i.e., astrogliosis), undergo hypertrophy and hyperplasia in reaction to CNS injury, contain **glial fibrillary acidic protein (GFAP)** and **glutamine synthetase,** which are good markers for astrocytes.

C. **MICROGLIA** are derived from monocytes and have phagocytic function.

D. **EPENDYMAL CELLS** line the central canal and ventricles of the brain. These cells are not joined by tight junctions, so that exchange between the cerebrospinal fluid (CSF) and CNS extracellular fluid occurs freely.

E. **CHOROID EPITHELIAL CELLS**
1. These cells are a continuation of the ependymal layer that is reflected over the choroid plexus villi, and they **secrete CSF** by selective transport of molecules from blood.
2. These cells are joined by tight junctions, which are the basis of the **blood-CSF barrier.**
3. CSF is normally **clear.** A **yellow color (xanthochromia)** indicates previous bleeding (subarachnoid hemorrhage) or increased protein concentration. A **pinkish color** is usually caused by a bloody tap. **Turbidity** is caused by the presence of leukocytes.
4. CSF normal values include:
   a. **CSF pressure = 70–80 mm H_2O**
   b. **CSF cell count = <6 lymphocytes/mm^3;** 0 neutrophils (presence of neutrophils is always pathologic)

    c. **CSF [protein] = 20–45 mg/dL** (serum proteins are generally too large to cross the blood-CSF barrier)

    d. **CSF [glucose] = 40–70 mg/dL**

  5. **In acute bacterial meningitis,** the CSF has the following characteristics: cloudy, ↑↑pressure, ↑↑neutrophils, ↑↑[protein], and ↓↓[glucose].

F. TANYCYTES are modified ependymal cells that project to both capillaries and neurons. They mediate transport between ventricles and the neuropil. They project to hypothalamic nuclei that regulate the release of gonadotropic hormones from the adenohypophysis.

G. SCHWANN CELLS produce myelin in the peripheral nervous system (PNS) and are derived from neural crest cells. One Schwann cell myelinates only one axon. Schwann cells invest all myelinated and unmyelinated axons of the PNS and are separated from each other by nodes of Ranvier.

VII THE BLOOD-BRAIN BARRIER (BB) represents an anatomic and physiologic separation of blood from the CNS extracellular fluid. The BB consists of **zonula occludens (tight junctions)** between nonfenestrated intracerebral capillary endothelial cells with few pinocytic vesicles, the surrounding **basal lamina,** and **astrocytic foot processes,** which promote the formation of tight junctions. Water, gases, and small lipid-soluble molecules freely diffuse across the BB. Glucose and amino acids cross via carrier-mediated transport mechanisms. The BB excludes many drugs from the CNS. Note: Dopamine does not cross the BB, but l-dopa (used to treat Parkinson disease) does cross the BB. The BB does not exist in some areas of the CNS, such as the median eminence, neurohypophysis, lamina terminalis, pineal gland, area postrema, and choroid plexus. Infarction of brain tissue destroys the BB and results in vasogenic edema.

VIII NERVE DEGENERATION AND REGENERATION

A. PNS

  1. **Degeneration. Anterograde (Wallerian) degeneration** of the axon and myelin sheath occurs distal to the site of injury. Macrophages infiltrate to remove cellular debris. **Chromatolysis** (loss of rER, movement of the nucleus to the periphery, and hypertrophy of the perikaryon) occurs. During this time, **muscle fasciculations** (small irregular contractions) occur, caused by release of ACh from the degenerating synaptic terminal.

  2. **Regeneration.** Schwann cells proliferate and form a cord that is penetrated by the growing axon. The axon grows at 3 mm/day until it reaches the skeletal muscle. If the axon does not penetrate the cord of Schwann cells, the axon will not reach the skeletal muscle. During this time, **muscle fibrillations** (spontaneous repetitive contractions) occur, caused by a supersensitivity of the muscle to ACh.

B. CNS

  1. **Degeneration.** Microglia phagocytose myelin and injured axons. Glial scars (astrogliosis) form.

  2. **Regeneration.** Effective regeneration does not occur in the CNS.

IX CLINICAL CONSIDERATIONS

A. HUNTINGTON DISEASE (HD). HD involves a 26–100+ unstable repeat sequence of $(CAG)_n$ located in an exon (or coding) sequence of the HD gene on chromosome 4p16.3. HD is an autosomal dominant genetic disorder caused by the CAG repeat sequence on chromosome 4p16.3. The HD gene encodes for a protein called **huntingtin,** which is a cytoplasmic protein present in neurons within the striatum, cerebral cortex, and cerebellum, although its precise function is unknown. A primary manifestation is movement jerkiness most apparent at movement termination. HD is also characterized by: chorea (dance-like movements), memory deficits, affective disturbances, personality changes, diffuse and marked atrophy of the neostriatum due to cell death of cholinergic neurons and GABA-ergic neurons within the striatum (caudate nucleus and putamen) and a relative increase in dopaminergic neuron activity, and neuronal intranuclear aggregates.

B. **PARKINSON DISEASE** is a degenerative disease that results in the **depletion of dopamine** and **loss of melanin-containing dopaminergic neurons** within the substantia nigra. This results clinically in bradykinesia, stooped posture, shuffling gait, and masked facies. Drug treatment includes:
1. **Levodopa (l-dopa; Dopar; Larodopa)** is converted to dopamine by dopa decarboxylase in many peripheral body tissues and the brain. L-Dopa crosses the blood-brain barrier.
2. **Levodopa plus carbidopa (Sinemet).** Carbidopa inhibits dopa decarboxylase only in peripheral body tissues. Carbidopa does not cross the blood-brain barrier.
3. **Selegiline (Eldepryl, Deprenyl)** inhibits type B MAO, which selectively metabolizes dopamine in preference to other catecholamines.
4. **Bromocriptine** is an ergot alkaloid that is a D_2 dopamine receptor agonist.
5. **Pergolide (Permax)** is a D_1 and D_2 dopamine receptor agonist.
6. **Amantadine (Symmetrel)** increases the synthesis and secretion of dopamine and delays the reuptake of dopamine.

C. **MOTORNEURON DISEASE** is a progressive disease caused by the death of motorneurons, the pathogenesis of which is not known. Death of upper motorneurons in the brainstem is called **progressive bulbar palsy.** Death of lower motorneurons in the spinal cord is called **progressive muscular atrophy.** Death of upper motorneurons of the corticospinal tract, corticobulbar tract, and brainstem along with lower motorneurons of the spinal cord is called **amyotrophic lateral sclerosis (ALS; Lou Gehrig disease).** ALS results clinically in hyperreflexia, spasticity, and Babinski reflex, along with muscle atrophy, weakness, and fasciculations.

D. **MULTIPLE SCLEROSIS** may be a type of autoimmune disease in which the myelin of the CNS is destroyed. This results clinically in paralysis, loss of sensation, and loss of coordination. The exact nature of the defect depends on the specific area of the CNS involved. Interferon β-1a (Avonex; Rebif) and interferon β-1b (Betaseron) are used clinically to ameliorate the autoimmune attack on myelin.

E. **ASTROCYTOMA** is a tumor of astrocytes that accounts for about 80% of adult primary brain tumors. Its hallmark is a proliferation of astrocytic cell processes of varying size that displace normal neurons. This results clinically in seizures, headaches, and focal neurologic deficits depending on the area of the CNS involved.

⊗ SELECTED PHOTOMICROGRAPHS

A. Neurons (Figure 9-2)
B. Peripheral nerve (Figure 9-3)
C. Neuroglia (Figure 9-4)
D. Blood-brain barrier and synapse (Figure 9-5)
E. Astrocytoma (Figure 9-6)
F. CNS pathology (Figure 9-7)

● **Figure 9-2 Neurons. (A)** A multipolar neuron showing the perikaryon (cell body; *CB*), axon (*Ax*), axon collaterals (*arrows*), and dendrites with dendritic spines (*D*). **(B)** LM of a multipolar neuron showing nucleus (*N*) and dendrites (*D*). **(C)** Diagram of a multipolar neuron showing nucleus (*N*), dendrites (*D*), microtubules (*Mt*), intermediate filaments (*IF*), rough endoplasmic reticulum (*rER*), Golgi (*G*), and axon hillock (*AH*). **(D)** LM·of a Purkinje neuron from the cerebellum. *CB* = cell body; *D* = dendrites. **(E)** LM of a multipolar neuron showing the nucleus with prominent nucleolus and axon hillock (*AH*). Note that most of the cytoplasmic staining is caused by rER and polyribosomes (Nissl substance). **(F)** LM of a neuron undergoing chromatolysis. Note the loss of rER and polyribosomes (*), movement of nucleus to the periphery (*arrow*), and hypertrophy·of the cell body. **(G)** Hurler disease is a lysosomal storage disease involving the l-iduronidase enzyme in which abnormal amounts of heparan sulfate and dermatan sulfate accumulate within the cytoplasm of neurons (*arrow*). **(H)** Parkinson disease involves the depigmentation of neurons in the substantia nigra and the appearance of round cytoplasmic inclusions called Lewy bodies (*arrow*). **(I)** LM of an atrophic neuron (*arrow*) that has a reduced amount of cytoplasm and an indistinct nucleus. A normal neuron is shown for comparison. **(J)** LM·of a neuron infected with the rabies virus showing the presence of a cytoplasmic inclusion called the Negri body (*arrow*).

● **Figure 9-3 Peripheral nerve.** A peripheral nerve contains both myelinated and unmyelinated axons. **(A)** LM of a cross section of a peripheral nerve stained with osmic acid. This area shows only myelinated axons of various diameters (*arrows*). Note the myelin sheath (*M; black*) and axon (*Ax; white*). **(B)** LM of a longitudinal section of a peripheral nerve stained with osmic acid. This area shows only myelinated axons of various diameters. Note the myelin sheath (*M; black*), axon (*Ax; white*), and node of Ranvier (*NR*). **(C)** EM of a cross section of a peripheral nerve. This area shows only a myelinated axon. Note the Schwann cell (*S*) nucleus and cytoplasm, myelin sheath (*M*), and axon (*Ax*) containing microtubules (*m*) and neurofilaments (*nf*). **(D)** EM of a longitudinal section of a peripheral nerve. Note the myelin sheath (*M*), axon (*Ax*) containing microtubules (*m*) and neurofilaments (*nf*), and the node of Ranvier (*NR; brackets*) where the myelin sheath is absent. The node of Ranvier is where action potentials are regenerated as a result of the presence of Na^+ ion channels that allow an influx of Na^+ to occur. **(E)** EM of a cross section of a peripheral nerve. This area shows only unmyelinated axons (*Ax, arrows*). Unmyelinated axons are embedded in the cytoplasm of a Schwann cell (*S*) but no myelin sheath is formed.

● **Figure 9-4 Neuroglial cells. (A)** Drawing of an oligodendrocyte. **(B)** EM of an oligodendrocyte (*OL*). Note the cell processes of the oligodendrocyte extending to two axons (*Ax*) within the CNS and forming a myelin sheath (*M*). Note that one oligodendrocyte can myelinate several axons. **(C)** Drawing of a protoplasmic astrocyte. **(D)** Drawing of a fibrous astrocyte. **(E)** Drawing of a microglial cell. **(F)** Drawing of an ependymal cell. **(G)** LM of the choroid plexus showing numerous villi with blood vessels in the connective tissue core. The choroidal epithelial cells secrete cerebrospinal fluid (*CSF; arrow*). Tight junctions at the apical portion of the choroidal epithelial cells form the blood-CSF barrier.

● **Figure 9-5 Blood-brain barrier and synapse. (A)** EM of a capillary within the CNS. A zonula occludens (*arrows*) between two endothelial cells prevents the escape of macromolecules into the brain. This is the basis of the blood-brain barrier. A paucity of pinocytotic vesicles and astrocytic foot processes also may play a role in the barrier. **(B)** High-magnification EM of the boxed area in A showing the zonula occludens (*zo; arrow*) between two endothelial cells. Note the basal lamina (*BL*) and the astrocytic foot process (*AF*). **(C)** EM of an axodendritic synapse (i.e., between an axon [*Ax*] and a dendrite [*D*]). Synaptic vesicles (*arrow 1*), mitochondria (*arrow 2*), and a postsynaptic density (*arrow 3*) are identified.

● **Figure 9-6 Astrocytoma (glioblastoma multiforme). (A)** Coronal brain section shows a glioma in the left frontal cortex containing pigmentation as a result of hemorrhage. This 65-year-old woman demonstrated personality and behavioral changes during a period of several months. Her condition became increasingly more serious and eventually led to institutionalization for the last 2 weeks of her life. **(B)** LM indicating areas of necrosis (*N*) that are surrounded by areas of hypercellularity with highly anaplastic tumor cells crowded along the edges of the necrotic regions producing so-called pseudopalisading (*PP*). **(C)** LM of the vascular proliferation associated with astrocytoma. Tufts of endothelium may bulge into the vascular lumen with extreme examples forming glomeruloid structures.

● **Figure 9-7 CNS pathology. (A)** Multiple sclerosis. A brain section is stained for myelin (*M*). Note the focal pale areas (*X*) where demyelination has occurred. **(B)** Dorsal column disease (tabes dorsalis) typically seen in neurosyphilis. A cross section of the spinal cord shows demyelination of the posterior columns (*). **(C)** Friedreich ataxia. A cross section of the spinal cord shows demyelination of the posterior columns (*) and lateral columns (*X*). **(D)** Subacute combined degeneration (vitamin B$_{12}$ neuropathy) is caused by pernicious (megaloblastic) anemia. A cross section of the spinal cord shows demyelination of the posterior columns (*), lateral columns (*X*), and anterior columns (+). **(E)** Pathologic lesions associated with Alzheimer disease. A senile plaque (*SP*) is shown that consists of a core of extracellular amyloid surrounded by a halo of dystrophic neurites (*arrowheads*). In addition, a number of dark-staining pyramidal neurons are present owing to the neurofibrillary tangles within the cytoplasm. A major component of neurofibrillary tangles is the tau protein, which enhances microtubule assembly. Normal pyramidal neurons are also present (*arrows*).

Heart and Blood Vessels

I **Heart Layers.** The heart consists of three layers.

A. ENDOCARDIUM. The endocardium is lined by endothelium and is underlain by the **subendocardial space,** which contains blood vessels, nerves, and Purkinje myocytes. The endocardium is continuous with the tunica intima of blood vessels.

B. MYOCARDIUM. The myocardium consists of cardiac myocytes, Purkinje myocytes, and myocardial endocrine cells that will be discussed below. The myocardium is continuous with the tunica media of blood vessels.

C. EPICARDIUM. The epicardium consists of connective tissue and a layer of mesothelium. In gross anatomy, the epicardium is called the **visceral layer of the pericardial sac** (or visceral pericardium). The visceral pericardium is reflected to form the **parietal layer of the pericardial sac** (or parietal pericardium).

II **Cardiac Myocytes** (Figure 10-1; also see Chapter 8). Cardiac myocytes contract through intrinsically generated action potentials, which are then passed on to neighboring myocytes by gap junctions; that is, the heartbeat is **myogenic.** There are two types of action potentials, which include:

A. SLOW ACTION POTENTIALS. Slow action potentials are observed in the sinoatrial node (SA node) and atrioventricular node (AV node). Slow action potentials are caused by the presence of **slow (funny) Na$^+$ channels** and are divided into three phases:

1. **Phase 0** is caused by **Ca^{2+} influx** into nodal cells through **L-type Ca^{2+} channels** (long-lasting type).
2. **Phase 3** is caused by **K$^+$ efflux** through **K$^+$ channels** out of nodal cells.
3. **Phase 4** is caused by **Ca^{2+} influx** into nodal cells through **T-type Ca^{2+} channels** (transient type) and **Na$^+$ influx** into nodal cells through **slow (funny) Na$^+$ channels.** Note that phase 4 is a gradual depolarization.

B. FAST ACTION POTENTIALS. Fast action potentials are observed in the atrial myocytes, bundle of His, Purkinje myocytes, and ventricular myocytes. Fast action potentials are caused by the presence of **fast Na$^+$ channels** and are divided into five phases.

1. **Phase 0** is caused by **Na$^+$ influx** into cardiac myocytes through **fast Na$^+$ channels.**
2. **Phase 1** is caused by **inactivation of fast Na$^+$ channels** and **K$^+$ efflux** out of cardiac myocytes through **K$^+$ channels.**
3. **Phase 2** is caused by **Ca^{2+} influx** into cardiac myocytes through **L-type Ca^{2+} channels.** This Ca^{2+} influx ("trigger Ca^{2+}") is involved in the contraction of cardiac myocytes.

● **Figure 10-1 Action potentials. (A)** Slow action potential and associated ion fluxes observed in the SA node. **Class IV Ca²⁺ channel blockers** (diltiazem and verapamil) block L-type Ca²⁺ channels and thus decrease SA node activity and AV nodal conduction. Adenosine binds to the P₁ purinergic receptors and acts by ↓ cAMP levels and stimulates a K⁺ channel protein so that the channel opens and K⁺ flows out of the cell, causing a hyperpolarization of the cell and thus decrease SA node and AV node activity. **(B)** Fast action potential and associated ion fluxes observed in ventricular myocytes. Various **antiarrhythmic drugs** are indicated along with their specific effect on ion channels. **Class I Na⁺ channel blockers** include class IA, IB, and IC. **Class IA** (quinidine, procainamide, disopyramide) blocks open Na⁺ channels and thus decreases phase 0 and phase 4 (increases QRS complex). **Class IB** (lidocaine, tocainide, mexiletine, phenytoin) blocks activated and inactivated Na⁺ channels and thus decreases phase 0. **Class IC** (flecainide, propafenone, moricizine) blocks Na⁺ channels and thus decreases phase 0. **Class III K⁺ channel blockers** (amiodarone and bretylium) block K⁺ channels, thus prolonging the action potential. **Cardiac glycosides** (digoxin and digitoxin) are Na⁺-K⁺ ATPase blockers that elevate intracellular Na⁺ ions. The elevated Na⁺ overwhelms the **Na⁺-Ca²⁺ exchanger** so that more Ca²⁺ can be reaccumulated by terminal cisternae (*TC*). During the next contraction, more Ca²⁺ is released from TC, increasing the force of contraction. Cardiac glycosides are used in congestive heart failure (CHF) to increase the strength of contraction. The antiarrhythmic effect of cardiac glycosides is a result of their indirect effect on the autonomic nervous system (increase parasympathetic activity and decrease sympathetic activity).

4. **Phase 3** is caused by **inactivation of Ca²⁺ channels** and **K⁺ efflux** out of cardiac myocytes through K⁺ channels.

5. **Phase 4** is caused by **high K⁺ efflux, removal of the excess Na⁺** that entered in phase 0 by **Na⁺-K⁺ ATPase,** and **removal of the excess Ca²⁺** that entered in phase 2 by the **Na⁺-Ca²⁺ exchanger.**

Ⅲ **Purkinje Myocytes** are modified cardiac myocytes that are specialized for conduction. Purkinje myocytes are *not* neurons. They are joined by gap junctions.

Ⅳ **Myocardial Endocrine Cells** are found in the right and left atria and have secretory granules containing **atrial natriuretic peptide (ANP).**

A. ANP is secreted in response to increased blood volume or increased venous pressure within the atria (e.g., atrial distention caused by left atrial failure). ANP functions include:

1. ANP increases glomerular filtration pressure and glomerular filtration rate (via vasoconstriction of the efferent arteriole) and decreases Na⁺ reabsorption by the medullary collecting ducts. These actions produce **natriuresis** (increased Na⁺ excretion) in a large volume of dilute urine.

2. ANP inhibits secretion of **antidiuretic hormone (ADH)** from the neurohypophysis.

3. ANP inhibits secretion of **aldosterone** from the adrenal cortex (zona glomerulosa).

4. ANP inhibits secretion of **renin** from juxtaglomerular cells.

5. ANP causes vasodilation of peripheral and renal blood vessels.

Ⅴ **Contraction of Cardiac Myocytes**

A. Cardiac myocytes demonstrate a **diad** that consists of a **T tubule** located at the Z disk and flanked by one **terminal cisterna** (TC). A T tubule is an invagination of the cell membrane. TC are dilated sacs of sarcoplasmic reticulum (SR) that store, release, and reaccumulate Ca²⁺.

B. The Ca²⁺ influx that occurs at the cell membrane and T tubule in **phase 2** of the action potential through **L-type Ca²⁺ channels** is *not* sufficient to cause contraction but acts as **trigger Ca²⁺** that stimulates the release of a large pool of Ca²⁺ stored in TC/SR through **fast Ca²⁺ release channel proteins (ryanodine receptor).**

C. Ca²⁺ binds to **troponin C,** which allows the myosin head–ADP–PO₄²⁻ complex to bind actin. From this point on, cardiac myocyte contraction resembles skeletal muscle contraction (see Figure 8-2).

D. ADP+PO₄²⁻ is released, leaving the myosin head bound to actin. Thick and thin filaments slide past each other (i.e., power stroke). The magnitude of the force of contraction is proportional to the intracellular [Ca²⁺].

E. The myosin head detaches from actin as a result of ATP binding.

F. ATP hydrolysis by **myosin ATPase** occurs, and the products (ADP + PO₄²⁻) remain bound to the myosin head, thereby reforming the myosin head–ADP–PO₄²⁻ complex.

G. As the influx of Ca²⁺ begins to decrease at the end of phase 2, Ca²⁺ is pumped from the cytoplasm back into the TC/SR by **Ca²⁺ ATPase** that is regulated by an intramembranous protein called **phospholamban** (i.e., relaxation). Troponin C is freed of Ca²⁺.

VI Conduction System (Figure 10-2)

A. SINOATRIAL (SA) NODE is the **pacemaker** of the heart and is located at the junction of the superior vena cava and right atrium just beneath the epicardium. From the SA node, the impulse spreads throughout the right atrium and to the AV node via

ECG	Heart Action
P wave	Represents atrial depolarization (0.08–0.1 sec)
PR interval	Is the interval from start of atrial depolarization to the start of ventricle depolarization (0.12–0.20 sec)
	Gets shorter as the heart rate increases
	Gets longer as conduction velocity through AV node is slowed (e.g., heart block)
QRS complex	Represents ventricle depolarization (0.06–0.10 sec)
QT interval	Represents the entire period of ventricle depolarization and ventricle repolarization (0.32 sec)
ST segment	Represents the period when the entire ventricle is depolarized
T wave	Represents ventricle repolarization (0.1–0.25 sec)

5mm = 0.5mV
1mm = 0.1mV

5mm = 0.2 sec
(1mm = 1 small box = 0.04 sec)

Paper speed: 25mm/sec

● **Figure 10-2 (A)** Diagram of the conduction system and innervation of the heart. Action potentials from various areas of the heart are shown. The electrocardiogram (ECG) is the body surface manifestation of all these action potentials. The various components of the ECG are indicated along with their associated heart function. Parasympathetic regulation of heart rate is solely a negative effect. **Atropine** is the classic cholinergic antagonist (mAChR blocker; muscarinic blocker; antimuscarinic). Sympathetic regulation of heart rate is solely a positive effect. **Class IIβ-blockers** (propanolol, metoprolol, esmolol, sotalol) block β-adrenergic receptors. The antiarrhythmic effect of β-blockers is caused by a decrease in phase 4 depolarization in nodal tissue resulting in a decrease in SA node activity and AV nodal conduction. The antianginal effect of β-blockers is caused by a decrease in heart rate (chronotropism) and a decrease in contractility (inotropism), which decreases myocardial oxygen demand. a = posterior internodal tract; b = middle internodal tract; c = anterior internodal tract; d = Bachmann bundle; e = posterior segment of left bundle branch; CN X = cranial nerve X.

II

1st degree heart block
• PR interval > 0.20 sec

II

2nd degree heart block (Wenckebach)
• PR interval gradually lengthens
• P wave but no QRS

II

3rd degree heart block (complete)
• P waves occur independently
  of QRS

B

● **Figure 10-2** *(continued)* **(B)** ECGs of first-, second-, and third-degree heart blocks.

the **anterior, middle,** and **posterior internodal tracts** and to the left atrium via the **Bachmann bundle.** If all SA node activity is destroyed, the AV node will assume the pacemaker role.

B. **ATRIOVENTRICULAR (AV) NODE** is located on the right side of the interatrial septum near the ostium of the coronary sinus in the subendocardial space.

C. **BUNDLE OF HIS, BUNDLE BRANCHES, PURKINJE MYOCYTES.** The **bundle of His** travels in the subendocardial space on the right side of the interventricular septum and divides into the **right and left bundle branches.** The left bundle branch is thicker than the right bundle branch. The left bundle branch further divides into an **anterior segment** and **posterior segment.** The right and left bundle branches both terminate in a complex network of intramural **Purkinje myocytes.**

D. **CLINICAL CONSIDERATIONS**
  1. **Ectopic pacemakers** are present in the normal heart, and their added activity may induce continuous rhythm disturbances, such as **paroxysmal tachycardias.** When the ectopic pacemaker stops functioning, the SA node may remain quiescent for a period of time (called SA node recovery time). In patients with **sick sinus syndrome,** the SA node recovery time is prolonged with a period of asystole (absence of heartbeat) and loss of consciousness.
  2. A **first-degree heart block** occurs when there is an abnormally long delay at the AV node. The delay between the start of the P wave (atrial depolarization) and the QRS complex (ventricular depolarization) occurs at the AV node. This normal delay allows for optimal ventricular filling during atrial contraction.
  3. A **second-degree heart block** occurs when only a portion of atrial impulses is conducted to the ventricles.
  4. A **third-degree heart block** occurs when no atrial impulses are conducted to the ventricles.

5. **Wolff-Parkinson-White syndrome** is a congenital disorder in which an **accessory conduction pathway** between the atria and ventricles exists. This syndrome is ordinarily asymptomatic. However, a reentry loop may develop in which impulses travel to the ventricles via the normal conduction pathway but return to the atria via the accessory pathway, causing **supraventricular tachycardia.**

VII Parasympathetic Regulation of Heart Rate

A. **EFFECTS**
   1. **Decreases heart rate** ("vagal arrest") by decreasing Na^+ influx associated with phase 4 depolarization in nodal tissue. This is also called a **negative chronotropism.**
   2. **Decreases conduction velocity through the AV node** (i.e., increases PR interval) by decreasing Ca^{2+} influx associated with phase 0 depolarization in nodal tissue. This is also called a **negative dromotropism.**
   3. **Decreases contractility of atrial myocytes** by decreasing Ca^{2+} influx associated with phase 2 in atrial myocytes. This is also called a **negative inotropism.**

B. **ORGANIZATION.** Preganglionic neuronal cell bodies are located in the **dorsal nucleus of the vagus** and **nucleus ambiguus** of the medulla. Preganglionic axons run in the **vagus (CN X) nerve.** Postganglionic neuronal cell bodies are located in the cardiac plexus and atrial wall. Postganglionic axons predominantly terminate on the **SA node, AV node,** and **atrial myocytes** (not ventricular myocytes). Postganglionic axons release **acetylcholine (ACh)** as a neurotransmitter. ACh binds to the M_2 muscarinic ACh receptor (mAChR), which is a G protein-linked receptor that inhibits adenylate cyclase, thereby ↓ cAMP levels and stimulating a K^+ channel protein so that the channel opens and K^+ flows out of the cell, causing a hyperpolarization of the cell. The SA node and AV node contain high levels of **acetylcholinesterase** (degrades ACh rapidly) such that any given vagal stimulation is **short-lived. Vasovagal syncope** is a brief period of lightheadedness or loss of consciousness caused by an intense burst of CN X activity.

VIII Sympathetic Regulation of Heart Rate

A. **EFFECTS**
   1. **Increases heat rate** by increasing Na^+ influx associated with phase 4 depolarization in nodal tissue. This is also called **positive chronotropism.**
   2. **Increases conduction velocity through the AV node** (i.e., increases PR interval) by increasing Ca^{2+} influx associated with phase 0 in nodal tissue. This is also called a **positive dromotropism.**
   3. **Increases contractility of atrial and ventricular myocytes** by increasing the Ca^{2+} influx associated with phase 2 of the action potential in atrial and ventricular myocytes and increases the activity of the Ca^{2+} **ATPase pump** by **phosphorylation of phospholamban** so that more Ca^{2+} reaccumulates during relaxation and therefore is available for release during later heartbeats. This is also called **positive inotropism.**

B. **ORGANIZATION.** Preganglionic neuronal cell bodies are located in the **intermediolateral columns** of the spinal cord. Preganglionic axons enter the paravertebral ganglion and travel to the stellate and middle cervical ganglia. Postganglionic neuronal cell bodies are located in the **stellate and middle cervical ganglia.** Postganglionic axons are distributed to the **SA node, AV node,** and **atrial and ventricular myocytes.** Postganglionic axons release **norepinephrine (NE)** as a neurotransmitter. NE binds to the β_1-**adrenergic receptor,** which is a G protein-linked receptor that stimulates adenylate cyclase and increases cAMP levels. Released NE is either carried away by the bloodstream or taken up by the nerve terminals so that sympathetic stimulation is relatively **long-lived.**

IX. Tunics of Blood Vessels

A. **TUNICA INTIMA** consists of endothelium, a basal lamina, loose connective tissue, and an internal elastic lamina.

B. **TUNICA MEDIA** consists of smooth muscle cells, type III collagen, elastic fibers, and an external elastic lamina. Many factors affect smooth muscle cells of the tunica media as indicated below:

1. **Sympathetic innervation** activity controls the **tonus.** Postganglionic sympathetic neurons release NE, which binds to $\alpha 1$-adrenergic receptors to cause vasoconstriction of skin, skeletal muscle, and visceral blood vessels. Doxazosin (Cardura), prazosin (Minipress), and terazosin (Hytrin) are $\alpha 1$-adrenergic receptor antagonists that cause vasodilation and are used to treat hypertension. Propranolol is a $\beta 1$ and $\beta 2$ adrenergic receptor antagonist that causes vasodilation and is used to treat hypertension.

2. **Thromboxane (TXA$_2$), endothelin-1, angiotensin II,** and **serotonin** are potent vasoconstrictors.

3. **Prostaglandins (PGE$_1$, PGE$_2$), prostacyclin (PGI$_2$), bradykinins, histamine,** and **nitric oxide (NO)** are potent vasodilators.

4. **Nifedipine (Procardia)** and **nicardipine (Cardene)** are L-type Ca^{2+} channel blockers ("afterload-reducing drugs" used to treat hypertension and angina) that block Ca^{2+} entry into smooth muscle cells. This causes relaxation of **arterial** smooth muscle (i.e., vasodilation) and therefore decreases peripheral vascular resistance (PVR).

5. **Vasodilators (e.g., hydralazine [Apresoline], minoxidil [Loniten]).** These drugs ("afterload-reducing drugs" used to treat hypertension) relax predominately **arteriolar** smooth muscle (i.e., vasodilation) leading to a decrease in PVR. The action of hydralazine is uncertain but may involve NO. Minoxidil is a K^+ channel agonist that causes an increased K^+ efflux, hyperpolarization, and relaxation of smooth muscle.

C. **Tunica adventitia** consists of fibroblasts, type I collagen, and some elastic fibers.

X. Types of Blood Vessels

A. **ELASTIC (CONDUCTING) ARTERIES** (e.g., pulmonary artery, aorta) have a tunica media with a prominent elastic fiber component that responds to the high systolic pressure generated by the heart.

B. **MUSCULAR (DISTRIBUTING) ARTERIES** have a tunica intima with a prominent internal elastic lamina and a tunica media with a prominent smooth muscle cell component.

C. **ARTERIOLES** have a tunica media that consists of only one to two layers of smooth muscle cells and play a major role in regulation of blood pressure.

D. **METARTERIOLES** are the smallest (or terminal) branches of the arterial system and flow directly into capillary beds. A **precapillary sphincter** plays a role in regulation of blood flow to capillary beds.

E. **ARTERIOVENOUS ANASTOMOSES (AVA)** allow arteriolar blood to bypass the capillary bed and empty directly into venules. AVA are found primarily in the skin to regulate body temperature. Constriction of the arteriolar component directs blood to the capillary bed, causing depletion of body heat. Dilation of the arteriolar component directs blood to the venules, causing conservation of body heat.

F. **CAPILLARIES** consist of a single layer of endothelial cells surrounded by a basal lamina and are the site of exchange (e.g., CO_2, O_2, water, glucose, amino acids, proteins) between blood and cells. Microvasculature damage associated with type 1 and type 2 diabetes is a result of **nonenzymatic glycosylation** of various proteins, which causes the release of harmful cytokines. The different types of capillaries include the following:

1. **Continuous capillaries** consist of a single layer of endothelial cells joined by a **zonula occludens** (a tight junction that extends around the entire perimeter of the cell) and contain no fenestrae (or pores). They are found in lung, muscle, and brain (blood-brain barrier).
2. **Fenestrated capillaries with diaphragms** consist of a single layer of endothelial cells joined by a **fascia occludens** (a tight junction that extends only partially around the perimeter of the cell creating slitlike **intercellular spaces**) and contain **fenestrae (or pores) with diaphragms.** They are found in endocrine glands, intestine, and kidney.
3. **Fenestrated capillaries without diaphragms** are found solely within the kidney glomerulus.
4. **Discontinuous capillaries** (sinusoids) consist of a single layer of endothelial cells that are separated by wide gaps (i.e., no zonula occludens present) and contain fenestrae. They are found in the liver, bone marrow, and spleen.

XI **Functions of Endothelium.** Although endothelial cells (ECs) are fairly unremarkable microscopically, they are very active physiologically as indicated below.

A. ECs maintain the subendothelial layer that prevents blood escape into the extravascular space by secretion of **basement membrane components, types III and IV collagen, elastin, mucopolysaccharides, vitronectin, fibronectin, proteases,** and **protease inhibitors.**

B. Normally, ECs act as a potent anticoagulant surface adjacent to blood by:
1. Expression of anticoagulant cell surface molecules: **glycosaminoglycans (GAGs). heparan sulfate–antithrombin III system, thrombin–thrombomodulin–protein C system,** and **plasminogen–plasmin activator system.**
2. Secretion of **prostacyclin (PGI$_2$) and endothelium-derived relaxing factor (EDRF),** which cause vasodilation and inhibit platelet adhesion and aggregation.
3. Secretion of **tissue plasminogen activator (TPA) and urokinase** that stimulate the conversion of plasminogen →plasmin.

C. On injury, ECs act as a potent procoagulation surface by the secretion of **tissue factor (TF), von Willebrand factor (vWF), factor V, plasminogen activator inhibitors (PAI-1, PAI-2), interleukin 1 (IL-1), tumor necrosis factor (TNF),** and **endothelin-1** (which affects smooth muscle cells of the tunica media and causes vasoconstriction).

D. Secretion of **von Willebrand factor (vWF),** which is stored in Weibel-Palade granules and promotes platelet adhesion to subendothelial collagen at an injury site and blood clotting. vWF combines with factor VIII secreted by hepatocytes to form a **factor VIII–vWF complex.** This complex circulates in the plasma as a unit and promotes blood clotting as well as platelet–vessel wall interactions necessary for blood clotting. **Von Willebrand disease** is a common bleeding disorder in humans.

E. Secretion of **nitric oxide (NO)**, which affects smooth muscle cells of the tunica media and causes vasodilation.

1. NO is synthesized by the reaction:

$$\text{Arginine} \xrightarrow{\text{NO synthase}} \text{NO} + \text{citrulline}$$

2. NO activates guanylate cyclase in smooth muscle cells causing **increased levels of cGMP** and vasodilation.

3. NO is involved in the vasodilation associated with penile erection. **Viagra** used in the treatment of erectile dysfunction is a cGMP phosphodiesterase inhibitor so that increased cGMP levels are maintained.

4. **Nitroglycerin, isosorbide dinitrate (Isordil), and amyl nitrite (Aspirols, Vaporole)** are metabolized by smooth muscle cells to NO, which relaxes **venous (main effect)** and arterial smooth muscle causing peripheral vasodilation. This results in decreased cardiac preload, decreased cardiac afterload, and decreased cardiac output. These drugs are used to treat **angina pectoris.**

F. Conversion of **angiotensin I to angiotensin II** (predominantly in lung capillaries), which causes vasoconstriction and secretion of both aldosterone and ADH.

G. Digestion of triacylglycerides (carried by very low-density lipoproteins [VLDL] and chylomicrons) into fatty acids and glycerol catalyzed by **lipoprotein lipase** attached to ECs of skeletal muscle and adipose tissue capillaries.

H. Passage of **lipid-soluble substances** (including O_2 and CO_2) by **diffusion, water-soluble substances** (including water, glucose, amino acids) through the slitlike **intercellular spaces,** and **large water-soluble substances** (e.g., proteins) by **pinocytosis.**

I. Exchange of fluid between blood and cells that is described by the **Starling equation.**

XII Blood Flow

A. **MODIFICATION.** Blood flow to an organ is modified in a number of ways.

1. **Autoregulation** is the phenomenon whereby blood flow to an organ remains constant over a wide range of pressures.

2. **Active hyperemia** is the phenomenon whereby blood flow to an organ is proportional to its metabolic activity.

3. **Reactive hyperemia** is the phenomenon whereby blood flow to an organ is increased after a period of occlusion.

B. **MODIFICATION THEORIES.** Modification of blood flow to an organ is explained by the following:

1. **The metabolic hypothesis** states that vasodilator metabolites are released upon an increase in tissue activity.

2. **The myogenic hypothesis** states that vascular smooth muscle contracts on stretching.

XIII Types of Circulation (Table 10-1)

TABLE 10-1		TYPES OF CIRCULATION	
Circulation	Percent of Cardiac Output	Blood Flow Demonstrates	Control
Coronary	15	Autoregulation Active hyperemia Reactive hyperemia	Hypoxia, adenosine, and NO cause vasodilation Increased O_2 demand is met by increased blood flow
Cerebral	15	Autoregulation Active hyperemia Reactive hyperemia	Increased Pco_2 or decreased pH causes vasodilation
Skeletal muscle	20	Autoregulation Active hyperemia Reactive hyperemia	During exercise, lactate, adenosine, and K^+ cause vasodilation At rest, sympathetic innervation through NE release stimulates α_1-adrenergic receptors, causing vasoconstriction At rest, sympathetic innervation through NE release stimulates β_2-adrenergic receptors, causing vasodilation
Kidney	25	Autoregulation	Renal blood flow remains constant from 100 to 200 mm Hg of arterial pressure Highest blood flow per gram of tissue
Respiratory	100	Hypoxic vasoconstriction	Hypoxia causes vasoconstriction so that blood is directed away from poorly ventilated areas to well-ventilated areas of the lung It is the only circulation that responds to hypoxia by vasoconstriction
Skin	5	Temperature regulation	Increase in temperature: sympathetic innervation causes vasodilation, directing blood to the surface

NE = norepinephrine; NO = nitric oxide.

XIV Selected Photomicrographs

A. Myocardial infarction (Figure 10-3)

B. Purkinje myocyte (Figure 10-4)

C. Muscular artery, arteriole, capillary, lymphatic, and fenestrated capillary (Figure 10-5)

D. Coronary artery atherosclerosis (Figure 10-6)

E. Kaposi sarcoma (Figure 10-7)

A

3
- Lateral wall of left ventricle

2
- Posterior wall of left ventricle
- Posterior part of septum
- Right ventricle

1
- Anterior wall of left ventricle
- Anterior part of septum

B

Troponin I
CK-MB
LDH₁

[serum]

MI pain

Days

1   2

C

Early Anterior MI (2–24hrs)
- ST segment elevated in V_3 and V_4

Recent Anterior MI (24–72hrs)
- Q waves in V_3 and V_4
- T Waves inverted in V_3 and V_4

Old Anterior MI
- Q waves persist in V_3 and V_4
- No T wave inversion

D

Day 1
- Coagulation necrosis
- Wavy myocytes
- Pyknotic nuclei
- Eosinophilic cytoplasm
- Contraction bands

Day 2–4
- Total coagulation necrosis
- Loss of nuclei
- Loss of striations
- Dilated vessels (hyperemia)
- Neutrophil infiltration

Day 5–10
- Macrophage infiltration
- Phagocytosis of necrotic myocytes

Week 7
- Collagenous scar

● **Figure 10-3 Myocardial infarction (MI). (A)** Transmural MIs are caused by thrombotic occlusion of a coronary artery. Infarction is localized to the anatomic area supplied by the occluded artery. Coronary artery occlusion occurs most commonly in the anterior interventricular artery ([*AIV*; also called the left anterior descending [LAD]), followed by the right coronary artery (*R*), and then the circumflex artery (*C*). This is indicated by the numbers 1, 2, and 3. **(B)** Serum markers of MI. **Troponin I** is a highly specific cardiac marker that can be detected within 4 hours and up to 7–10 days after MI pain. **Creatine kinase** (*CK*) consists of M and B subunits. CK-MM is found in skeletal muscle and cardiac muscle. **CK-MB** is found mainly in cardiac muscle. **CK-MB is the test of choice in the first 24 hours after MI pain.** CK-MB begins to rise 4–8 hours after MI pain, peaks at 24 hours, and returns to normal within 48–72 hours. This sequence is important because skeletal muscle injury or non-MI conditions may raise serum CK-MB but do not show this pattern. It is common to calculate the ratio **CK-MB/total CK.** A **CK-MB/total CK >2.5%** indicates MI. **Lactate dehydrogenase** (LDH) consists of H and M subunits. LDH-HHHH (or **LDH₁**) and LDH-HHHM (or **LDH₂**) are found in cardiac muscle. **LDH₁ is the test of choice 2–3 days after MI pain because CK-MB levels have already returned to normal at this time.** It is common to calculate the ratio **LDH₁/LDH₂.** An LDH₁/LDH₂ >1.0 indicates MI. **(C)** Electrocardiographs. An acute MI is associated with ST elevation. A recent MI (within 1–2 days) is associated with deep Q waves and inverted T waves. An old MI (weeks later) is associated with persistence of deep Q waves but no T-wave inversion. **(D)** Evolution of an MI. The histologic changes of an MI are indicated.

● **Figure 10-4 Purkinje cell. (A)** LM of Purkinje cells (*P*) traveling within the myocardium (*my*). By light microscopy, Purkinje cells appear pale because the large amount of glycogen that is normally contained in the cytoplasm is lost during histologic processing. **(B)** EM of a Purkinje cell (*P*) showing a large amount of glycogen (*gly*) and few myofilaments (*mf*). A portion of a cardiac myocyte within the myocardium (*my*) is also shown.

A

VASOCONSTRICTORS	VASODILATORS

α_1 antagonists
- Doxazosin (Cardura)
- Prazosin (Minipress)
- Terazosin (Hytrin)

β_1 antagonists
- Propanolol (β_1 and β_2)

Hydralazine
Minozidil

TXA$_2$, endothelin 1, angiotensin II, serotonin
Hypoxia (lung vessels)

IEL

α_1

β_2

NE

K$^+$

Ca^{2+}

M

EEL

AD

Sympathetic tonus

Nifedipine (Procardia)
Nicardipine (Cardene)

Antihypertensive drugs

PGE$_1$, PGE$_2$, PGI$_2$, bradykinins, histamine, NO
Hypoxia, adenosine, NO (coronary vessels)
↑PCO$_2$, ↓pH (cerebral vessels)
Lactate, adenosine, K$^+$ (skeletal muscle vessels)

B

Arteriole

Capillary

Venule

Lymphatic

C

endo
L
B

D

L
endo
I

● **Figure 10-5 Blood vessels. (A)** LM of a muscular artery. The tunica intima (*I*), tunica media (*M*), and tunica adventitia (*Ad*) are indicated by the brackets. A typical smooth muscle cell with α$_1$-adrenergic receptors, K$^+$ channels, and Ca^{2+} channels is drawn within the tunica media. The various vasoconstrictors and vasodilators are indicated. The drugs that act as vasodilators are important clinically as antihypertensive drugs. *EEL* = external elastic lamina; *IEL* = internal elastic lamina; *NE* = norepinephrine; *TXA$_2$* = thromboxane A$_2$; *PG* = prostaglandin; *NO* = nitric oxide. **(B)** LM of an arteriole, capillary, venule, and lymphatic vessel. **(C)** EM of a fenestrated capillary within the pancreatic islets of Langerhans (an endocrine gland) adjacent to a beta cell. The fenestrae with diaphragms are indicated at the *arrows*. *L* = lumen of the capillary; *B* = beta cell; *endo* = endothelial cell. **(D)** High-magnification EM of a fenestrated capillary showing insulin (*I*) within a secretory granule and its route of release through the fenestra (*large arrow*) into the lumen (*L*) of the capillary. The *small arrow* indicates fenestra with diaphragm. *endo* = endothelial cell.

● **Figure 10-6 Coronary artery with atherosclerosis. (A)** The entire coronary artery is shown with an eccentric, narrow lumen (*L*) because of the presence of an atheromatous plaque (tunica intima thickening). Atherosclerosis is considered an **intimal disease. (B, C, and D)** High magnification of the boxed areas (shown in **A**) of the **atheromatous plaque.** The fibrous cap (*fc*) is composed of smooth muscle cells, a few leukocytes, and a relatively dense deposition of collagen. The deeper necrotic core **(C)** consists of a disorganized mass of lipid material, cholesterol crystals (*cc*), cell debris, and foam cells (macrophages digesting modified LDL) of the fatty streak. *Ad* = tunica adventitia; *M* = tunica media. An atheromatous plaque may undergo many histologic changes, such as (1) **plaque calcification** that turns arteries into brittle pipes, (2) **hemorrhage into the plaque** that induces focal rupture or ulceration, and (3) **focal plaque rupture** at the luminal surface that results in **thrombus formation,** whereby the thrombus may partially or completely occlude the lumen, leading to approximately 90% of all myocardial infarctions. In this situation, thrombus formation is initiated by platelet aggregation induced by **thromboxane** (TXA_2). TXA_2 is synthesized from arachidonic acid using the enzyme cyclooxygenase. **Aspirin** covalently inhibits cyclooxygenase, and **nonsteroidal anti-inflammatory drugs (NSAIDs) such as ibuprofen and acetaminophen** reversibly inhibit cyclooxygenase and thereby block the synthesis of TXA_2. Consequently, low doses of aspirin and NSAIDs are effective in prevention of myocardial infarction. Thrombolysis is stimulated by **tissue plasminogen activator** (TPA) treatment, which successfully decreases the extent of ischemic damage caused by myocardial infarction. TPA stimulates the **conversion of plasminogen to plasmin.** Plasmin is a protease that digests fibrin within the thrombus.

● **Figure 10-7 Kaposi sarcoma.** Kaposi sarcoma is a relatively rare vascular tumor but has come to the forefront because of its high frequency of occurrence in AIDS patients. Multiple red-to-purple skin plaques are observed clinically. **(A, B)** Low- and high-magnification LMs show an intact epidermis (*epi*) of the skin covering the malignant vascular lesion in the dermis consisting of numerous vascular channels (*vc*), spindle-shaped neoplastic stromal cells (*), and extravasated red blood cells (*arrows*).

Chapter 11

Blood

I **Plasma** is the fluid portion of blood that contains many different proteins, which include: **albumin**, which maintains blood colloidal osmotic (oncotic) pressure; **gamma globulins; beta globulins**, which participate in the transport of hormones, metal ions, and lipids; and **fibrinogen**, which participates in blood clotting. Plasma without fibrinogen is called **serum**.

II **Red Blood Cells** (RBCs or erythrocytes)

A. **CHARACTERISTICS**
1. RBCs do not contain a nucleus or mitochondria.
2. RBCs use **glucose** as the primary fuel source (i.e., **glycolysis** or **hexose monophosphate shunt** during stress).
3. RBCs are biconcave-shaped disks (shape maintained by **spectrin**) and contain both **hemoglobin** and **carbonic anhydrase**.
4. Erythropoiesis (RBC formation) is regulated by **erythropoietin (EPO),** which is a glycoprotein hormone secreted by endothelial cells of the peritubular capillary network of the kidney. Serum EPO levels can be extremely high (normal value, 4–16 IU/L) in patients with severe anemias (e.g., aplastic anemia, severe hemolytic anemia, and hematologic cancers).
5. RBCs have a lifespan of **100 to 120 days**.
6. The cell membrane of the RBC is well characterized and includes the following proteins (Figure 11-1):
   a. **Spectrin** maintains the biconcave shape of the RBC. The tail ends of spectrin bind to **actin** and **band 4.1 protein**.
   b. **Ankyrin** attaches to spectrin and **band 3 protein**.
   c. **Band 3 protein** is an anion transporter that allows HCO_3^- to cross the RBC membrane in exchange for Cl^-.
   d. **Glycophorin** is the first transmembrane protein for which a complete amino acid sequence was determined. Its hydrophilic NH_2-terminal end is exposed to the extracellular space, its hydrophobic portion (22 amino acids long arranged in an alpha helix) spans the lipid bilayer, and its hydrophilic COOH-terminal end is exposed to the cytoplasm.

B. **LAYERS.** If blood is centrifuged (and clotting is prevented), three layers are separated:
1. **Top layer:** plasma
2. **Middle layer:** buffy coat containing leukocytes and platelets
3. **Bottom layer:** RBCs

A

Plasma   Cytoplasm

Band 4.1

Actin

Glycophorin

Spectrin

Ankyrin

Band 3

B

↓$PaCO_2$
↓H^+(alkalosis)
↓ Body temp
↓ 2, 3 BPG
Stored blood
HbF

↑$PaCO_2$
↑H^+(acidosis)
↑ Body temp
↑ 2, 3 BPG
Exercise
High altitude

CO poisoning

Hemoglobin saturation %

100

75

50

PO_2 in blood (mm Hg)

0   25 40   60   100

C

$CO_2 + H_2O$ —CA→ $H^+ + HCO_3^-$

Chloride shift

Cl^-

oxyHb → deoxyHb → deoxyHb·H^+

HCO_3^- in plasma

Cl^-

HCO_3^- —CA→ $CO_2 + H_2O$

deoxyHb·H^+ → oxyHb

CO_2

O_2

O_2 inhaled

CO_2 exhaled

Cell

Tissue

PO_2=40 mm Hg

Alveolus

Lung

PO_2=100 mm Hg

● **Figure 11-1 Red blood cells. (A)** Diagram of the red blood cell (RBC) cell membrane depicting the well-characterized protein component. **(B)** Hemoglobin (*Hb*)–O_2 dissociation curve. Note the sigmoid shape of the curve. At a PO_2 of 100 mm Hg found in arterial blood and lung alveoli, Hb is 100% saturated (*square*). At a PO_2 of 40 mm Hg found in mixed venous blood and tissues, Hb is 75% saturated (*triangle*). At a PO_2 of 25 mm Hg, Hb is 50% saturated (P_{50}; *circle*). Note the conditions that cause a shift to the left and right. In carbon monoxide (*CO*) poisoning, the curve is shifted to the left and plateaus well below 100% saturation. *HbF* = fetal hemoglobin; *2,3 BPG* = 2,3-bisphosphoglycerate. **(C)** Blood gas exchange in tissues and lung alveoli. In tissues, CO_2 is generated and freely diffuses into RBCs. In RBCs, CO_2 combines with H_2O to form H^+ and HCO_3^- in a reaction catalyzed by **carbonic anhydrase** (*CA*). HCO_3^- leaves the RBC in exchange for Cl^- (called the **chloride shift**) using **band III protein** (*solid black dot*). CO_2 is transported to the lung as HCO_3^- in the plasma. The PO_2 within tissues is 40 mm Hg and favors O_2 dissociation from oxyHb to form deoxyHb. The O_2 freely diffuses to tissues. The H^+ is buffered by combining with deoxyHb to form deoxyHb·H^+. In the lung, HCO_3^- enters the RBC and combines with H^+ from deoxyHb·H^+ to form CO_2 and H_2O in a reaction catalyzed by CA. CO_2 diffuses to lung alveoli and is exhaled. The PO_2 within lung alveoli is 100 mm Hg and favors saturation of deoxyHb with O_2 to form oxyHb.

C. HEMATOCRIT is the percent volume of a blood sample occupied by RBCs. A normal hematocrit value is 45%. Hematocrit values <45% may indicate **anemia**.

D. ENVIRONMENT
1. **A hypotonic environment** causes RBCs to swell, rupture (thereby forming ghosts), and release hemoglobin. This process is called **hemolysis**.
2. **A hypertonic environment** causes RBCs to shrink so that spiny projections protrude from the surface. This process is called **crenation**.

E. BLOOD GROUP ANTIGENS. The **A, B, and O** blood group antigens are carbohydrates linked to lipids of the RBC membrane. Because these carbohydrate antigens are genetically determined, an individual who receives mismatched blood will mount an immune reaction. Type O blood is the **universal donor**. Type AB blood is the **universal recipient**.

F. THE Rh FACTOR is clinically important in pregnancy. If the mother is Rh−, she will produce Rh antibodies if the fetus is Rh+. This situation will not affect the first pregnancy, but will affect the second pregnancy with an Rh+ fetus. In the second pregnancy with an Rh+ fetus, a hemolytic condition of RBCs occurs known as **Rh-hemolytic disease of newborn (erythroblastosis fetalis). Rh_0 (D) immune globulin (RhoGAM, MICRhoGAM)** is a human immunoglobulin (IgG) preparation that contains antibodies against Rh factor and prevents a maternal antibody response to Rh+ cells that may enter the maternal bloodstream of an Rh− mother. This drug is administered to Rh− mothers within 72 hours after the birth of an Rh+ baby to prevent erythroblastosis fetalis during subsequent pregnancies.

G. KERNICTERUS, which is a pathologic deposition of bilirubin in the basal ganglia, may develop as a result of the jaundice from the RBC hemolysis.

III Hemoglobin (Hb)

A. CHARACTERISTICS
1. Hb is a globular protein consisting of **four subunits**.
   a. **Adult Hb (HbA)** consists of two alpha globin subunits and two beta globin subunits designated **Hb $\alpha_2\beta_2$**.
   b. **Fetal Hb (HbF)** consists of two alpha globin subunits and two gamma globin subunits designated **Hb $\alpha_2\gamma_2$**. HbF is the **major form of Hb during fetal development** because the O_2 affinity of HbF is higher than the O_2 affinity of HbA and thereby "pulls" O_2 from the maternal blood into fetal blood. The higher O_2 affinity of HbF is explained by **2,3-bisphosphoglycerate (BPG)**. When 2,3-BPG binds HbA, the O_2 affinity of HbA is lowered. However, 2,3-BPG does not bind HbF, and therefore, the O_2 **affinity of HbF is higher**.
2. Hb contains a **heme moiety**, which is an **iron (Fe)-containing porphyrin**. Fe^{2+} (ferrous state) binds O_2, forming **oxyhemoglobin**. Fe^{3+} (ferric state) does not bind O_2, forming **deoxyhemoglobin**. The heme moiety is synthesized partially in mitochondria and partially in cytoplasm.
3. The **Hb–O_2 dissociation curve** is **sigmoid-shaped** because each successive O_2 that binds to Hb increases the affinity for the next oxygen (i.e., binding is cooperative). Therefore, the affinity for the fourth O_2 is the highest.

4. Concentration of Hb
    a. In males, the normal concentration of Hb is **13.5 to 17.5 g/dL.**
    b. In females, the normal concentration of Hb is **12.0 to 16.0 g/dL.**

B. **CLINICAL CONSIDERATIONS**
1. **Thalassemia syndromes** are a heterogeneous group of genetic defects characterized by the lack of or decreased synthesis of either α-globin (**α-thalassemia**) or
   β-globin (**β-thalassemia**).
    a. **Hydrops fetalis** is the most severe form of α-thalassemia and causes severe
       pallor, generalized edema, and massive hepatosplenomegaly, and invariably
       leads to intrauterine fetal death.
    b. **β-Thalassemia major** is the most severe form of β-thalassemia and causes a
       severe, transfusion-dependent anemia. It is most common in Mediterranean
       countries, parts of Africa, and Southeast Asia.
2. **Types 1 and 2 diabetes.** The amount of **glycosylated Hb (HbA$_{1c}$)** is an indicator
   of blood glucose normalization during the previous 3 months (because the half-life
   of RBCs is 3 months) in patients with type 1 and type 2 diabetes. Long periods of
   elevated blood glucose levels result in an **HbA$_{1c}$ of 12% to 20%,** whereas normal
   levels of HbA$_{1c}$ are 5%.

IV. Blood Gas Exchange (Figure 11-1)

A. **CHARACTERISTICS**
1. O_2 is transported mainly by Hb because it is not very soluble in plasma. Each Hb
   molecule can carry up to four O_2 molecules, which is described by the **Hb–O$_2$ dissociation curve.**
2. CO_2 is transported mainly as HCO_3^- in plasma.
3. The rate-limiting step in the utilization of O_2 by a cell is at the **ADP level.**

B. **CLINICAL CONSIDERATIONS**
1. **A shift to the left** of the Hb–O$_2$ dissociation curve occurs when the **affinity of Hb
   for O$_2$ is increased.** This makes the unloading of O_2 from arterial blood to tissues
   more difficult. A shift to the left is caused by a number of different factors:
   decreased Paco$_2$, decreased arterial H$^+$ (e.g., alkalosis), **decreased body temperature, and decreased 2,3-BPG** (e.g., stored blood, HbF). Stored blood loses
   2,3-BPG. HbF does not bind 2,3-BPG.
2. **A shift to the right** of the Hb–O$_2$ dissociation curve occurs when the **affinity of
   Hb for O$_2$ is decreased.** This makes the unloading of O_2 from arterial blood to tissues easier. A shift to the right is caused by a number of different factors: **increased
   Paco$_2$, increased arterial H$^+$** (e.g., acidosis), **increased body temperature** (e.g.,
   exercise), and **increased 2,3 BPG** (e.g., living at high altitude).
3. **Carbon monoxide (CO) poisoning.** CO binds to Hb with an affinity 200-fold
   greater than that of O_2, forming **carboxyhemoglobin (HbCO)** that gives blood
   a characteristic **cherry-red color.** CO poisoning **decreases the O$_2$ content** of
   the blood and causes a **shift to the left** of the Hb–O$_2$ dissociation curve.
   Patients with CO poisoning are given 100% O_2 to breathe to competitively
   displace CO from Hb and to increase the amount of dissolved O_2 content in the
   blood.

V White Blood Cells (WBCs or leukocytes)

A. NEUTROPHILS (POLYS, SEGS, OR PMNs)

1. Neutrophils are the most abundant leukocyte in the peripheral circulation (**50%–70%**).
2. Neutrophils have a multilobed nucleus.
3. Neutrophils have primary (azurophilic) granules, which are lysosomes that contain **acid hydrolases** and **myeloperoxidase** (produces hypochlorite ions).
4. Neutrophils have secondary granules that contain: **lysozyme, lactoferrin, alkaline phosphatase,** and other **bacteriostatic and bacteriocidal substances.**
5. Neutrophils have **respiratory burst oxidase** (a membrane enzyme), which produces hydrogen peroxide (H_2O_2) and superoxide, which kill bacteria.
6. Neutrophils are the first to arrive at an area of tissue damage (within 30 minutes; **acute inflammation**), being attracted to the site by complement C5a and leukotriene B_4.
7. Neutrophils are highly adapted for **anaerobic glycolysis** with large amounts of **glycogen** to function in a devascularized area.
8. Neutrophils play an important role in **phagocytosis of bacteria and dead cells** by using **antibody receptors (Fc portion), complement factors,** and **bacterial polysaccharides** to bind to the foreign material. Neutrophils must bind to the foreign material to begin phagocytosis.
9. Neutrophils impart **natural (or innate) immunity** along with macrophages and natural killer (NK) cells.
10. Neutrophils have a lifespan of **6 to 10 hours; 2 to 3 days in tissues.**

B. EOSINOPHILS

1. Eosinophils comprise **0% to 4%** of the leukocytes in the peripheral circulation.
2. Eosinophils have a bilobed nucleus.
3. Eosinophils have highly eosinophilic granules that contain **major basic protein, eosinophil cationic protein, histaminase,** and **peroxidase.**
4. Eosinophils have **immunoglobulin E (IgE) antibody receptors.**
5. Eosinophils play a role in **parasitic infection** (e.g., schistosomiasis, ascariasis, trichinosis).
6. Eosinophils play a role in **reducing the severity of allergic reactions** by secreting histaminase and PGE_1 and PGE_2, which degrade histamine (secreted by mast cells) and inhibit mast cell secretion, respectively.
7. Eosinophils have a lifespan of **1 to 10 hours; up to 10 days in tissues.**

C. BASOPHILS

1. Basophils comprise **0% to 2%** of the leukocytes in the peripheral circulation (i.e., the least abundant leukocyte).
2. Basophils have highly basophilic granules that contain **heparin, histamine, 5-hydroxytryptamine,** and **sulfated proteoglycans.**
3. Basophils have **IgE antibody receptors.**
4. Basophils play a role in immediate (type I) hypersensitivity reactions (anaphylactic reactions) causing **allergic rhinitis (hay fever), some forms of asthma, urticaria,** and **anaphylaxis.**
5. Basophils have a lifespan of **1 to 10 hours; variable in tissues.**

D. MONOCYTES

1. Monocytes comprise **2% to 9%** of the leukocytes in the peripheral circulation.
2. Monocytes are members of the **monocyte–macrophage system,** which includes: Kupffer cells in liver, alveolar macrophages, histiocytes in connective tissue, microglia in brain, Langerhans cells in skin, osteoclasts in bone, and dendritic antigen-presenting cells.
3. Monocytes have granules that are lysosomes that contain **acid hydrolases, aryl sulfatase, acid phosphatase,** and **peroxidase.**
4. Monocytes respond to dead cells, microorganisms, and inflammation by leaving the peripheral circulation to enter tissues and are then called macrophages.
5. Monocytes impart natural (innate) immunity along with neutrophils and NK cells.
6. Monocytes have a lifespan of **1 to 3 days; variable in tissue.**

E. NATURAL KILLER (NK) CELL is a member of the **null cell population** (i.e., lymphocytes that do not express the T cell receptor or cell membrane immunoglobulins that distinguish lymphocytes as either T cells or B cells, respectively). NK cells are $CD16^+$ and capable of cytotoxicity without prior antigen sensitization. NK cells attack damaged cells, virus-infected cells, and tumor cells by release of **cytolysin** (a cytokine that causes cell membrane porosity) and endonuclease-mediated **apoptosis** (i.e., **cell-mediated cytotoxicity**). They impart natural (innate) immunity along with neutrophils and macrophages.

F. T LYMPHOCYTES (see Chapter 12)

G. B LYMPHOCYTES AND PLASMA CELLS (see Chapter 13)

VI Platelets (Thrombocytes)

A. CHARACTERISTICS

1. Platelets are cell fragments derived from **megakaryocytes.**
2. Platelets are involved in **hemostasis (blood clotting).** Exposure of subendothelial collagen as a result of endothelial cell injury causes platelet adhesion mediated by von Willebrand factor (vWF). This stimulates platelet cell membrane phospholipases to free arachidonic acid, which is converted to thromboxane A_2 (TXA_2). TXA_2 contracts the platelet tubular system, which facilitates the release of platelet granules.
3. Platelets have α-granules that contain: **platelet factor 4, platelet-derived growth factor (PDGF), factor V,** and **fibrinogen.**
4. Platelets have δ-granules that contain: **serotonin, ADP,** and Ca^{2+}.
5. Platelets have a lifespan of **9 to 10 days.**

B. PHARMACOLOGY OF ANTIPLATELET DRUGS. These drugs increase bleeding time by inhibiting platelet aggregation.

1. **Aspirin (acetylsalicylic acid, Bayer, Bufferin)** is a nonsteroidal anti-inflammatory drug (NSAID) that irreversibly inhibits cyclooxygenase, thereby decreasing the production of TXA_2.
2. **Ticlopidine (Ticlid)** inhibits ADP-induced binding of fibrinogen to the platelet membrane.
3. **Dipyramidole (Dipridacot)** may increase adenosine levels thereby inhibiting platelet aggregation. It is used clinically to prevent thromboemboli in patients with a prosthetic heart valve.

VII   Hemostasis (Blood Clotting) (Figure 11-2)

A. TWO PATHWAYS

1. **Extrinsic pathway** follows this sequence of events: damaged tissue releases **thromboplastin**; thromboplastin initiates a cascade involving **factors VII, X, and V and prothrombin activator**; prothrombin activator converts **prothrombin (factor II)** → **thrombin (factor IIa)**; thrombin converts **fibrinogen (factor I)** → **fibrin**; fibrin, along with RBCs, platelets, and plasma, forms a **blood clot (or thrombus)**.

2. **Intrinsic pathway** follows this sequence of events: RBC trauma or RBC contact with subendothelial collagen initiates a cascade involving **factors XII, XI, IX, VIII, X, and V** and **prothrombin activator**; prothrombin activator converts **prothrombin (factor II)** → **thrombin (factor IIa)**; thrombin converts **fibrinogen (factor I)** → **fibrin**; fibrin, along with RBCs, platelets, and plasma, forms a **blood clot (or thrombus)**.

B. VITAMIN K

VITAMIN K is essential for hemostasis because it acts as a cofactor for an enzyme involved in the posttranslational carboxylation of glutamic acid forming **γ-carboxyglutamate residues** in certain blood factor proteins (e.g., factors X, IX, VII, and II). This allows factor proteins to bind to cell membranes because γ-carboxyglutamate residues have a high affinity for Ca^{2+}. **Vitamin K deficiency** can result in hemorrhage. However, adult vitamin K deficiency is rare because intestinal bacteria produce 50% of the required vitamin K.

C. PHARMACOLOGY OF ANTICOAGULANTS

1. **Heparin** stimulates the proteolytic action of **antithrombin III**, which inactivates thrombin (factor IIa) and other blood factor proteins. It is used clinically as an anticoagulant during pregnancy because heparin does not cross the placenta, to treat deep vein thrombosis, and to treat pulmonary thromboembolism.

2. **Warfarin (Coumadin, Dicumarol)** inhibits the synthesis of **vitamin K** thereby preventing the vitamin K-mediated formation of γ-carboxyglutamate residues in prothrombin (factor II) and other blood factor proteins. It is used clinically as an anticoagulant to treat deep vein thrombosis and pulmonary thromboembolism. It is contraindicated during pregnancy because it crosses the placenta and may interfere with fetal bone development.

D. PHARMACOLOGY OF THROMBOLYTICS

1. **Streptokinase (Streptase, Kabikinase)** is an indirect thrombolytic drug that combines with plasminogen to form an activator complex that converts plasminogen to plasmin.

2. **Tissue plasminogen activator (TPA, Alteplase) and urokinase (Abbokinase)** are direct thrombolytic drugs that directly convert plasminogen to plasmin.

E. CLINICAL CONSIDERATIONS

1. **Thrombocytopenia** (reduction in the number of circulating platelets) is the most common cause of abnormal bleeding. Bleeding time is prolonged when platelet count is $<100 \times 10^9$/L. Bleeding may occur at the skin, mucous membranes, genitourinary (GU) tract, and gastrointestinal (GI) tract. **Petechiae** (pinhead size hemorrhage in the skin) and **purpura** (small reddish-purple blotches in the skin) are apparent.

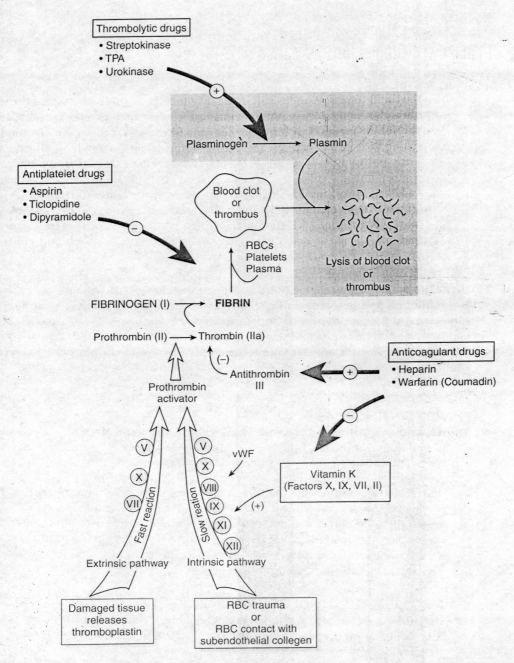

Thrombolytic drugs
• Streptokinase
• TPA
• Urokinase

(+)

Plasminogen → Plasmin

Antiplatelet drugs
• Aspirin
• Ticlopidine
• Dipyramidole

(−)

Blood clot
or
thrombus

Lysis of blood clot
or
thrombus

RBCs
Platelets
Plasma

FIBRINOGEN (I) → **FIBRIN**

Prothrombin (II) → Thrombin (IIa)

(−)

Antithrombin
III

Anticoagulant drugs
• Heparin
• Warfarin (Coumadin)

(+)

Prothrombin
activator

(−)

vWF

Vitamin K
(Factors X, IX, VII, II)

(+)

Ⓥ Ⓥ
      Ⓧ
Ⓧ Ⓥ̲Ⓘ̲Ⓘ̲Ⓘ̲
      Ⓘ̲Ⓧ
Ⓥ̲Ⓘ̲Ⓘ̲ Ⓧ̲Ⓘ̲
      Ⓧ̲Ⓘ̲Ⓘ̲

Fast reaction   Slow reation

Extrinsic pathway   Intrinsic pathway

Damaged tissue
releases
thromboplastin

RBC trauma
or
RBC contact with
subendothelial collegen

● **Figure 11-2 Diagram of hemostasis.** The extrinsic and intrinsic pathways are depicted, both of which lead to the production of prothrombin activator. Prothrombin activator converts prothrombin to thrombin. Thrombin subsequently converts fibrinogen to fibrin. Vitamin K is essential for hemostasis. The shaded box indicates the mechanism for lysis of the blood clot or thrombus. Plasmin initiates lysis. Note the action of thrombolytic, antiplatelet, and anticoagulant drugs. *TPA* = tissue plasminogen activator; *vWF* = von Willebrand factor.

2. **Idiopathic thrombocytopenic purpura (ITP)** is caused by antibody-mediated destruction of platelets. The **acute form** is associated with viral infection in children and resolves spontaneously. The **adult form** is chronic, occurs particularly in women of child-bearing age, and may be associated with other autoimmune diseases.

3. **Thrombotic thrombocytopenic purpura (TTP)** is a platelet consumption syndrome that usually affects **young women** and has a **viral prodrome.** TTP is characterized by the presence of **hyaline thrombi** in arterioles (without inflammation) leading to microvascular disease. TTP presents with a pentad of symptoms: thrombocytopenia, microangiopathic hemolytic anemia, neurologic abnormalities, renal dysfunction, and fever.

4. **Hemophilia A (factor VIII deficiency)** is an **X-linked recessive** disease and is the most common hereditary coagulopathy. The procoagulant portion of the factor VIII protein (**factor VIII^{pro}**) is deficient, whereas the antigenic portion of the factor VIII protein (**factor VIII^{ag}**) is present in normal amounts. Clinical features include: positive family history; usually affects men; bleeding into soft tissues, muscles, and weight-bearing joints; hematuria; after injury, bleeding may persist for weeks leading to compartment syndrome.

5. **von Willebrand disease (vWD)** is an **autosomal dominant** disease. **Factor VIII^{pro}** and **factor VIII^{ag}** are deficient. Because factor VIII^{ag} is necessary for normal platelet aggregation, lack of factor VIII^{ag} causes symptoms similar to defective platelet function. Clinical features include a mixed bleeding picture (mucocutaneous bleeding and soft tissue bleeding); affects men and women.

VIII Red Bone Marrow (Myeloid Tissue)

A. The bone marrow is the main site of hematopoiesis; it removes aged and defective RBCs by macrophage phagocytosis (along with the liver and spleen), and is the site of B lymphocyte formation.

B. In the adult, red bone marrow is present in vertebrae, sternum, ribs, skull, pelvis, and proximal femur. Bone marrow aspirates or biopsies are obtained from the superior iliac crest (posterior or anterior), sternum, or upper end of tibia (in children).

C. The bone marrow consists of stromal (1%), myeloid (granulocytes, 65%), erythroid (RBC, 20%), and lymphoid (14%) components. The **myeloid:erythroid (M:E) ratio is 3:1 to 5:1** normally.

IX Selected Photomicrographs

A. Hereditary spherocytosis, β-thalassemia major, sickle cell disease, and glucose-6-phosphate dehydrogenase (G6PD) deficiency (Figure 11-3)

B. Vitamin B_{12} deficiency, lead poisoning, iron deficiency, Howell-Jolly bodies (Figure 11-4)

C. Spur cells in alcoholic cirrhosis, burr cells in kidney failure, target cells (Figure 11-5)

D. Chronic myeloid leukemia (CML), chronic lymphocytic leukemia (CLL) (Figure 11-6)

E. Hairy cell leukemia, Reed-Sternberg cells, Chediak-Higashi syndrome (Figure 11-7)

F. Erythropoiesis (Figure 11-8)

G. Granulopoiesis (neutrophilic) (Figure 11-9)

H. Various blood cells (Figure 11-10)

I. Complete blood count (CBC) normal values for peripheral blood (Table 11-1)

● **Figure 11-3 Red blood cell disorders. (A)** Hereditary spherocytosis, a genetic disease characterized by a deficiency in the spectrin protein that helps stabilize the RBC membrane, usually is caused by a mutation of the ankyrin gene. This results in anisocytosis (variation in size of RBCs) and spherocytes with no central pallor zone. The osmotic fragility test is the confirmatory test for hereditary spherocytosis. **(B)** β-Thalassemia major is shown with some large, polychromatic RBCs that are newly released from the bone marrow in response to the anemia. However, most RBCs are small (microcytic) and colorless (hypochromic). Also apparent are many irregular-shaped RBCs (poikilocytes) that have been traumatized or damaged during passage through the spleen. **(C)** Sickle cell anemia is shown with sickle RBCs (drepanocytes) as a result of the rod-shaped polymers of the inherited abnormal hemoglobin S (HbS). The RBC does not become sickled until it has lost its nucleus and has its full complement of HbS. Sickle cells are thin, elongated, and well filled with HbS. The main clinical manifestations of sickle cell disease are chronic hemolytic anemia and occlusion of microvasculature (called vasoocclusive disease). Vasoocclusive crisis may occur in the brain, liver, lung, or spleen. Factors that induce sickling are Po_2 (e.g., high altitude) or a concentration of 60% HbS or greater in RBCs. **(D)** Glucose-6-phosphate dehydrogenase (G6PD) deficiency is a genetic disease in which the deficiency reduces the ability of RBCs to protect themselves from oxidative injury. This leads to a denaturation of Hb, which forms Hb precipitates within the RBC (see inset) called Heinz bodies. As these RBCs percolate through the spleen, splenic macrophages "chew" the Heinz bodies so that RBCs have a "bite" of cytoplasm removed and are called bite cells. However, the majority of RBCs are normocytic and normochromatic.

● **Figure 11-4 Red blood cell disorders in deficiences, poisoning, and splenectomy. (A)** Pernicious anemia as a result of vitamin B_{12} deficiency caused by atrophic gastritis with decreased intrinsic factor production. Some RBCs are deformed as they pass through the splenic sinuses and appear teardrop-shaped (dacryocytes), **macrocytic,** and **hyperchromic.** In addition, large neutrophils with a hypersegmented nucleus (five to six lobes) can be observed (inset). A **Schilling test** is where an oral dose of "hot" vitamin B_{12} tagged with ^{57}Co is given along with an intramuscular injection of "cold" vitamin B_{12}. Normally, >7% of the hot vitamin B_{12} is collected in the urine within 24 hours (in pernicious anemia <1%). Sensory neuropathy (tingling, numbness) associated with pernicious anemia reflects impairment of methylcobalamin-dependent methionine synthesis. Patients respond favorably after a 2-week regimen of intramuscular vitamin B_{12} injections. **(B)** Lead (Pb^{2+}) poisoning is shown in which the RBCs are **microcytic and hypochromic** and show basophilic stippling, which probably represents breakdown of ribosomes. Lead denatures sulfhydryl (SH) groups in ferrochelatase within mitochondria that bind iron to protoporphyrin to form heme, thus inhibiting hemoglobin synthesis. As a result, unbound iron accumulates in mitochondria and forms ringed sideroblasts. **(C)** Iron (Fe^{2+}) deficiency anemia is shown with RBCs that are **microcytic and hypochromic** with a thin rim of Hb at the periphery. Iron deficiency is probably the most common nutritional disorder in the world. Iron is stored in the body as ferritin within the cytoplasm of cells and as hemosiderin within lysosomes. Some ferritin normally circulates in the plasma and is a good indicator of iron stores (iron deficiency = <12 mg/L; iron overload = 5,000 mg/L). Iron is transported in the body mainly by transferrin, which is synthesized by the liver. The main function of transferrin is to deliver iron to cells, particularly to RBC precursors, which need iron for Hb synthesis. **(D)** Howell-Jolly bodies after splenectomy. Howell-Jolly bodies represent nuclear fragments that are normally removed from RBCs as they pass through the splenic sinuses. After splenectomy, increased numbers of RBCs with these inclusions are observed.

● **Figure 11-5 Red blood cells in various pathologies. (A and B)** Hemolytic anemia associated with alcoholic cirrhosis shows RBCs with a periphery consisting of sharp points called spur cells. **(C)** Anemia associated with kidney failure (or renal insufficiency) shows RBCs with a periphery consisting of bumps called burr cells. **(D)** Target cells (or codocytes) have a central dark area of Hb that is surrounded by a colorless ring followed by a peripheral rim of Hb. Target cells can be found in a number of pathologic states, including thalassemia, obstructive liver disease, and iron deficiency.

● **Figure 11-6 (A and B) Chronic myeloid leukemia (CML). (A)** Low-power LM showing an increased number of granulocytes in all stages of maturation and many mature neutrophils. **(B)** Higher-power LM showing neutrophils (*N*), metamyelocytes (*M*), myelocytes (*ML*), and promyelocytes (*P*). A characteristic finding in CML is the absence of alkaline phosphatase in granulocytes. The absence of alkaline phosphatase activity is used to distinguish CML from a leukemoid reaction. In 90% of CML cases, the Philadelphia (Ph) chromosome, which is a reciprocal translocation of DNA involving band q34 on chromosome 9 and band q11 on chromosome 22 [t(9;22)(q34;q11)], is found. This translocation results in the *bcr-c-abl* fusion gene, which codes for a protein with tyrosine kinase activity. **(C and D) Chronic lymphocytic leukemia (CLL). (C)** Low-power LM showing an increased number of small, mature-looking B lymphocytes. **(D)** Higher-power LM showing B lymphocytes with condensed nuclear chromatin and a high nucleus to cytoplasm ratio. CLL, which is the most common leukemia, is a disorder of mature (virgin) B cells that are unable to differentiate into plasma cells, causing hypogammaglobulinemia.

● **Figure 11-7. (A and B) Hairy cell leukemia. (A)** B lymphocytes are shown with prominent cytoplasmic projections. **(B)** Nomarski interference illumination clearly showing B lymphocytes with prominent cytoplasmic projections. Hairy cell leukemia is a relatively rare but distinctive form of chronic B lymphocyte leukemia that receives its name because of the distinctive feature of the cytoplasmic projections of the B lymphocyte. Massive splenomegaly is the most common physical finding. A positive tartrate-resistant acid phosphatase stain is a key to confirming the diagnosis. **(C)** A Reed-Sternberg cell is a distinctive giant cell that is considered an essential neoplastic element in Hodgkin disease. The Reed-Sternberg cell is often binucleate or bilobed with a prominent nucleolus. **(D)** Chediak-Higashi syndrome is a genetic disease characterized by neutropenia and impaired phagocytosis of bacteria as a result of a defect in microtubule polymerization. Large abnormal lysosomes can be observed in the cytoplasm of a neutrophil.

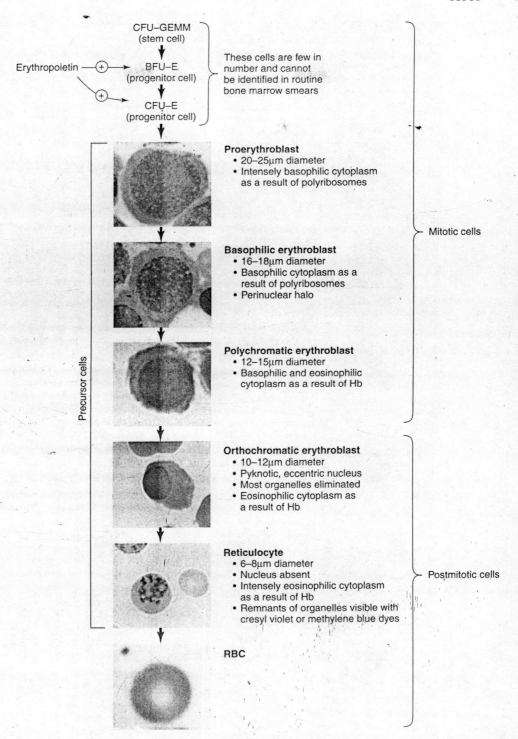

CFU–GEMM
(stem cell)

Erythropoietin ⟶ ⊕ ⟶ BFU–E
(progenitor cell)

⊕ ⟶ CFU–E
(progenitor cell)

These cells are few in
number and cannot
be identified in routine
bone marrow smears

Proerythroblast
- 20–25μm diameter
- Intensely basophilic cytoplasm
  as a result of polyribosomes

Basophilic erythroblast
- 16–18μm diameter
- Basophilic cytoplasm as a
  result of polyribosomes
- Perinuclear halo

Polychromatic erythroblast
- 12–15μm diameter
- Basophilic and eosinophilic
  cytoplasm as a result of Hb

Orthochromatic erythroblast
- 10–12μm diameter
- Pyknotic, eccentric nucleus
- Most organelles eliminated
- Eosinophilic cytoplasm as
  a result of Hb

Reticulocyte
- 6–8μm diameter
- Nucleus absent
- Intensely eosinophilic cytoplasm
  as a result of Hb
- Remnants of organelles visible with
  cresyl violet or methylene blue dyes

RBC

Mitotic cells

Precursor cells

Postmitotic cells

● **Figure 11-8 Erythropoiesis (RBC formation).** The various cells and characteristics involved in the formation of a mature RBC are shown. The colony-forming unit–granulocyte/erythroid/monocyte/megakaryocyte (*CFU-GEMM*) stem cells give rise to burst-forming unit–erythroid (*BFU-E*) progenitor cells that form "bursts" of erythroid cells in culture. The BFU-E cells give rise to colony-forming unit–erythroid (*CFU-E*) progenitor cells. Note the action of erythropoietin. The CFU-E cells give rise to the various precursor cells leading to the mature RBCs. Note the mitotic activity of the various cells.

● Figure 11-9 Granulopoiesis (neutrophilic). The various cells and characteristics involved in the formation of a mature neutrophil are shown. The colony-forming unit–granulocyte/erythroid/monocyte/megakaryocyte (*CFU-GEMM*) stem cells give rise to colony-forming unit–granulocyte/monocyte (*CFU-GM*) progenitor cells. The CFU-GM cells give rise to colony-forming unit–granulocyte (*CFU-G*) progenitor cells. The CFU-G cells give rise to the various precursor cells leading to the mature neutrophil. Note the action of granulocyte-monocyte colony-stimulating factor (*GM-CSF*) and granulocyte colony-stimulating factor (*G-CSF*), which are glycoproteins secreted by the endothelial cells and macrophages within the bone marrow. Note the mitotic activity of the various cells.

● **Figure 11-10 LM of various blood cells. (A)** Neutrophil. **(B)** Eosinophil. **(C)** Basophil. **(D)** Monocyte. **(E)** Small lymphocyte. **(F)** Plasma cell. B lymphocytes differentiate into plasma cells, whose main function is the synthesis and secretion of immunoglobulins. Plasma cells have an eccentric nucleus with a clock-face chromatin pattern, a perinuclear clear area (Hof area) corresponding to the Golgi, and a basophilic cytoplasm as a result of rER for protein synthesis. **(G)** Platelets. **(H)** Diagram of a platelet. Note the microtubules, actin cortex, membranous canalicular network (*cn*), dense tubular system (*dts*), lysosomes (*lys*), glycogen (*gly*), mitochondria (*mt*), α-granules, and δ-granules. **(I)** Megakaryocyte.

TABLE 11-1	COMPLETE BLOOD COUNT (CBC) VALUES FOR PERIPHERAL BLOOD

Complete Blood Count (CBC)	Normal Values
RBC count	
Men	$4.5–6.5 \times 10^{12}/L$
Women	$3.9–5.6 \times 10^{12}/L$
Hemoglobin (Hb)	
Men	13.5–17.5 g/dL
Women	12.0–16.0 g/dL
Hematocrit (Hct)	
Men	40%–52%
Women	35%–47%
Mean corpuscular volume (MCV)	80–100 fL
Mean corpuscular Hb (MCH)	27–34 pg
Mean corpuscular Hb concentration (MCHC)	30–35 g/dL
RBC distribution width (RDW)	11%–14%
Reticulocyte count	0.5%–2.0% of normal RBCs
Platelet count	$150–440 \times 10^9/L$
WBC count	$3.2–9.8 \times 10^9/L$
Differential count	
Promyelocytes	0
Myelocytes	0
Metamyelocytes	0%–1%
Band neutrophils	$0.1–0.6 \times 10^9/L$ (2%–6%)
Mature neutrophils (segs)	$2.5–7.5 \times 10^9/L$ (50%–70%)
Eosinophils	$0.0–0.4 \times 10^9/L$ (0%–4%)
Basophils	$0.0–0.2 \times 10^9/L$ (0%–2%)
Monocytes	$0.1–1.0 \times 10^9/L$ (2%–9%)
Lymphocytes	$1.0–5.0 \times 10^9/L$ (20%–45%)

Case Study

A 60-year-old man comes to your office complaining that "I've been feeling really tired lately and get out of breath just walking around the house." He also tells you that "my feet always go to sleep on me; they feel like pins and needles." After some discussion, he informs you that his tongue feels "kind of big and beefy" and that he has been falling down a lot. When questioned about his alcohol consumption, he emphatically denies being an alcoholic but admits that "I do like to have a glass of whiskey every day." In addition, you noticed that he walked very stiffly as he came into the examining room. What is the most likely diagnosis?

Differentials

- Beri beri, diabetes, folate deficiency caused by alcoholism or poor diet, lead poisoning, uremia

Relevant Physical Exam Findings

- Conjunctiva and nail beds are pale
- Skin is colored lemon yellow
- Auscultation reveals a 2/6 systolic flow murmur over the left sternal border
- A stiff, unsteady gait; hyperreflexia; loss of positional and vibratory sense in the lower limbs

Relevant Lab Findings

- Blood chemistry: Hgb = 10.5 μg/L (Low); Mean corpuscular volume (MCV) = 120fL (High); Leukocyte count = 3,400/mm³ (Low); Platelet count = 78,000/mm³ (Low); B_{12} = 85 pg/mL (Low); Methylmalonic acid = High; parietal cell autoantibodies = High BUN = Normal; Creatinine = Normal
- Peripheral blood smear: megaloblastic anemia; neutrophils with hypersegmented nuclei
- Schilling test: Positive

Diagnosis

Pernicious anemia. Pernicious anemia is an autoimmune disease that is associated with a predisposition to other autoimmune disorders (particularly of the adrenal and thyroid glands). Parietal cell autoantibodies develop, which causes a chronic fundal (Type A) gastritis and parietal cell destruction. Parietal cells normally produce HCl and intrinsic factor (which is necessary for vitamin B_{12} absorption). The lack of intrinsic factor causes vitamin B_{12} deficiency, which leads to megaloblastic anemia and subacute combined degeneration of the posterior and lateral spinal tracts. Vitamin B_{12} deficiency may also be caused by: surgical resection of the stomach or ileum; Crohn disease; strict vegan diet; bacterial overgrowth; *D. lactum* infection. Beri beri is a disease caused by thiamine deficiency often resulting from alcoholism. Dry beri beri (first stage) is characterized by peripheral neuropathy. Wet beri beri (second stage) is characterized by high output heart failure. Wernicke-Korsakoff syndrome (final stage) is characterized by confusion, ataxia, ophthalmoplegia, and confabulation. Clinical findings of diabetes include: diabetic peripheral neuropathy, gastroparesis, and the inability to regulate heart rate. Folate deficiency may be caused by alcoholism, certain diets, pregnancy, celiac sprue, giardiasis, phenytoin, oral contraceptives, antifolate chemotherapeutic agents. Clinical findings of folate deficiency include: megaloblastic anemia but not subacute combined degeneration of the posterior and lateral spinal tracts. Clinical findings of lead poisoning include motor neuropathy leading to wrist or foot drop; microcytic, hypochromic anemia; basophilic stippling of RBCs; encephalopathy; Fanconi syndrome; and a lead line deposit in the gums. Uremia is defined as elevated BUN and creatinine levels in the blood, usually as a result of renal failure. Clinical findings of uremia include anemia, peripheral neuropathy, bleeding, heart failure, pericarditis, esophagitis, pruritus, and encephalopathy.

Case Study

A 16-year-old girl is sent to your office because she had a nosebleed during class and this was not the first time. The girl comes to your office saying that "I get these nosebleeds once in a while but they're no big deal because they stop after about 10 minutes. But, I think I bleed a lot more during my period than my girlfriends do." She also tells you that "my mother has some kind of bleeding problem, but she never speaks about it." After some discussion, she informs you that her brother was in the Betty Ford Clinic for cocaine addiction. You ask her if she is using and she says "I've tried it a few times but I'm no crackhead like my silly brother." What is the most likely diagnosis?

Differentials

- Coagulation disorders (secondary hemostasis), disorders with increased vascular fragility

Relevant Physical Exam Findings

- Physical exam is unremarkable
- No history of vomiting blood (hematemesis), passage of bloody stools (hematochezia), or black, tarry stools (melena)
- No signs of ecchymoses (small hemorrhagic spots)

Relevant Lab Findings

- Blood chemistry: Platelets = 250,000 μL (Normal); prothrombin time (PT) = 13 seconds (Normal); partial thromboplastin time (PTT) = 65 seconds (High); bleeding time = 10 minutes (High)
- Ristocetin assay = no aggregation of platelets

Diagnosis

Von Willebrand disease (vWD). vWD is a type of primary hemostasis disorder and is the most common inherited bleeding disorder (autosomal dominant). vWD is due to low levels of von Willebrand factor (vWF). Endothelial cells secrete vWF, which combines with Factor VIII secreted by hepatocytes to form a Factor VIII–vWF complex (this increases the half-life of Factor VIII). This complex promotes blood clotting as well as platelet-subendothelial connective tissue interactions necessary for blood clotting. Platelets attach to the subendothelial connective tissue when the Gp1b glycoprotein receptor located on the cell membrane of the platelet binds to the Factor VIII–vWF complex. Since vWF forms a complex with Factor VIII, vWD patients have a qualitative (not quantitative) deficiency of factor VIII that leads to a prolonged PTT. Clinical findings of vWD include excessive bleeding from superficial cuts, bleeding from mucous membranes (e.g., gums, nasal mucosa), prolonged bleeding after dental work, menorrhagia, internal GI bleeding, and easy bruising. Primary hemostasis disorders with a platelet count below 150,000/μL (quantitative) include bone marrow failure, Wiskott-Aldrich syndrome, idiopathic thrombocytopenic purpura, thrombotic thrombocytopenic purpura, hemolytic uremic syndrome, multiple transfusions, and splenic sequestering. Primary hemostasis disorders with a normal platelet count (qualitative) include vWD, Bernard-Soulier disease, Glanzmann thrombasthenia, aspirin overdose, and uremia. A prolonged bleeding time is diagnostic of a primary hemostasis disorder. Coagulation disorders (secondary hemostasis) are clotting factor deficiencies involved in the coagulation cascade. Coagulation disorders include hemophilia A, hemophilia B (Christmas disease), and vitamin K deficiency. A prolonged PTT is diagnostic of a coagulation disorder. Clinical findings of coagulation disorders include: severe bleeding from large blood vessels with hemarthrosis, large hematomas after trauma, and prolonged wound healing. Diseases with increased vascular fragility include: scurvy, Henoch-Schonlein purpura, rickettsial and meningococcal infections, Ehlers-Danlos syndrome, and Cushing syndrome. Clinical findings of disorders with increased vascular fragility include symptoms similar to primary hemostasis disorders but with a normal bleeding time.

Ch

Th

geal
migra
origin
amou
rema
gland
Histo

Chapter 12

Thymus

I **General Features.** The thymus is derived embryologically from **endodermal pharyngeal pouch 3,** which forms thymic epitheliocytes and becomes populated by T stem cells that migrate in from the **mesodermal bone marrow.** Therefore, the thymus has a dual embryologic origin. At birth, the thymus weighs 10 to 15 g and increases to 20 to 40 g by puberty. Although the amount of lymphoid tissue decreases with age, being replaced by adipose tissue, the thymus remains a source of T cells throughout life. In the adult, the thymus is a soft, bilobed, encapsulated gland that lies in the anterior mediastinum. The thymus is the main site of T cell differentiation. Histologically, the thymus is divided into the **cortex** and **medulla.**

II **Thymic Cortex** (Figure 12-1) consists of:

A. THYMIC EPITHELIOCYTES (endodermal origin; also called thymic nurse cells) contain **cytokeratin** intermediate filaments and form a cellular meshwork joined by **desmosomes** into which thymocytes are tightly packed. They secrete **thymotaxin,** which attracts T stem cells from the bone marrow into the thymus, and **thymosin, serum thymic factor, and thymopoietin,** which transform immature T cells into mature T cells.

B. THYMOCYTES (mesodermal origin), which include: **T stem cells, pre-T cells, and immature T cells.**

C. MACROPHAGES

III **Thymic Medulla** (Figure 12-1) consists of:

A. THYMIC EPITHELIOCYTES

B. MATURE T CELLS (CD4+ HELPER T CELLS, CD4+ OR CD8+ SUPPRESSOR T CELLS, CD8+ CYTOTOXIC T CELLS)

C. THYMIC (HASSALL'S) CORPUSCLES, which are whorl-like structures composed of keratinized thymic epitheliocytes

IV **T Cell Lymphopoiesis** (T cell formation) (Figure 12-2)

V **Types of Mature T Cells**

A. CD4+ HELPER T CELLS, whose functions include: recognition of antigen in association with **class II MHC,** release of lymphokines that stimulate proliferation of B lymphocytes

● **Figure 12-1 LM Features of the thymus. (A)** Diagram of the thymus. Note the various cell types within the cortex and medulla. *T* = thymocytes; *TE* = thymic epitheliocytes; *HC* = Hassall's corpuscle. **(B)** LM of thymus showing the darkly stained cortex (C) and pale medulla (M). **(C)** LM of thymic cortex shows a large number of densely packed thymocytes (T) of various sizes. In addition, thymic epitheliocytes (TE; arrows) are apparent. **(D)** LM of thymic medulla showing the whorl-like Hassall's corpuscles (HC), which are keratinized thymic epitheliocytes surrounded by mature T cells. Bar = blood-thymus barrier; Mac = macrophage.

and antibody production, stimulation of proliferation of T cells, regulation of hemopoiesis, and activation of macrophages.

B. **CD4⁺ OR CD8⁺ SUPPRESSOR T CELLS,** whose function is to downregulate the immune response.

C. **CD8⁺ CYTOTOXIC T CELLS,** whose functions include: recognition of antigen in association with **class I MHC;** killing of allogeneic cells, virus-infected cells, and fungi; and release of **cytolysin** that causes membrane porosity and endonuclease-mediated apoptosis.

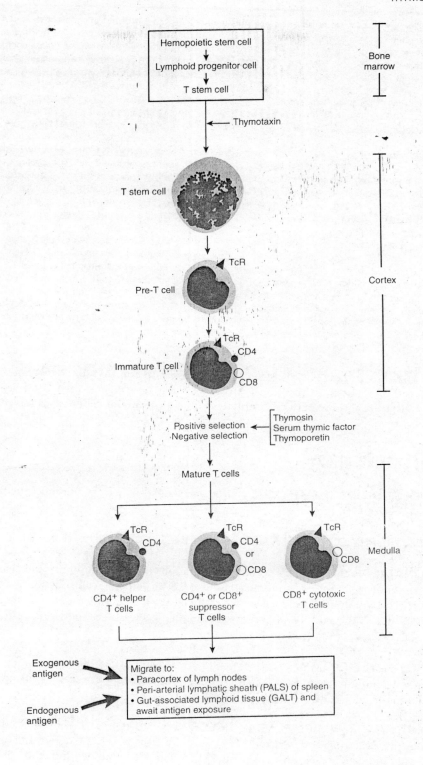

● **Figure 12-2 T cell lymphopoiesis. Hemopoietic stem cells** differentiate into **lymphoid progenitor cells** that form **T stem cells** within the bone marrow. Under the influence of **thymotaxin,** T stem cells leave the bone marrow and enter the thymic cortex where they differentiate into **pre-T cells.** Pre-T cells begin T cell receptor (T*c*R) gene rearrangement and express TcR. **Immature T cells** express **TcR, CD4, and CD8** and undergo positive or negative selection under the influence of **thymosin, serum thymic factor, and thymopoietin. Positive selection** is a process whereby CD4+/CD8+ T cells bind with a certain affinity to MHC proteins expressed on thymic epitheliocytes such that the CD4+/CD8+ T cells become **"educated";** all other CD4+/CD8+ T cells undergo apoptosis. This means that a mature T cell will respond to antigen only when presented by an MHC protein that it encountered at this stage in its development. This is known as **MHC restriction of T cell responses. Negative selection** is a process whereby CD4+/CD8+ T cells interact with thymic dendritic cells at the corticomedullary junction of the thymus such that CD4+/CD8+ T cells that recognize "self" antigens undergo apoptosis (or are somehow inactivated), leaving only CD4+/CD8+ T cells that recognize only foreign antigens. **Mature T cells** down regulate CD4 or CD8 to form either **CD4+ helper T cells, CD4+ or CD8+ suppressor T cells, or CD8+ cytotoxic T cells.** Mature T cells migrate to the **paracortex (thymic-dependent zone)** of all lymph nodes and the **periarterial lymphatic sheath (PALS) in the spleen** to await antigen exposure. **Exogenous protein antigens** (circulating in the bloodstream) are phagocytosed by APCs and undergo lysosomal degradation in **endolysosomes** to form antigen peptide fragments. The antigen peptide fragments become associated with **Class II MHC** and are transported and exposed on the cell surface of the APC. The antigen peptide fragment + Class II MHC on the surface of the APC is recognized by **CD4+ helper T cells,** which secrete **IL-2** (stimulates proliferation of B and T cells), **IL-4 and IL-5** (activate antibody production by causing B cell differentiation into plasma cells and promote isotype switching and hypermutation), **TNF-α** (activates macrophages), and **IFN-γ** (activates macrophages and natural killer cells). **Endogenous antigens** (intracellular virus or bacteria) undergo proteosomal degradation in **proteosomes** within the infected cell to form antigen peptide fragments. The antigen peptide fragments become associated with the **Class I MHC** and are transported and exposed on the cell surface of the infected cell. The antigen peptide fragment + class I MHC on the surface of the infected cell is recognized by **CD8+ cytotoxic T cells,** which secrete **perforins, cytolysins, lymphotoxins,** and **serine esterases,** which cause membrane porosity and endonuclease-mediated apoptosis of the infected cell.

VI ## Blood-Thymus Barrier. This barrier is found **only in the thymic cortex** and ensures that immature T cells undergo positive and negative selection in an antigen-free environment. This barrier consists of **tight junctions between nonfenestrated endothelial cells, basal lamina, and thymic epitheliocytes.**

VII ## Clinical Considerations

A. **INVOLUTION OF THE THYMUS** can be accelerated by: stress, adrenocorticotrophic hormone (ACTH), or steroids.

B. **HYPERTROPHY OF THE THYMUS** can be caused by: T_3, prolactin, or growth hormone.

C. **NEONATAL THYMECTOMY** severely impairs cell-mediated immunity and also somewhat diminishes humoral immunity because CD4+ helper T cell function is compromised. The lymph nodes and spleen are **reduced in size** because the thymic-dependent zone of the lymph nodes and periarterial lymphatic sheath of the spleen, respectively, do not become populated with T cells.

D. **ADULT THYMECTOMY** causes less severe impairment of cell-mediated immunity and humoral immunity because the lymph nodes and spleen are already well populated with long-lived T cells.

E. **CONGENITAL THYMIC APLASIA (DIGEORGE SYNDROME)** is a disorder characterized by hypocalcemia and recurrent infections with viruses, bacteria, fungi, and protozoa. It occurs in infants when **pharyngeal pouches 3 and 4** fail to develop embryologically, which results in the absence of the **thymus** and **parathyroid glands.** These infants have **no T cells.** Many infants even fail to mount an immunoglobulin response that requires CD4+ helper T cells.

F. **ACQUIRED IMMUNE DEFICIENCY SYNDROME (AIDS)** is a disorder that slowly weakens the immune system through selective destruction of **CD4+ helper T cells.**

VIII **Pharmacology of Immunosuppressive Drugs.** These drugs are used clinically with organ transplantation.

A. **CYCLOSPORINE (SANDIMMUNE)** blocks T cell activation by binding to cyclophilin (an intracellular receptor) and decreasing activity of calcineurin (a protein phosphatase). This ultimately prevents production of interleukin 2 (IL-2) and γ-interferon (γ-IFN). Cyclosporine is a peptide produced by the fungus *Tolypocladium inflatum Gams.*

B. **TACROLIMUS (FK506)** blocks T cell activation by binding to FK506 (a protein) and decreasing the activity of calcineurin. This ultimately prevents production of IL-2 and γ-IFN.

C. **MUROMONAB CD3 (OKT-3)** blocks T cell function by binding the CD3 component of the T cell antigen receptor complex. OKT-3 is a murine (mouse) monoclonal antibody directed against CD3.

D. **ANTILYMPHOCYTIC GLOBULIN (ALG; ATGAM)** induces T cell destruction by binding to T cells and inducing complement-mediated destruction of T cells. ALG is a purified immunoglobulin preparation of hyperimmune serum of horses, rabbits, or goats that have been immunized with human T cells.

IX **Selected Photomicrograph**

A. Thymoma (Figure 12-3).

● **Figure 12-3 LM of a thymoma.** A thymoma is a tumor of thymic epitheliocytes. A huge proliferation of thymic epitheliocytes is shown (compare with normal thymus in Figure 12-1C). Inset shows high magnification of thymic epitheliocytes. Note that thymic epitheliocytes may exist in three different states: normal (in Figure 12-1C), keratinized (in Figure 12-1D), and tumorous as shown here.

Chapter 13

Lymph Node

I **General Features** (Figure 13-1). A lymph node is a small, encapsulated, ovoid (bean-shaped) gland that lies in the course of lymphatic vessels draining various anatomic regions. Histologically, a lymph node is divided into the **cortex** and **medulla.**

II **Outer Cortex** consists of:

A. **MATURE (VIRGIN) B CELLS,** which are organized into **lymphatic follicles** that may contain **germinal centers.** Germinal centers are evidence of activated B cells that begin the transformation into plasma cells.

B. **FOLLICULAR DENDRITIC CELLS,** which have an antigen-presenting function

C. **MACROPHAGES**

D. **FIBROBLASTS** (reticular cells), which secrete **type III collagen** (reticular fibers) that form a stromal meshwork.

III **Inner Cortex** (paracortex; thymic-dependent zone) consists of:

A. **MATURE T CELLS**

B. **DENDRITIC CELLS,** which have an antigen-presenting function

C. **MACROPHAGES**

D. **FIBROBLASTS** (reticular cells), which secrete type III collagen (reticular fibers) that form a stromal meshwork

IV **Medulla** consists of:

A. **LYMPHOCYTES**

B. **PLASMA CELLS:** In antigen-stimulated nodes, the medulla becomes increasingly populated by plasma cells and their precursors and therefore is a **major site of immunoglobulin secretion.**

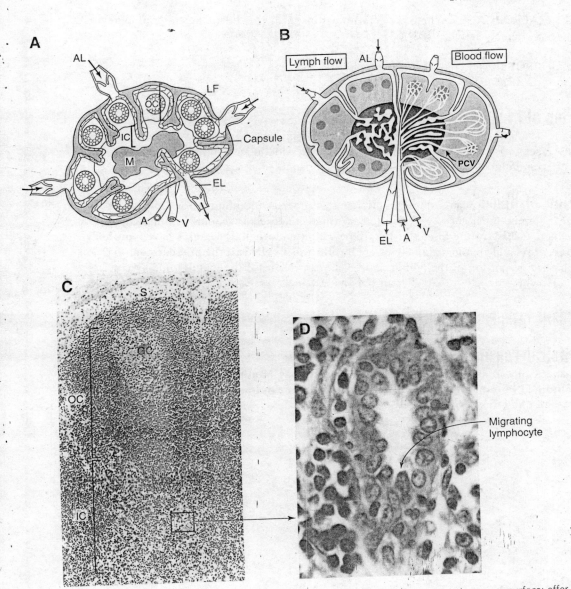

● **Figure 13-1 (A)** Diagram of a lymph node. Note the afferent lymphatic vessels (*AL*) along the convex surface; efferent lymphatic vessel (*EL*) at the hilus; outer cortex (*OC*) with lymphatic follicles (*LF*), many of which contain germinal centers; inner cortex (*IC*); and medulla (*M*). **(B)** Diagram showing the flow of lymph and blood through the lymph node. *PCV* = postcapillary venule; *AL* = afferent lymphatic vessel; *EL* = efferent lymphatic vessel; *A* = artery; *V* = vein. **(C)** LM of a normal lymph node showing the subcapsular sinus (*s*), outer cortex (*OC*), inner cortex (*IC*), and germinal center (*GC*) of a lymphatic follicle. **(D)** EM of the boxed area in C showing a postcapillary venule within the inner cortex. Note the lymphocytes exiting the bloodstream to repopulate the lymph node.

C. MACROPHAGES, which are very numerous in the medulla (therefore, **phagocytosis is extremely active)**

D. FIBROBLASTS (reticular cells), which secrete type III collagen (reticular fibers) that form a stromal meshwork

V Flow of Lymph occurs through: afferent lymphatic vessels with valves entering at the convex surface → subcapsular (marginal) sinus → cortical sinuses → medullary sinuses → efferent lymphatic vessel with valves exiting at the hilum. Sinuses contain sinus macrophages, veiled cells, reticular cells, and reticular fibers that crisscross the lumen in a haphazard fashion.

VI Flow of Blood occurs through: arteries that enter at the hilum → a capillary network within the outer and inner cortex → postcapillary (high endothelial) venules within the inner cortex → veins that leave at the hilus. **Postcapillary (high endothelial) venules** have **lymphocyte homing receptors** and are the major site where **B cells and T cells exit the bloodstream** to repopulate their specific portion of the lymph node. Lymphocytes leave the lymph node by entering a nearby sinus, which drains into an efferent lymphatic vessel.

VII B Cell Lymphopoiesis (B Cell Formation) (Figure 13-2)

VIII Clinical Consideration (Figure 13-3). The population of lymphocytes within lymph nodes changes in certain clinical states, such as **agammaglobulinemia, DiGeorge syndrome, severe combined immunodeficiency (SCID), adenosine deaminase deficiency (ADA; "bubble boy" disease),** and **late-stage AIDS.**

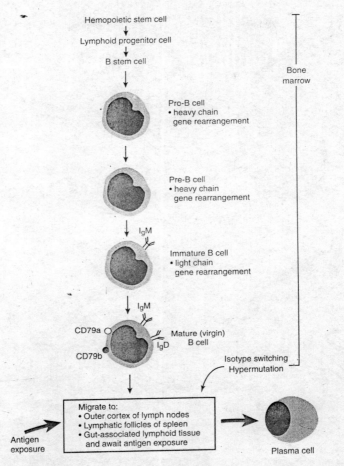

Hemopoietic stem cell

Lymphoid progenitor cell

B stem cell

Pro-B cell
• heavy chain
  gene rearrangement

Pre-B cell
• heavy chain
  gene rearrangement

IgM

Immature B cell
• light chain
  gene rearrangement

IgM

CD79a

Mature (virgin)
B cell

IgD

CD79b

Bone
marrow

Isotype switching
Hypermutation

Migrate to:
• Outer cortex of lymph nodes
• Lymphatic follicles of spleen
• Gut-associated lymphoid tissue
  and await antigen exposure

Antigen
exposure

Plasma cell

● **Figure 13-2 B cell lymphopoiesis.** In early fetal development, B cell lymphopoiesis occurs in the **fetal liver.** In later fetal development and throughout the rest of adult life, B cell lymphopoiesis occurs in the bone marrow. In humans, the **bone marrow is considered the primary site of B cell lymphopoiesis. Hemopoietic stem cells** originating in the bone marrow differentiate into **lymphoid progenitor cells,** which later form **B stem cells.** B stem cells form **pro-B cells** that begin heavy chain gene rearrangement. **Pre-B cells** continue heavy chain gene rearrangement. **Immature B cells** (IgM⁺) begin light chain gene rearrangement and express **antigen-specific IgM** (i.e., will recognize only one antigen) on their cell surface. **Mature (or virgin) B cells** (IgM⁺/IgD⁺) express **antigen-specific IgM and IgD** on their cell surface. Mature B cells migrate to the outer cortex of lymph nodes, lymphatic follicles in the spleen, and gut-associated lymphoid tissue (tonsils, Peyer's patches, etc.) and lie in wait for antigen exposure. Early in the immune response, mature B cells bind antigen using IgM and IgD. As a consequence of antigen binding, two transmembrane proteins **(CD79a and CD79b)** that function as signal transducers cause proliferation and differentiation of B cells into **plasma cells that secrete either IgM or IgD.** Later in the immune response, **antigen-presenting cells (APCs; macrophages)** phagocytose the antigen, where it undergoes lysosomal degradation in **endolysosomes** to form antigen peptide fragments. The **antigen peptide fragments** become associated with the **class II MHC (major histocompatibility complex)** and are transported and exposed on the cell surface of the APC. The antigen peptide fragment + class II MHC on the surface of the APC is recognized by **CD4⁺ helper T cells,** which secrete **IL-2** (stimulates proliferation of B and T cells), **IL-4 and IL-5** (activate antibody production by causing B cell differentiation into plasma cells and promote isotype switching and hypermutation), **TNF-α** (activates macrophages), and **INF-γ** (activates macrophages and natural killer cells). Under the influence of IL-4 and IL-5, mature B cells undergo **isotype switching** and **hypermutation. Isotype switching** is a gene rearrangement process whereby the μ (mu and δ (delta) **constant segments** of the heavy chain (C_H) are spliced out and replaced with γ (gamma), ε (epsilon), or α (alpha) C_H segments. This allows mature B cells to differentiate into **plasma cells that secrete IgG, IgE, or IgA. Hypermutation** is a mutation process whereby a high rate of mutations occur in the **variable segments** of the heavy chain (V_H) and light chain (V_κ or V_λ). This allows mature B cells to differentiate into plasma cells that secrete IgG, IgE, or IgA that will bind antigen with greater and greater affinity. B cells, plasma cells, and immunoglobulins are the basis of **humoral response. B memory cells** are programmed to react to the same antigen on reexposure to that antigen, resulting in a faster immune response called the **secondary immune response.** The immunoglobulin secreted by B memory cells has a higher affinity for the antigen than the immunoglobulin produced during the initial exposure because of hypermutation. This is the **basis of immunization.**

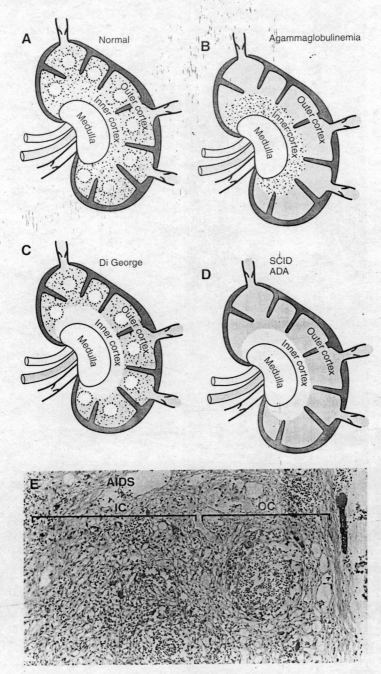

● **Figure 13-3 Diagram of lymph nodes in various clinical states. (A)** Normal lymph node with B cells (outer cortex) and T cells (inner cortex) that impart a humoral immune response and cell-mediated immune response to the individual, respectively. **(B)** Lymph node in X-linked infantile (Bruton's) agammaglobulinemia with B cells absent but T cells present, so that humoral immune response is absent but cell-mediated immune response is present. **(C)** Lymph node in DiGeorge syndrome with B cells present but T cells absent, so that humoral immune response is present but cell-mediated immune response is absent. **(D)** Lymph node in severe combined immunodeficiency disease (*SCID*) or adenosine deaminase deficiency (*ADA*; "bubble boy" disease) with B cells and T cells absent, so that both humoral and cell-mediated immune response are absent. **(E)** Lymph node in late-stage AIDS showing a marked reduction of lymphocytes, especially in the inner cortex (*IC*). OC = outer cortex.

Case Study

A 38-year-old woman who is a manicurist comes to your office complaining that "My back hurts real bad, especially when I bend over or turn to the side. I bought a new chair with a lumbar support for work but it hasn't helped." She also tells you that she has always worked very hard (6 days a week) because she had a lot of energy and loves her job, but lately she feels very fatigued and can't work as much. After some discussion, she informs you that she has had recent bouts of confusion, weakness, polyuria, constipation, and has smoked cigarettes (2 packs a day) for 24 years. The woman is clearly worried and says, "if I don't get better, I will lose my business and I have three kids to support all by myself." What is the most likely diagnosis?

Differentials

- Herniated disk, metastatic bone lesions, osteoarthritis, fibromyalgia

Relevant Physical Exam Findings

- Tenderness to palpation in the thoracic and lumbar spine
- Limited range of motion because of pain

Relevant Lab Findings

- Blood chemistry: Pancytopenia; RBC rouleaux formation; monoclonal M spike on electrophoresis; $Ca^{2+} = 15$ mg/dL (High); RBC sedimentation rate = 50 mm/h (High)
- Bone marrow sample: atypical plasma cells
- Urinalysis: Bence-Jones proteins
- Radiograph: diffuse lytic lesions of the skull, vertebrae, and long bones

Diagnosis

Multiple myeloma. Multiple myeloma is a disorder characterized by malignant monoclonal plasma cells that proliferate in the bone marrow and produce immunoglobulins (usually IgG or IgA). The plasma cell proliferation causes a space-occupying lesion in the marrow, resulting in myelosuppressive anemia and pancytopenia. Clinical findings of multiple myeloma include osteolytic lesions, pathologic fractures, anemia, renal insufficiency, and recurrent bacterial infections. A herniated disk will produce a sharp, localized pain at a specific dermatome. A metastatic bone lesion caused by breast cancer or lung cancer is a possibility, but the bone marrow sample showed no infiltration of metastatic cancer cells. Osteoarthritis is a noninflammatory, "wear and tear" disease caused by mechanical injury and affects the interphalangeal joints in the hand. Clinical findings of fibromyalgia include widespread musculoskeletal pain, stiffness, paresthesia, fatigue, sleep problems, and multiple tender points.

Chapter 14

Spleen

I   General Features. The spleen is the largest lymphoid organ, weighing about 150 g, and is covered by a connective tissue **capsule** that sends a **trabecular network** into the parenchyma of the gland. The parenchyma is divided into the **white pulp** and **red pulp,** each of which has different functions. On the cut surface of the fresh spleen, the unaided eye can distinguish white pulp, which appears as small, pale islands of lymphoid tissue, and red pulp, which appears bright red because of the large number of RBCs. The splenic artery, splenic vein, and efferent lymphatics (the spleen has no afferent lymphatics) are found at the **hilus.**

II   White Pulp (Figure 14-1). The white pulp immunologically monitors the blood (unlike lymph nodes, which monitor lymph) where T cells and B cells interact to form a large number of plasma cells that migrate to the red pulp and produce immunoglobulins. The white pulp consists of the following:

    A.   MATURE (VIRGIN) B CELLS, which are organized into **lymphatic follicles** that are closely associated with the central artery

    B.   MATURE T CELLS, which are organized into a sheath around a central artery called the **periarterial lymphatic sheath (PALS),** which is a thymic-dependent zone similar to the inner cortex of a lymph node

III   Marginal Zone is located between the white pulp and red pulp. The marginal zone is the **site where the immune response is initiated** (which occurs in the spleen as foreign antigens encounter antigen-presenting cells) and where **lymphocytes exit the bloodstream** to repopulate the spleen. The marginal zone consists of the following:

    A.   MACROPHAGES

    B.   ANTIGEN-PRESENTING CELLS (APCs)

IV   Red Pulp. The red pulp removes senescent, damaged, or genetically altered (e.g., sickle cell disease) RBCs and particulate matter from the circulation by macrophages. The iron ($Fe2+$) portion of hemoglobin is stored as ferritin and eventually recycled. The heme moiety of hemoglobin is broken down into bilirubin, transferred to the liver, and becomes a component of bile. The red pulp also stores platelets and is the site of immunoglobulin production released from plasma cells. The red pulp is organized into **splenic (Billroth) cords** that are separated by **splenic venous sinusoids.**

● **Figure 14-1 General features of the spleen. (A)** Diagram of normal splenic architecture and vascular pattern. The trabecular artery (*TA*) branches into a central artery (*CA*), which becomes ensheathed by T cells forming the periarterial lymphatic sheath (*PALS*). Some branches of the CA, called radial arterioles (*RA*), terminate in the marginal zone (*M*), where the immune response in the spleen is initiated and where lymphocytes exit the bloodstream to repopulate the spleen. The CA branches into penicillar arterioles (*PA*) that may open directly into the red pulp, forming an extensive extravascular compartment of blood (open circulation), or empty directly into splenic venous sinusoids (*VS*; closed circulation). Splenic venous sinusoids empty into trabecular veins (*TV*). Along the central artery, lymphatic follicles (*LF*) consisting of B cells are apparent. *SC* = splenic cords. **(B)** A closer view of a venous sinusoid (boxed area in A). The venous sinusoid consists of long, narrow endothelial cells (*endo*) with wide gaps at the lateral margins. Connecting rings of basement membrane (*BM*) are present. An RBC is shown migrating from the splenic cord through the wide gaps between the endothelial cells. Macrophages (*M*) in close association with the venous sinusoids will phagocytose defective RBCs or particulate matter.

A. SPLENIC (BILLROTH) CORDS consist of the following:

   1. **Macrophages**
   2. **Plasma cells**
   3. **Lymphocytes**
   4. **RBCs**
   5. **Fibroblasts** (reticular cells), which secrete type III collagen (reticular fibers) that form a stromal meshwork

B. SPLENIC VENOUS SINUSOIDS are lined by specialized endothelial cells that are long and narrow and have wide gaps between their lateral margins with connecting rings of basement membrane for support. This microanatomy resembles the metal hoops (i.e., basement membrane) that support the wooden staves (i.e., endothelial cells) of a barrel. These cells provide an effective filter between the splenic cords and lumen of the sinusoids. Defective RBCs, dead leukocytes, senescent platelets, and particulate matter are phagocytosed by macrophages as they try to negotiate the filter.

V **Blood Flow** the spleen involves: the splenic artery → trabecular arteries → central arteries → radial arterioles → penicillar arterioles → splenic venous sinusoids → trabecular veins → and splenic vein.

VI **Clinical Considerations**

A. **HOWELL-JOLLY BODIES** are found after splenectomy and represent **nuclear fragments** that are normally removed from RBCs as they pass through the splenic sinuses. After splenectomy, increased numbers of RBCs with Howell-Jolly bodies are observed.

B. **OVERWHELMING POSTSPLENECTOMY SEPSIS.** Postsplenectomy patients (especially children) are at great risk for **bacterial septicemia** because of decreased opsonic production, decreased IgM levels, and decreased clearance of bacteria from blood. The most commonly involved pathogens are *Streptococcus pneumoniae, Haemophilus influenzae,* and *Neisseria meningitidis.* Patients with **sickle cell anemia** usually undergo "autosplenectomy" as a result of multiple infarcts caused by stagnation of abnormal RBCs and are therefore prime targets for postsplenectomy sepsis. Clinical signs include influenzalike symptoms that progress to high fever, shock, and death.

C. **CONGESTIVE SPLENOMEGALY** is usually a result of portal hypertension caused by cirrhosis. The spleen is frequently covered by a "sugar-coated" capsule and focal areas of fibrosis containing iron and calcium called **Gandy-Gamna nodules.**

D. **FELTY SYNDROME** is a syndrome with the combined features of rheumatoid arthritis, splenomegaly, and neutropenia.

VII **Hypersensitivity Reactions.** The thymus, lymph nodes, and spleen are the major organs of the immune system. In addition to providing protection, the immune system may also produce deleterious reactions called **hypersensitivity or allergic reactions,** which include the following:

A. **TYPE I ANAPHYLACTIC REACTIONS** are mediated by **IgE (i.e., antibody-mediated),** which binds to antibody receptors on basophils and mast cells. When cross-linked by antigens, IgE triggers basophils and mast cells to release their contents. Reaction occurs within **minutes.** Clinically, this type of reaction occurs in a wide spectrum ranging from **rashes and wheal-and-flare reactions to anaphylactic shock.**

B. **TYPE II CYTOTOXIC REACTIONS** are mediated by **IgG or IgM (i.e., antibody-mediated),** which binds to antigen on the surface of a cell and kills the cell through complement activation. Clinically, this type of reaction occurs in **blood transfusion reactions, Rh incompatibility, transplant rejection via antibodies, drug-induced thrombocytopenia purpura, hemolytic anemia, and autoimmune diseases.**

C. **TYPE III IMMUNE COMPLEX REACTIONS** are mediated by **antigen–antibody complexes (i.e., antibody-mediated)** that activate complement, which in turn activates neutrophils and macrophages to cause tissue damage. Reaction occurs within **hours.** Clinically, this type of reaction occurs in **serum sickness, chronic glomerulonephritis, poststreptococcal glomerulonephritis, rheumatoid arthritis, systemic lupus erythematosus, polyarteritis nodosa, Farmer's lung, and the Arthus reaction.**

D. **TYPE IV DELAYED-TYPE REACTIONS** are mediated by **T cells (i.e., cell-mediated).** This type of reaction takes longer to mount **(1–2 days)** than antibody-mediated reactions (types I–III) because of the time it takes to mobilize T cells through a cascade of activation events. Clinically, this type of reaction occurs in **poison ivy dermatitis (contact sensitivity),** whereby Langerhans cells (antigen-presenting cells) in the skin respond to urushiol (an oil); **transplant rejection** via cells; **tuberculin reaction** (*Mycobacterium tuberculosis;* **purified protein derivative skin test); sarcoidosis; Crohn disease; and ulcerative colitis.**

Chapter 15

Stomach

I **General Features.** The function of the stomach is to macerate, homogenize, and partially digest the swallowed food to produce a semisolid paste called **chyme.** The stomach is organized into a **mucosa** (consisting of an epithelium, glands, lamina propria, and muscularis mucosae), **submucosa** (connective tissue containing blood vessels, nerves, Meissner plexus), **muscularis externa** (smooth muscle randomly arranged containing Auerbach plexus), and **serosa.** The inner luminal surface of the stomach contains longitudinal ridges of mucosa and submucosa called **rugae** and is dotted with millions of openings called **gastric pits or foveolae.**

II **Gastric Mucosa** (Figure 15-1). The epithelium of the gastric mucosa lines the lumen of the stomach and consists of **surface mucous cells** that are attached to each other by juxtaluminal tight junctions. Surface mucous cells secrete **mucus and HCO_3^-** to protect the mucosa from the acid pH and hydrolytic enzymes contained in the gastric juice.

III **Gastric Glands** (Figure 15-1). The epithelium of the gastric mucosa also invaginates to form gastric glands that contain the following cell types:

A. **STEM CELLS** demonstrate a high rate of **mitosis.** They migrate upward to replace surface mucous cells every 4 to 7 days and downward to replace other cell types.

B. **MUCOUS NECK CELLS** secrete **mucus.**

C. **PARIETAL CELLS** secrete the following:
   1. **HCl** into the gastric lumen. HCl is produced through the action of **carbonic anhydrase** and **H^+-K^+ ATPase** (an H^+ pump). Because **Cl^-** is secreted along with H^+, the secretion product of parietal cells is HCl.
   2. HCO_3^- into the bloodstream, causing a rise in the pH called the **"alkaline tide."**
   3. **Intrinsic factor,** which is necessary for **vitamin B_{12}** absorption. **Pernicious anemia** may result from vitamin B_{12} deficiency caused by atrophic gastritis with decreased intrinsic factor production (see Figure 11-4A).

D. **CHIEF CELLS** secrete **pepsinogen** (inactive) that is converted to **pepsin** (active) on contact with the acid pH of the gastric juice.

E. **ENTEROENDOCRINE CELLS**
   1. **G cells** secrete **gastrin (in response to a meal)** that stimulates HCl secretion from parietal cells. They are found predominantly in the antrum of the stomach so that, in the case of ulcers, the antrum may be resected to reduce the amount of HCl secretion.

● **Figure 15-1 A diagram of the cell types that line the stomach lumen and the gastric pits (surface mucous cells) and the cell types that constitute a typical gastric gland.** A **surface mucous cell** contains rER, a well-developed Golgi, and numerous mucus-containing granules that are oriented toward the lumen of the stomach. A **mucous neck cell** is a flower bouquet–shaped cell that contains rER, a well-developed Golgi, and large, spherical mucus-containing granules oriented toward the gastric gland lumen. A **parietal cell** is a large, triangular-shaped, acidophilic cell that contains numerous mitochondria and an **intracellular canalicular system** that is continuous with the cell membrane and related to an elaborate **tubulovesicular network.** A **chief cell** is an intensely basophilic cell that contains extensive rER, Golgi, and granules that are oriented toward the gastric gland lumen. An **enteroendocrine cell** contains rER, Golgi, and numerous secretory granules that are oriented toward capillaries within the lamina propria (i.e., away from the gastric gland lumen).

2. **EC cells** secrete **serotonin,** which increases gut motility, and **histamine,** which stimulates HCl secretion.
3. **D cells** secrete **somatostatin,** which inhibits secretion of nearby enteroendocrine cells.

IV **Clinical Considerations**

A. **GASTRIC ULCERS** (Figure 15-2). Ulcers are a breach in the mucosa that extend into the submucosa or deeper. They occur where exposure to the aggressive action of gastric juice is high (e.g., stomach, duodenum, or esophagus). **Sucralfate (Carafate or Sulcrate)** is a drug that forms a polymer in an acidic environment that protects ulcers from further irritation and damage. The bacterium *Helicobacter pylori* plays a causative role in ulcers. The antibiotic regimens of **bismuth subsalicylate (Pepto-Bismol),**

● Figure 15-2 Control of hydrochloric acid *(HCl)* secretion from the parietal cell and its role in gastric ulcers. Note the site of action of the various drugs used to treat a gastric ulcer.

tetracycline, and metronidazole or **amoxicillin and clarithromycin** are effective in eradication of *H. pylori*. Other treatments of ulcers include ways to reduce HCl secretion:

1. **Surgical resection of the pyloric antrum** to remove G cells that secrete gastrin (which stimulates HCl secretion).
2. **Omeprazole (Prevacid, Nexium, Prilosec)** is an irreversible H^+-K^+ ATPase inhibitor that inhibits HCl secretion from parietal cells.

3. **Atropine** is an mAChR antagonist that blocks the stimulatory effects of ACh released from postganglionic parasympathetic neurons (CN X) on HCl secretion.

4. **Cimetidine (Tagamet), ranitidine (Zantac), nizatidine (Axid),** and **famotidine (Pepcid)** are H_2-receptor antagonists that block the stimulatory effects of histamine released from EC cells or mast cells on HCl secretion. The H_2-receptor is a G protein–linked receptor that increases cAMP levels.

5. **Misoprostol (Cytotec)** is a prostaglandin E (PGE_1) analogue that inhibits HCl secretion and stimulates secretion of mucus and HCO_3^-.

B. **GASTRINOMA (ZOLLINGER-ELLISON SYNDROME).** A gastrinoma is a malignant tumor consisting of G cells and is generally associated with the MEN I syndrome. A gastrinoma secretes **excess gastrin,** thereby producing hyperacidity (HCl) and peptic ulcer disease. In most cases, a single peptic ulcer is observed, but multiple ulcers may occur also. A gastrinoma should always be suspected if a peptic ulcer is found in an unusual site. Clinical findings include abdominal pain caused by peptic ulcer; diarrhea (malabsorption since enzymes can not work in an acid pH); markedly increased basal acid output (BAO) test; secretin test is confirmatory (secretin administration results in an elevation of gastrin levels in patients with a gastrinoma); and, serum gastrin levels >600 pg/mL. Other causes of elevated serum gastrin levels include use of H_2 blockers (e.g., Tagamet, Zantac, etc.), which decrease HCl production and thereby elevate gastrin; and atrophic gastritis, which decreases HCl production (by destruction of parietal cells) and thereby elevates gastrin.

Chapter 16

Small Intestine

I. General Features. The functions of the small intestine are **to continue digestion of the chyme** received from the stomach using enzymes of the glycocalyx, pancreatic enzymes, and liver bile and **to absorb the nutrients** derived from the digestive process. The small intestine is organized into a **mucosa** (consisting of an epithelium, glands, lamina propria, and muscularis mucosae), **submucosa** (connective tissue containing blood vessels, nerves, and Meissner plexus), **muscularis externa** (smooth muscle arranged as an inner circular layer and outer longitudinal layer and containing Auerbach plexus), and **serosa.** The inner luminal surface of the small intestine contains semilunar ridges of mucosa and submucosa called **plica circulares (or valves of Kerckring)** and is dotted with millions of openings, where the intestinal glands open to the surface, and fingerlike projections of the epithelium and lamina propria called **villi.**

II. Intestinal Mucosa (Figure 16-1). The epithelium of the intestinal mucosa covers the villi and consists of the following cell types:

A. **SURFACE ABSORPTIVE CELLS (ENTEROCYTES)** are joined by juxtaluminal tight junctions and possess **microvilli** that are coated by filamentous glycoproteins called the **glycocalyx.** The glycocalyx contains important enzymes, which include: **maltase, α-dextrinase, sucrase, lactase, trehalase, aminopeptidases, and enterokinase** (which converts the inactive form [e.g., trypsinogen] of pancreatic enzymes to the active form [e.g., trypsin]). Enterocytes absorb carbohydrates, protein, lipids, vitamins, Ca^{2+}, and Fe^{2+} from the intestinal lumen and transport them to the blood or lymph.

1. **Carbohydrates** are digested to monosaccharides (glucose, galactose, fructose; only monosaccharides can be absorbed). Glucose and galactose enter enterocytes by secondary active transport using the **Na^+-glucose cotransporter (SGLT-1).** Fructose enters enterocytes by facilitated diffusion using the **GLUT5 transporter.** Glucose, galactose, and fructose exit enterocytes by facilitated diffusion using the **GLUT2 transporter** and are delivered to **portal blood.**

2. **Proteins** are digested to amino acids, dipeptides, and tripeptides. Most amino acids, dipeptides, and tripeptides enter enterocytes by secondary active transport using **Na^+-amino acid cotransporters** (there are four separate cotransporters for neutral, basic, acidic, and amino amino acids). Dipeptides and tripeptides are then further digested to amino acids by **cytoplasmic peptidases.** Amino acids exit enterocytes by facilitated diffusion and are delivered to **portal blood.**

3. **Triacylglycerols** (the main fat in a human diet) are emulsified by bile salts and digested to fatty acids and monoacylglycerols.

    a. Long-chain fatty acids (>12 carbons), monoacylglycerols, cholesterol, and fat-soluble vitamins (A, D, E, and K) are packaged into **micelles** and enter enterocytes by diffusion assisted by **fatty acid–binding proteins (FABPs).** Within the enterocyte, **resynthesis of triacylglycerols** occurs in the **sER,** which contains acyl-CoA synthetase and acyltransferases. Subsequently, the triacylglycerols,

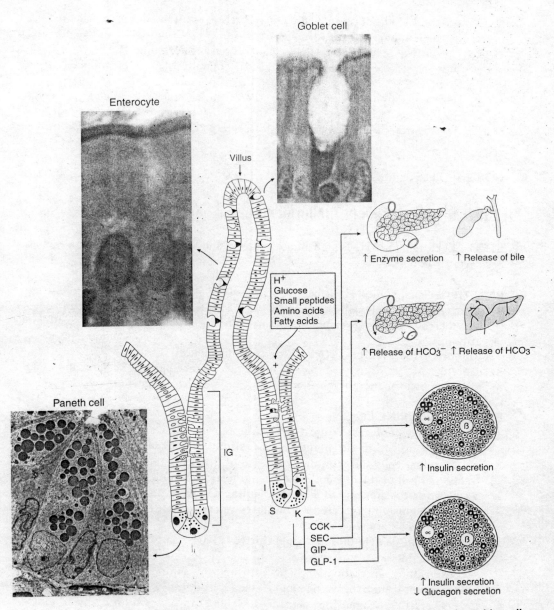

Goblet cell

Enterocyte

Villus

Paneth cell

H⁺
Glucose
Small peptides
Amino acids
Fatty acids

↑ Enzyme secretion   ↑ Release of bile

↑ Release of HCO₃⁻   ↑ Release of HCO₃⁻

IG

I   L

S   K

↑ Insulin secretion

CCK
SEC
GIP
GLP-1

↑ Insulin secretion
↓ Glucagon secretion

● **Figure 16-1** **Diagram of a villus and intestinal gland (*IG*) along with photomicrographs of a Goblet cell, surface absorptive cell (enterocyte), and Paneth cell.** The hormonal secretion from intestinal glands and their actions is also indicated. Note that H⁺, glucose, small peptides, amino acids, and fatty acids within the lumen of the intestinal gland stimulate I cells (*I*), S cells (*S*), K cells (*K*), and L cells (*L*) to secrete cholecystokinin (*CCK*), secretin (*SEC*), gastric inhibitory peptide (*GIP*), and glucagon-like peptide–1 (*GLP*-1), respectively. Note action of various hormones.

cholesterol, and fat-soluble vitamins are packaged by the **Golgi** with **apoproteins** into **chylomicrons**, which are delivered to **lymph** via **lacteals**.

b. Short- and medium-chain fatty acids (<12 carbons) and glycerol enter the enterocyte directly by diffusion (no micelle packaging), exit the enterocyte by diffusion (no chylomicron packaging), and are delivered to **portal blood.**

c. **Xenical** is a drug used in the treatment of morbid obesity that blocks about 30% of dietary fat from being absorbed.

4. **Water-soluble vitamins** enter the enterocyte by diffusion, although some require a **Na$^+$-dependent cotransporter**. Vitamin B$_{12}$ is absorbed in the **ileum** and requires **intrinsic factor** secreted by parietal cells of the stomach.
   a. **Ca^{2+}** is absorbed and requires 1,25 (OH)$_2$ vitamin D, which is produced by the kidney.
   b. **Fe^{2+}** enters the enterocyte as **heme Fe^{2+}** (Fe^{2+} bound to hemoglobin or myoglobin) or as **free Fe^{2+}**. Within the enterocyte, heme Fe^{2+} is degraded to release free Fe^{2+}. Free Fe^{2+} is released into the blood and circulates in the blood bound to **transferrin**.

B. **GOBLET CELLS** synthesize **mucinogen**, which is stored in membrane-bound granules.

III Intestinal Glands (Crypts of Lieberkuhn) (Figure 16-1)

A. **STEM CELLS** demonstrate a high rate of mitosis and replace enterocytes and goblet cells every 3 to 6 days.

B. **PANETH CELLS** are found at the base of the intestinal glands and secrete the following:
   1. **Lysozyme** is a proteolytic enzyme that degrades the peptidoglycan coat of bacteria, thereby increasing membrane permeability of bacteria so that they swell and rupture.
   2. **Tumor necrosis factor-α (TNF-α)** is a proinflammatory substance.
   3. **Defensins (cryptidins)** increase the membrane permeability of bacteria and other parasites by formation of ion channels.

C. **ENTEROENDOCRINE CELLS**
   1. **I cells** secrete **cholecystokinin (CCK)** in response to small peptides, amino acids, and fatty acids within the gut lumen. CCK **stimulates enzyme secretion** from pancreatic acinar cells and **stimulates release of bile** from the gall bladder (by contraction of gall bladder smooth muscle and relaxation of the sphincter of Oddi).
   2. **S cells** secrete **secretin (called nature's antacid)** in response to H$^+$ and fatty acids within the gut lumen. Secretin **stimulates release of HCO$_3^-$** from the pancreas and the liver biliary tract.
   3. **K cells** secrete **gastric-inhibitory peptide (GIP)** in response to orally administered glucose, amino acids, and fatty acids in the gut lumen. GIP **stimulates insulin secretion** from pancreatic islets. This explains why an oral glucose load produces higher serum insulin levels than an IV glucose load.
   4. **L cells** secrete **glucagon-like peptide–1 (GLP-1)** in response to orally administered glucose, amino acids, and fatty acids in the gut lumen. GLP-1 **stimulates insulin secretion in the presence of hyperglycemia** and **inhibits postprandial glucagon secretion** from pancreatic islets. GLP-1 may be an effective therapeutic agent for **type 2 diabetes** because the stimulatory effect of GLP-1 on insulin secretion is preserved in type 2 diabetic patients.
   5. There are basically three stimuli for insulin secretion: glucose, GIP, and GLP-1. A drug called **Byetta** (which is GLP-1) increases insulin secretion in both normal physiology and type 2 diabetes. Byetta is the first in a new class of drugs called **incretin-mimetics** for the treatment of type 2 diabetes. **Incretins** are gut peptides that increase insulin secretion. Incretin-mimetics are drugs that mimic the insulin secretion activity of the two gut peptides, GIP and GLP-1.

IV **Gut-Associated Lymphatic Tissue** (GALT; **Peyer patches**) are lymphatic follicles found in the intestinal mucosa and submucosa that are covered by an epithelial lining containing **M cells**. M cells are **antigen-transporting cells** that have **microfolds** on their luminal surface.

A. M cells endocytose antigens into protease-containing vesicles at their apical domain. These vesicles are transported across the M cell to the basolateral domain where the antigen is discharged into the intercellular space in close vicinity to **mature (or virgin) B lymphocytes** (see Chapter 13; Figure 13–2).

B. Under the influence of CD4$^+$ helper T cells and interleukins (IL-2, IL-4, IL-5) mature B lymphocytes differentiate into **plasma cells** that secrete antigen-specific **IgA** into the lamina propria.

C. IgA within the lamina propria binds to the **poly-Ig receptor** on the basal domain of the enterocyte to form an **IgA + poly-Ig receptor complex** that is endocytosed and transported across the enterocyte. At the apical domain, the complex is cleaved such that IgA is released into the intestinal lumen joined with the **secretory piece** of the receptor and is known as **secretory IgA (sIgA)**.

D. A significant amount of IgA also enters the bloodstream and is processed by hepatocytes in the liver using the same mechanism as enterocytes mentioned above. The secretory IgA is released into bile canaliculi and travels to the intestinal lumen with bile.

E. sIgA binding to microorganisms or antigens reduces their ability to penetrate the epithelial lining.

V **Clinical Considerations** (Figure 16-2)

A. CELIAC DISEASE (CE; SPRUE) is a **hypersensitivity to gluten and gliadin** protein found in wheat and other grains. On ingestion of gluten-containing foods, a large number of lymphocytes, plasma cells, macrophages, and eosinophils accumulate within the lamina propria of the intestinal mucosa and result in loss of villi. Gliadin antibodies are generally detectable in the blood. These factors may contribute to the immunologic damage of the mucosa. Clinical findings include: chronic diarrhea, flatulence, weight loss, and fatigue.

B. CROHN DISEASE (CR) is a chronic inflammatory bowel disease that most commonly affects the **ileum** and involves an abundant accumulation of lymphocytes forming a **granuloma** (a typical feature of CR) within the submucosa that may further extend into the muscularis externa. Neutrophils infiltrate the intestinal glands and ultimately destroy them, leading to ulcers. With progression of CR, the ulcers coalesce into long, **serpentine ulcers (linear ulcers)** oriented along the long axis of the bowel. A classic feature of CR is the clear demarcation between diseased bowel segments located directly next to uninvolved normal bowel and a cobblestone appearance that can be seen grossly and radiographically. The etiology of CR is unknown. Clinical findings include: intermittent bouts of diarrhea, weight loss, and weakness. Complications include: strictures of the intestinal lumen, formation of fistulas, and perforation.

C. CHOLERA is caused by the Gram-negative bacteria *Vibrio cholerae,* which produces an enterotoxin called **cholera toxin.** Cholera toxin is an enzyme that catalyzes **ADP ribosylation** of the α_s chain of G_s protein. This effectively raises cAMP levels that activate Cl$^-$ channels of enterocytes to secrete Cl$^-$ into the lumen; Na$^+$ and H$_2$O

● **Figure 16-2 Normal and pathological features of small intestine. (A)** LM of normal small intestine showing villi (*V*) and intestinal glands (*IG*). Dotted line indicates boundary of villi and intestinal glands. Compare with celiac disease in **B** and note the loss of villi in celiac disease. **(B)** LM pathology of celiac disease (sprue). Note the chronic inflammation of the lamina propria adjacent to intestinal glands along with the loss of villi (compare with normal in **A**). Inflammation is generally confined to the mucosa. A gluten-free diet will eliminate the inflammation and allow villi to return to normal. **(C, D)** Crohn disease. **(C)** Gross specimen of ileum from a patient with Crohn disease. Note the prominent cobblestoning (*arrow*) caused by multiple transverse and linear ulcers. The other portion of the ileum is normal (***). **(D)** LM pathology of Crohn disease showing a submucosal granuloma (*arrow*) that may extend into the muscularis externa.

follow. Clinical findings include a severe, watery diarrhea. Certain strains of *Escherichia coli* produce toxins that cause traveler's diarrhea by a similar mechanism.

D. LACTOSE INTOLERANCE is caused by the absence of the enzyme **lactase** from the glycocalyx so that lactose cannot be digested to glucose. The unabsorbed lactose within the lumen results in osmotic diarrhea. **Congenital lactase deficiency** is a rare condition that becomes apparent in infants at the start of milk feeding. **Acquired lactase deficiency** is generally caused by rotavirus, gastroenteritis, kwashiorkor, or old age. Clinical findings include abdominal distention and explosive, watery diarrhea.

Case Study

A 22-year-old man comes to your office complaining that "I have bouts of diarrhea in the morning that come and go; I have a fever, and pain on the lower right side near my appendix." After some discussion, he informs you that he has not noticed any blood in the diarrhea and that he has lost 20 pounds this past year. What is the most likely diagnosis?

Differentials

- Acute appendicitis, irritable bowel syndrome, ulcerative colitis

Relevant Physical Exam Findings

- Middle Eastern heritage
- Fever
- Palpable, tender mass in the lower right quadrant
- Guarding is not present
- Psoas and obturator signs are negative
- Rectal exam: negative for occult blood

Relevant Lab Findings

- Blood chemistry: Hgb = 10 g/dL (Low); Hct = 32% (Low); WBCs = 15,000/mm³ (H); Albumin = 3g/L (Low)
- Stool sample: Culture = negative; Occult blood = negative
- Barium enema radiograph: reflux of barium into terminal ileum; luminal narrowing ("string sign"); cobblestone pattern; wall thickening
- Colonoscopy: ulceration; strictures in the colonic mucosa

Diagnosis

Crohn Disease (CR). Crohn disease (CR) is a chronic inflammatory bowel disease that most commonly affects the ileum and involves an abundant accumulation of lymphocytes forming a granuloma (a typical feature of CR) within the submucosa that may further extend into the muscularis externa. Neutrophils infiltrate the intestinal glands and ultimately destroy them leading to ulcers. With progression of CR, the ulcers coalesce into long, serpentine ulcers ("linear ulcers") oriented along the long axis of the bowel. A classic feature of CR is the clear demarcation between diseased bowel segments located directly next to uninvolved normal bowel and a cobblestone appearance that can be seen grossly and radiographically. The etiology of CR is unknown but occurs most frequently in Ashkenazi Jews 20–40 years of age. Clinical findings of CR include intermittent bouts of diarrhea, weakness, abdominal pain, arthritis, ankylosing spondylitis, iritis, and erythema nodosum. Acute appendicitis is most often caused by inflammation of the lymphoid tissue or the presence of a fecalith. Clinical findings of acute appendicitis include diffuse periumbilical pain that migrates to the lower right quadrant; anorexia; guarding of the lower right quadrant is present; tenderness at the McBurney point; psoas sign (passive extension of right hip is painful) is positive; obturator sign (passive flexion and inward rotation of right hip is painful) is positive. Irritable bowel syndrome (IBS) is the most common gastrointestinal tract disease in the general population and involves an abnormality in colonic motility that is precipitated by stress or high-fat meals. Clinical findings of IBS include cramps, constipation, alternating bouts of constipation and diarrhea, or chronic diarrhea. IBS is more common in females and occurs before 30 years of age. Ulcerative colitis is a type of idiopathic inflammatory bowel disease. Ulcerative colitis always involves the rectum and extends proximally for varying distances. The inflammation is continuous, i.e., there are no "skip areas" as in Crohn disease. The etiology of ulcerative colitis is unknown. Clinical signs of ulcerative colitis include bloody diarrhea with mucus and pus, malaise, fever, weight loss, anemia, and may lead to toxic megacolon.

Case Study

A 60-year-old man comes to your office complaining that "I have real bad watery diarrhea that seems to be getting worse over the last 6 months; sometimes when I have diarrhea I feel nauseated and vomit a lot." He also tells you that "I'm getting hot flashes just like my wife did during menopause and awhile back I remember having black, tarry stools." After some discussion, he informs you that he has been trying to lose a few pounds and started the Atkins' high carbohydrate diet. What is the most likely diagnosis?

Differentials

- Crohn disease, infectious diarrhea, irritable bowel syndrome, VIPoma

Relevant Physical Exam Findings

- Auscultation reveals diffuse wheezes over both lungs and a pulmonic ejection murmur over the right sternal border at intercostal space 2
- Liver is palpable well below the costal margin
- Hyperactive bowel sounds are apparent

Relevant Lab Findings

- Blood chemistry: WBCs = 7000/μL (Normal); Hgb = 14 g/dL (Normal); Hematrocit = 42% (Normal); Platelet count = 153,000/mm^3 (Normal); K$^+$ = 4.2 mEq/L (Normal); pH = 7.42 (Normal)
- Stool sample showed positive for heme and no evidence of parasites
- Urinalysis: positive for 5-hydroxyindoleacetic acid (5-HIAA)
- CT scan: nodular masses in the duodenum and liver

Diagnosis

Carcinoid tumor (CAR). CARs account for ≈50% of all malignant tumors of the small intestine and arise from neuroendocrine cells, which are most numerous in the appendix and terminal ileum. CARs found in the appendix almost never metastasize. However, CARs found in other regions of the small intestine may metastasize to the liver. CARs secrete serotonin (5-HT), which is broken down by monoamine oxidase to 5-HIAA. 5-HT in the systemic circulation causes carcinoid syndrome. Clinical findings of CARs include diarrhea, episodic flushing, bronchospasm, cyanosis, telangiectasia, and fibrosis of the valves on the right side of the heart. CARs are composed of small, round cells containing cytoplasmic granules arranged in nests, cords, or rosettes located within the submucosa. Crohn disease (CR) is a chronic inflammatory bowel disease that most commonly affects the ileum and involves an abundant accumulation of lymphocytes forming a granuloma (a typical feature of CR) within the submucosa that may further extend into the muscularis externa. Neutrophils infiltrate the intestinal glands and ultimately destroy them, leading to ulcers. With progression of CR, the ulcers coalesce into long, serpentine ulcers ("linear ulcers") oriented along the long axis of the bowel. A classic feature of CR is the clear demarcation between diseased bowel segments located directly next to uninvolved normal bowel and a cobblestone appearance that can be seen grossly and radiographically. The etiology of CR is unknown but occurs most frequently in Ashkenazi Jews 20–40 years of age. Clinical findings of CR include intermittent bouts of diarrhea, weakness, abdominal pain, arthritis, ankylosing spondylitis, iritis, and erythema nodosum. Infectious diarrhea may be caused by *Giardia lamblia* or *Entamoeba histolytica* that can be identified in a stool sample. Infectious diarrhea rarely lasts for 6 months (except in the cases of certain parasites). Irritable bowel syndrome (IBS) is the most common gastrointestinal tract disease in the general population and involves an abnormality in colonic motility that is precipitated by stress or high-fat meals. Clinical findings of IBS include cramps, constipation, alternating bouts of constipation and diarrhea, or chronic diarrhea. IBS is more common in females and occurs before 30 years of age. VIPoma is a rare tumor of the pancreatic islets. Clinical findings of VIPoma include watery diarrhea, hypokalemia, and achlorhydria. The Atkins' high carbohydrate has nothing to do with his condition.

Chapter 17

Large Intestine (Colon)

I   **General Features.** The functions of the large intestine are to absorb Na^+, Cl^-, and H_2O from the lumen, to soften fecal matter by addition of mucus, and to eliminate fecal matter. The large intestine is organized into a **mucosa** (consisting of an epithelium, glands, lamina propria, and muscularis mucosae), **submucosa** (connective tissue containing blood vessels, nerves, and Meissner plexus), **muscularis externa** (smooth muscle arranged as an inner circular layer and three outer longitudinal bands called **teniae coli** and containing Auerbach plexus; contraction of teniae coli forms sacculations called **haustra**), and **serosa** (contains fatty tags called **appendices epiploicae**). The inner luminal surface is smooth (i.e., no rugae, plicae circulares, no villi) and is dotted with millions of openings where intestinal glands open to the surface.

II   **Large Intestinal Mucosa.** The epithelium of the mucosa consists of the following cell types:

    A.   **SURFACE ABSORPTIVE CELLS (ENTEROCYTES)** absorb Na^+, Cl^-, and H_2O by facilitated diffusion using ion channels under the regulation of aldosterone. Aldosterone increases the number of Na^+ ion channels, thereby increasing the amount of Na^+ absorbed. **Sedatives, anesthetics, and steroids** are also absorbed, which is clinically important when medication cannot be delivered orally.

    B.   **GOBLET CELLS** synthesize mucinogen, which is stored in membrane-bound granules.

III   **Intestinal Glands** contain:

    A.   **SURFACE ABSORPTIVE CELLS (ENTEROCYTES)**

    B.   **GOBLET CELLS**

    C.   **STEM CELLS,** which demonstrate a high rate of mitosis and replace surface absorptive cells and goblet cells every 5 to 6 days

    D.   **ENTEROENDOCRINE CELLS**

IV   **Gut-Associated Lymphatic Tissue (Galt)** is prominent within the lamina propria throughout the large intestine.

Upper Anal Canal	Lower Anal Canal
Venous drainage is by the superior rectal vein → portal vein. Varicosities of the superior rectal vein are called **internal hemorrhoids.**	Venous drainage is by the inferior rectal vein → inferior vena cava. Varicosities of the inferior rectal vein are called **external hemorrhoids.**
Tumors will drain to **deep** lymphatic nodes (not palpable).	Tumors will drain to **superficial** lymphatic nodes (palpable).
Sensory innervation is for stretch sensation. No pain sensation is present. Therefore, internal hemorrhoids or tumors in this area will **not** be accompanied by patient complaints of pain.	Sensory innervation is for pain, temperature, and touch. Therefore, external hemorrhoids or tumors in this area will be accompanied by patient complaints of pain.
Motor innervation involves autonomic control of the internal anal sphincter (smooth muscle).	Motor innervation involves voluntary control of the external anal sphincter (skeletal muscle).

● **Figure 17-1 (A–D)** Anal canal. The anal canal is divided into the upper and lower anal canal by the pectinate line. The upper anal canal is lined by a typical simple columnar (colonic) epithelium arranged as intestinal glands **(B).** The colonic epithelium undergoes a transition at the pectinate line to a nonkeratinized stratified squamous epithelium lining the lower anal canal **(C).** The anal verge is lined by a keratinized stratified squamous epithelium **(D).** The upper anal canal is derived embryologically from the hindgut, whereas the lower anal canal is derived embryologically from the proctodeum. This dual embryologic origin has important clinical considerations as indicated in the table.

V **Anal Canal** (Figure 17-1) is divided into the upper and lower anal canal by the pectinate line.

A. **UPPER ANAL CANAL** (Figure 17-1). The mucosa extends into longitudinal folds called the **anal columns (or columns of Morgagni).** The base of the anal columns defines the **pectinate line.** The anal columns are connected at their bases by transverse folds of mucosa called the **anal valves.** Behind the anal valves are small, blind pouches called the **anal sinuses** into which mucous **anal glands** open. The upper anal canal is lined by a typical simple columnar epithelium (colonic epithelium) and intestinal glands called the **colorectal zone.** The colonic epithelium undergoes a complete transition to a stratified squamous epithelium at the pectinate line called the **transitional zone.** The upper anal canal is derived embryologically from the **hindgut (endoderm).**

B. **LOWER ANAL CANAL** is lined by a **nonkeratinized stratified squamous epithelium** called the **squamous zone.** It is derived embryologically from the **proctodeum (ectoderm).**

C. **ANAL VERGE** is the point at which the perianal skin begins and is lined by a **keratinized stratified squamous epithelium.**

VI **Clinical Considerations**

A. **HIRSCHSPRUNG DISEASE (COLONIC AGANGLIONOSIS)** is a congenital defect that results from the failure of neural crest cells to migrate and form the myenteric plexus within the sigmoid colon and rectum. This results in a loss of peristalsis in the colon segment **distal** to the normal innervated colon. The **RET gene** (a tyrosine kinase receptor required for neural crest migration) and **endothelin-3** and its receptor **endothelin B** have been implicated in Hirschsprung disease. Clinical findings include absence of peristalsis, fecal retention, and abdominal distention.

B. **FAMILIAL ADENOMATOUS POLYPOSIS COLI (FAPC)** (Figure 17-2) is the archetype of adenomatous polyposis syndromes whereby patients develop 500 to 2,000 polyps that carpet the mucosal surface of the colon and invariably become malignant. FAPC accounts for about 1% of all colorectal cancer cases and involves a mutation in the **APC anti-oncogene.**
   1. The progression from a small polyp to a large polyp is associated with a mutation in the *ras* **proto-oncogene.**
   2. The progression from a large polyp to metastatic carcinoma is associated with mutations in the **DCC anti-oncogene** (deleted in colon carcinoma) and the **p53 anti-oncogene.**

C. **GARDNER SYNDROME** is a variation of FAPC in which patients demonstrate adenomatous polyps and multiple osteomas.

D. **TURCOT SYNDROME** is a variation of FAPC in which patients demonstrate adenomatous polyps and gliomas.

E. **ADENOCARCINOMAS** (Figure 17-2) account for 98% of all cancers in the large intestine. Mutations in the **HNPCC gene** (hereditary nonpolyposis colorectal cancer), which codes for a DNA repair enzyme, have been implicated in some cases. Clinical findings include fatigue, weakness, change in bowel habits, weight loss, and iron-deficiency anemia. In fact, it is a clinical maxim that iron-deficiency anemia in an older man means adenocarcinoma of the colon until shown otherwise.

● **Figure 17-2 Normal and pathological features of the colon. (A)** LM of normal colon. The mucosa shows typical simple columnar (colonic) epithelium arranged as intestinal glands, lamina propria (*lp*), and muscularis mucosa (*mm*). Note the straight, regular arrangement of the intestinal glands, which terminate at the basement membrane intact at the muscularis mucosa. **(B, C)** LM of an adenomatous polyp. A polyp is a tumorous mass that extends into the lumen of the colon. Note the convoluted, irregular arrangement of the intestinal glands with the basement membrane intact. The epithelium is transformed into a pseudostratified epithelium with mitotic figures apparent (*arrows;* C is a high magnification of the boxed area in B). **(D, E)** LM of an adenocarcinoma of the colon. Note the convoluted, irregular arrangement of the intestinal glands that have breached the basement membrane to extend deep into the submucosa or muscularis externa (*bracket*). The epithelium is transformed into a pseudostratified epithelium, which grows in a disorderly pattern, extending into the lumen of the gland (*arrows;* E is a high magnification of a typical area in D).

Chapter 18

Liver and Gall Bladder

⓵ Hepatocytes. Hepatocytes contain the Golgi complex, rER, sER, mitochondria, lysosomes, peroxisomes, lipid, and glycogen. The functions of hepatocytes include:

A. Conversion of NH_4^+ to urea

B. Production of 50% of the lymph found within the thoracic duct

C. Production of bile. The cell membrane of the hepatocytes lining the bile canaliculus contains the:
1. **Multidrug resistance 1 transporter (MDR1),** which transports cholesterol into the bile canaliculus.
2. **Multidrug resistance 2 transporter (MDR2),** which transports phospholipids (mainly lecithin) into the bile canaliculus.
3. **Multispecific organ anionic transporter (MOAT),** which transports bilirubin glucuronide (bile pigment) and glutathione conjugates into the bile canaliculus.
4. **Biliary acid transporter (BAT),** which transports bile salts (cholic acid and chenodeoxycholic acid conjugated to glycine or taurine) into the bile canaliculus.
5. **Ion exchanger,** which allows passage of HCO_3^- and Cl^- into the bile canaliculus.
6. **Ectoenzymes,** which generate nucleosides and amino acids that enter the bile canaliculus.
7. **Tight junctions** surrounding the bile canaliculus are relatively "leaky," which allows passage of H_2O and Na^+ into the bile canaliculus.
8. **Secretory IgA** is also released into the bile canaliculus.

D. Conjugation of bilirubin. Bilirubin (water-insoluble) is derived from the breakdown of hemoglobin (i.e., senescent RBCs) by macrophages and in the spleen and Kupffer cells. Bilirubin travels in the blood as an **albumin–bilirubin complex** (Note: free bilirubin is toxic to the brain, e.g., **kernicterus**). Bilirubin is endocytosed by hepatocytes and conjugated to glucuronide by **UDP-glucuronyl transferase** in the sER to form **bilirubin-glucuronide** (a water-soluble bile pigment), which is released into bile canaliculi. Within the distal small intestine and colon, bilirubin-glucuronide is broken down to **free bilirubin** by intestinal bacterial flora. Free bilirubin is reduced to **urobilinogen** and excreted in feces. **Crigler-Najjar disease** is a genetic disease involving UDP-glucuronyl transferase resulting in a failure to conjugate bilirubin. **Dubin-Johnson syndrome** is a familial disease involving failure to release bilirubin-glucuronide into bile canaliculi.

E. Maintenance of blood glucose levels by glucose uptake and glycogen synthesis.

F. Glycogen storage and degradation to glucose.

G. Gluconeogenesis, i.e., conversion of amino acids and lipids into glucose.

H. Synthesis of cholesterol.

I. Synthesis of plasma proteins (e.g., albumin, fibrinogen, prothrombin, vitamin K–dependent clotting factors).

J. Uptake of IgA and release of secretory IgA into the bile canaliculus.

K. Uptake and inactivation of steroids, lipid-soluble drugs (e.g., phenobarbital), vitamins A and D, T_3 and T_4 by removal of iodine, and nonpolar carcinogens by enzymes in the sER (e.g., cytochrome P_{450} mono-oxygenase).

L. Metabolism of ethanol. After absorption in the stomach, most ethanol is metabolized in the liver by **alcohol dehydrogenase (ADH pathway)** to produce **acetaldehyde** and **excess H^+** in the cytoplasm. An excess of acetaldehyde is toxic, causing mitochondrial damage, microtubule disruption, and protein alterations that induce an autoimmune response. With chronic ethanol intake, ethanol is metabolized in the liver by the **microsomal ethanol-oxidizing system (MEOS)** to produce **acetaldehyde** and **excess oxygen free radicals** in the cytoplasm. Free radicals cause lipid peroxidation, resulting in cell membrane damage.

M. 25-Hydroxylation of vitamin D.

N. Storage of Fe^{2+} as **ferritin** or **hemosiderin** (degradation product of ferritin). **Hemochromatosis** is an extreme accumulation of Fe^{2+} associated with liver and pancreas damage.

O. Secretion of angiotensinogen.

P. Secretion of α_1-antitrypsin, which is a serum protease inhibitor. Methionine 358 in the reactive center of α_1-antitrypsin acts as a "bait" for elastase where elastase is trapped and inactivated. This protects the physiologically important **elastic fibers** present in the lung from destruction. α_1-antitrypsin deficiency is an autosomal recessive disorder caused by a missense mutation where methionine 358 is replaced with arginine (i.e., the **Pittsburgh variant**), which destroys the affinity for elastase. This results in **pulmonary emphysema** because tissue-destructive elastase is allowed to act in an uncontrolled manner in the lung.

Q. Maintenance of blood lipid levels by fatty acid uptake, fatty acid esterification to triglycerides in the sER, and combination of triacylglycerides with protein in the Golgi to form **lipoproteins** (Figure 18-1), which include:
  1. **VLDL (very low-density lipoprotein)** is rich in triacylglycerides and travels to adipose tissue and skeletal muscle where the triacylglycerides are hydrolyzed by lipoprotein lipase to fatty acids.
  2. **LDL (low-density lipoprotein)** is rich in cholesterol and distributes cholesterol to cells throughout the body that have specific LDL receptors. LDL is called **"bad cholesterol"** and is the target in lipid-lowering therapy.
  3. **HDL (high-density lipoprotein)** plays a role in the hydrolysis of triacylglycerides in chylomicrons and VLDL by providing **apoprotein C** for the activation of lipoprotein lipase. HDL facilitates the flow of excess plasma triacylglycerides and cholesterol back to the liver; hence, HDL is called **"good cholesterol."** The enzyme **lecithin-cholesterol acyl transferase (LCAT)** is associated with HDL and converts cholesterol → cholesterol ester (i.e., cholesterol + a fatty acid).

	Density	Electrophoretic Mobility	Triacylglyceride (%)	Cholesterol (%)
Chylomicrons	<0.95	– – –	85	6
VLDL	0.95–1.006	Pre-beta	60	20
LDL	1.006–1.063	Beta	7	50
HDL	1.063–1.210	Alpha	5	20

A

Normal Lipoprotein Profile (mg/dL)

Total Cholesterol	Triacylglycerides	VLDL	LDL "bad cholesterol"	HDL "good cholesterol"
<200	<200	<35	<170	<80

B

● **Figure 18-1 Features of Blood Lipids. (A)** Characteristics of lipoproteins. Lipoproteins may be classified according to their density separation by ultracentrifugation or electrophoretic mobility, both of which are not routinely used in clinical practice. Cholesterol is assayed by the cholesterol oxidase method; triacylglycerides are assayed by an enzymatic method after hydrolysis and release of glycerol; HDL is measured as cholesterol in the supernatant after precipitation of other lipoproteins; LDL is calculated by the Friedman equation [LDL = total cholesterol − (TG/5 + HDL)]. Note that chylomicron composition is 85% triacylglycerides, VLDL composition is 60% triacylglycerides, and LDL composition is 50% cholesterol. **(B)** Normal lipoprotein profile values.

II **Kupffer Cells** are **macrophages** derived from circulating monocytes that are found in the liver sinusoids. These cells secrete proinflammatory cytokines: **TNF-α** (causes a slowdown in bile flow called cholestasis), **interleukin 6** (causes synthesis of acute-phase proteins by hepatocytes), and **TGF-β** (causes synthesis of type I collagen by hepatic stellate cells).

III **Hepatic Stellate Cells (Fat-Storing Cells; Ito Cells)** are found in the perisinusoidal space (space of Disse). These cells contain **fat, store and metabolize vitamin A,** and secrete **type I collagen.** In liver cirrhosis, increased deposition of type I collagen (along with laminin and proteoglycans) in the perisinusoidal space narrows the diameter of the sinusoid, causing **portal hypertension.**

IV **Classic Liver Lobule** (Figure 18-2). The classic liver lobule is roughly hexagon-shaped with a **central vein** at its center and six **portal triads** at its periphery. A portal triad consists of a:

A. **HEPATIC ARTERIOLE.** The hepatic arterioles (terminal branches of the **right and left hepatic arteries**) carry oxygen-rich blood and contribute **20%** of the blood within the liver sinusoids. The blood flows from the periphery to the center of the lobule (i.e., **centripetal flow**).

B. **PORTAL VENULE.** The portal venules (terminal branches of the **portal vein**) carry nutrient-rich blood and contribute **80%** of the blood within the liver sinusoids. The blood flows from the periphery to the center of the lobule (i.e., **centripetal flow**).

C. **BILE DUCTULE.** Bile follows this route: bile canaliculi → cholangioles → canals of Hering → bile ductules in the portal triad → right and left hepatic ducts → common hepatic duct → common bile duct. Bile flows from the center of the lobule to the periphery (i.e., **centrifugal flow**). **Cholestasis** is a general term that defines the impaired production and semisecretion of bile at the level of the hepatocyte (**intrahepatic cholestasis**), or a structural blockage (e.g., tumor of pancreas or biliary tract) or mechanical blockage (e.g., **cholelithiasis** [presence of gallstones]) in the excretion of bile (**extrahepatic cholestasis**).

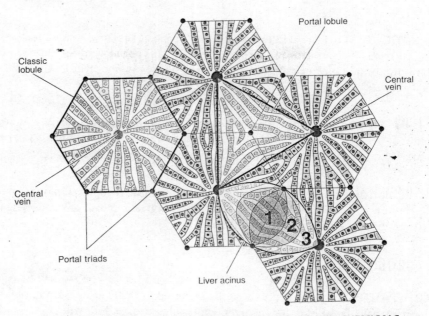

Classic lobule

Portal lobule

Central vein

Central vein

Portal triads

Liver acinus

VARIOUS TYPES OF LIVER DAMAGE CAUSED BY DRUGS AND CHEMICALS

Morphologic Appearance	Drug/Chemical
Acute hepatitis	Isoniazid (10%–20% liver damage; acetyl hydrazine is the active metabolite), salicylate, halothane (symptoms occur after 1 week, fever precedes jaundice, and metabolites form via action of P_{450} system); methyldopa (positive Coombs test), phenytoin, and ketoconazole
Chronic active hepatitis	Methyldopa, acetaminophen, aspirin, isoniazid, nitrofurantoin, and halothane
Zonal necrosis	**Zone 1:** Undergo necrosis in poisoning caused by yellow phosphorus, manganese, ferrous sulfate, allyl alcohol, and endotoxin of *Proteus vulgaris*
	Undergo necrosis due to: chronic hepatitis, primary biliary cirrhosis, bile duct occlusion, and pre-eclampsia/eclampsia (Note: Hepatic disease is very common in preeclamptic women and monitoring of platelet count and serum liver enzymes is standard practice.)
	Are exposed to blood high in nutrients and oxygen; synthesize glycogen and plasma proteins actively
	Zone 2: Undergo necrosis caused by yellow fever
	Are exposed to blood intermediate in nutrients and oxygen
	Zone 3: Undergo necrosis caused by ischemic injury, right-sided cardiac failure, and bone marrow transplantation
	Undergo necrosis in poisoning caused by carbon tetrachloride, chloroform, L-amanitin, pyrrolizidine alkaloids (bush tea), tannic acid, copper, acetaminophen (free radicals formed; acetylcysteine therapy replaces glutathione to neutralize free radicals)
Intrahepatic cholestasis	**Non-inflammatory:** Oral contraceptives and anabolic steroids
	Inflammatory: Erythromycin estolate, amoxicillin-clavulanic acid, chlorpromazine, and thiazides
Fatty change	**Single droplet:** ethanol, corticosteroids, amiodarone (looks like alcoholic hepatitis)
	Microvesicular: Tetracycline, valproic acid
Fibrosis	Methotrexate, hypervitaminosis A
Vascular lesions	**Budd-Chiari syndrome:** Oral contraceptives
	Peliosis hepatic: Oral contraceptives, anabolic steroids
	Angiosarcoma: Vinyl chloride, arsenic, Thorotrast
Tumors	**Nodular hyperplasia:** Azathioprine, anticancer agents
	Benign tumors: Oral contraceptives
	Malignant tumors: Oral contraceptives
Granulomatous hepatitis	Allopurinol, hydralazine, sulfonamides, phenylbutazone

● **Figure 18-2 Diagram of a classic liver lobule and liver acinus.** The classic liver lobule contains a central vein at its center with six portal triads at the periphery. The liver acinus defines three zones (zones 1, 2, and 3) on the basis of the location of hepatocytes to incoming blood. Hepatocytes in zone 1 are nearest the incoming blood, hepatocytes in zone 2 are intermediate, and hepatocytes in zone 3 are farthest from the incoming blood.

D. **LYMPHATIC VESSEL.** Lymph follows this route: space of Disse → lymphatic vessels in the portal triad → lymphatic vessels that parallel the portal vein → thoracic duct. Lymph flows from the center of the lobule to the periphery of a liver lobule (i.e., **centrifugal flow**).

V   Liver Acinus (Figure 18-2). The liver acinus is divided into **zone 1, zone 2,** and **zone 3** based on the location of hepatocytes to incoming blood. Hepatocytes within each zone have specific characteristics as indicated.

VI   Repair (Regeneration). Hepatocytes are a relatively stable cell population under normal circumstances (i.e., not under continual renewal). After partial surgical removal or damage by toxic substances, hepatocytes demonstrate a high rate of mitosis.

VII   Clinical Considerations

A. **VIRAL HEPATITIS** is a term used to describe infection of the liver by a group of viruses that have a particular affinity for the liver, which includes the following:
    1. **Hepatitis A virus** is a self-limiting disease that does not lead to chronic hepatitis or fulminant hepatitis. It is commonly referred to as **"infectious hepatitis."**
    2. **Hepatitis B virus** leads to acute and chronic hepatitis, fulminant hepatitis, and hepatocellular carcinoma. It is transmitted by transfusions, dialysis, and IV drug abuse. It is commonly referred to as **"serum hepatitis."**
    3. **Hepatitis C virus** leads to chronic hepatitis, cirrhosis, and hepatocellular carcinoma. It may be the leading cause of chronic hepatitis in the Western world.
    4. **Hepatitis D virus** leads to hepatitis only in the presence of hepatitis B virus.
    5. **Hepatitis E virus** is a self-limiting disease that does not lead to chronic hepatitis or fulminant hepatitis. It is transmitted through the water. A characteristic feature is the high mortality rate among pregnant women.

B. **PRIMARY BILIARY CIRRHOSIS** is caused by a granulomatous destruction of medium-sized **intrahepatic bile ducts** with cirrhosis appearing late in the course of the disease. It is characterized by **mitochondrial pyruvate dehydrogenase autoantibodies,** the role of which is not clear.

C. **PRIMARY SCLEROSING CHOLANGITIS** is caused by inflammation, fibrosis, and segmental dilatation of both **intrahepatic and extrahepatic bile ducts.** It is characterized by **anti-neutrophil cytoplasmic autoantibodies.** It is frequently seen in association with chronic ulcerative colitis of the bowel.

D. **ANTIHYPERLIPIDEMIC DRUGS**
    1. **Lovastatin (Mevacor), dimvastatin (Zocor), pravastatin (Pravachol), and fluvastatin (Lescol)** lower serum cholesterol levels by competitively inhibiting 3-hydroxy-3-methylglutaryl-coenzyme A reductase (HMG-CoA reductase), which catalyzes the rate-limiting step in cholesterol synthesis (HMG-CoA → mevalonate).
    2. **Niacin (nicotinic acid; vitamin B$_3$)** decreases hepatic production of VLDL.
    3. **Gemfibrozil (Lopid) and clofibrate (Atromid-S)** lower serum triglyceride levels by decreasing hepatic production of VLDL and increase lipoprotein lipase activity in capillary endothelial cells.
    4. **Probucol (Lorelco)** lowers serum cholesterol levels by increasing LDL catabolism.

● Fig
hepa
of a
ic sin
ted l
the
lymp

VIII **Selected Photomicrographs**

A. Electron micrographs of hepatocytes, Kupffer cell, space of Disse, and bile canaliculus and light micrograph of portal triad (Figure 18-3).

B. Light micrograph of normal liver and alcoholic liver cirrhosis (Figure 18-4).

C. Light micrograph of normal gall bladder and cholecystitis (Figure 18-5).

● **Figure 18-3 General features of the liver. (A–C)** EM of the liver. **(A)** A Kupffer cell (*K*) is shown within the lumen of a hepatic sinusoid (*sin*). The sinusoid is lined by a discontinuous endothelium (*endo*). *H* = hepatocyte. **(B)** The basolateral border of a hepatocyte (*H*) is shown projecting microvilli into the space of Disse (*SD*). The space of Disse is separated from the hepatic sinusoid (*sin*) by a discontinuous endothelium (*endo*). **(C)** Two adjacent hepatocytes (*H*) are shown abutting each other (*dotted lines*) to form a bile canaliculus (*bc*) that is bounded by tight junctions (*arrows*) that serve to contain the bile. **(D)** LM of the liver showing the components of a portal tract: hepatic arteriole (*HA*), portal venule (*PV*), bile ductule (*BD*), and a lymphatic vessel (*LYM*).

● **Figure 18-4 Normal liver and liver cirrhosis. (A)** LM of normal liver. The classic liver lobules (*outlined*) with central vein (*circle*) are clearly delineated. **(B–D)** LM of alcoholic liver cirrhosis. **(B)** Broad bands of fibrous septae (*fib*), present in alcoholic liver cirrhosis, bridge regions of the liver from central vein to portal triad and from portal triad to portal triad. This fibrotic activity will entrap sections of hepatic parenchyma, which undergo regeneration to form nodules (*nod*). **(C)** Neutrophil, lymphocyte, and macrophage infiltration (*) is prominent at the periphery of the liver lobule. **(D)** Some hepatocytes accumulate tangled masses of cytokeratin intermediate filaments within the cytoplasm known as **Mallory bodies** (*arrow*). Alcoholism results in a **fatty liver, steatohepatitis** (fatty liver plus inflammation), **cirrhosis** (collagen proliferation and fibrosis), and **hepatocellular carcinoma.**

● **Figure 18-5 Normal gall bladder and cholecystitis. (A)** LM of normal gall bladder. The main function of the gall bladder is storage, concentration, and release of bile. The gall bladder consists of a mucosa, muscularis externa, and adventitia. There is no submucosa in the gall bladder. Numerous mucosal folds lined by a simple columnar epithelium, which project into the lumen of the gall bladder, are shown. These mucosal folds flatten out as the gall bladder is distended. At times, the mucosa may penetrate deep into the muscularis externa to form **Rokitansky-Aschoff sinuses,** which are early indicators of pathologic changes within the mucosa. **(B)** LM of cholecystitis (inflammation of the gall bladder). Acute or chronic cholecystitis is generally associated with the presence of gallstones. In this case, the mucosal epithelium is completely obliterated, and there is focal hemorrhage (*hem*) and lymphocyte infiltration (*) of the lamina propria.

Exocrine Pancreas and Islets of Langerhans

I. Exocrine Pancreas

A. The functional unit of the exocrine pancreas is the pancreatic **acinus,** which consists of **acinar cells** that contain rER, Golgi, and zymogen granules. Acinar cells secrete digestive enzymes, which include: **trypsinogen, chymotrypsinogen, procarboxypeptidase, lipase, amylase, elastase, ribonuclease, deoxyribonuclease, cholesterol esterase,** and **phospholipase.** The secretion of digestive enzymes is stimulated by cholecystokinin (CCK) released by I-cells of the small intestine.

B. The exocrine pancreas also contains a **network of ducts:** centroacinar cells of the intercalated duct → intralobular duct → interlobular duct → main pancreatic duct (duct of Wirsung) → joins the common bile duct at the hepatoduodenal ampulla (ampulla of Vater) → duodenum. The duct network delivers digestive enzymes to the duodenum and secretes HCO_3^-. Secretion of HCO_3^- by the intercalated and intralobular ducts is stimulated by secretin (SEC) released by S-cells of the small intestine.

C. **CLINICAL CONSIDERATION. Pancreatitis** is inflammation of the pancreas that is almost always associated with acinar cell injury. **Chronic pancreatitis** is relapsing inflammation of the pancreas, causing pain and eventually irreversible damage in which **pancreatic calcifications** (pathognomonic) are frequently diagnosed by imaging procedures. **Acute pancreatitis** is an acute condition associated with abdominal pain and raised levels of pancreatic enzymes in the blood and urine. Increased levels of amylase in the pleural fluid are pathognomonic of acute pancreatitis. About 80% of acute pancreatitis cases are associated with **biliary tract disease** or **alcoholism.** Its most severe form is known as **acute hemorrhagic pancreatitis.** The ultimate pathologic process is the destructive effect of pancreatic enzymes released from damaged acinar cells, resulting in **autodigestion** of the pancreas.

II. Endocrine Pancreas (Figure 19-1).

The endocrine pancreas comprises only 2% of the entire pancreas and consists of the **islets of Langerhans** that are scattered throughout the pancreas. The islets of Langerhans consists mainly of the following cell types:

A. **ALPHA (α) CELLS** (20% of the islet) secrete **glucagon** (29 amino acids; 3.5 kDa) in response to hypoglycemia, which will elevate blood glucose, free fatty acid, and ketone levels. Glucagon binds to the **glucagon receptor,** which is a **G protein-linked receptor** present on hepatocytes and adipocytes. Glucagon is derived from a large precursor protein called **preproglucagon,** whose gene is present on chromosome 2. About 30%–40% of glucagon within the blood is derived from α cells; the remainder of the glucagon (called **enteroglucagon**) is derived from enteroendocrine cells within the gastrointestinal tract.

GLUCAGON

Liver

↑ Glycogen degradation
(↑*glycogen phosphorylase*)

↑ Gluconeogenesis
(↑*fructose 1, 6 bisphosphatase*)
(↓*pyruvate kinase*)

Adipose

↑ Lipolysis (*thormone = sensitive lipase*)

↑ β-Oxidation of free fatty acids

Elevates blood glucose,
free fatty acids, and
ketone levels

INSULIN

Liver

↑ Glycogen synthesis
(↑*glycogen synthase*)

↑ Glycolysis
(↑*phosphofructokinase*)
(↓*pyruvate dehydrogenase*)

↑ Fatty acid synthesis

Skeletal
muscle

↑ Glucose uptake (GLUT 4)

↑ Glycogen synthesis
(↑*glycogen synthase*)

↑ Glycolysis
(↑*phosphofructokinase*)
(↓*pyruvate dehydrogenase*)

Adipose

↑ Glucose uptake (GLUT 4)

↑ Triacylglyceride synthesis

Lowers blood glucose,
free fatty acids, and
ketone levels

● **Figure 19-1 The effect of glucagon and insulin on target tissues.** The target tissues of glucagon are the liver and adipose. The target tissues of insulin are liver, adipose, and skeletal muscle. The main biochemical pathways and enzymes (in parentheses) that are affected by glucagon and insulin are indicated. The alpha (α) cells (*shaded*), beta (β) cells (*white*), and delta (δ) cells (*black*) are shown within the islet of Langerhans.

B. BETA (β) CELLS (75% of the islet) secrete **insulin** [51 amino acids consisting of **chain A** (21 amino acids) and **chain B** (30 amino acids) held together by **disulfide bonds;** 6 kilodaltons] in response to hyperglycemia, which will lower blood glucose, free fatty acid, and ketone levels. Insulin binds to the **insulin receptor,** which is a **receptor tyrosine kinase** present on hepatocytes, skeletal muscle cells, and adipocytes. Insulin is derived from a large precursor protein called **preproinsulin,** whose gene is present on chromosome 11. Preproinsulin is converted to proinsulin by removal of the **signal sequence** in the rER. **Proinsulin** (86 amino acids; 9 kDa; consists of the **C peptide** connecting chain A and chain B together) is transferred to the Golgi where it is packaged into secretory granules. Within secretory granules, proinsulin is cleaved by a protease to release the C peptide (35 amino acids) from insulin. Within the secretory granule, insulin organizes as a **hexamer** associated with Zn^{2+}. Insulin secretion is triggered when glucose enters the beta cell via **glucose transporter 2 (GLUT2).**

C. DELTA (δ) CELLS (5% of the islet) secrete **somatostatin** (14 amino acids), which inhibits hormone secretion from nearby cells in a paracrine manner. Somatostatin binds to the **somatostatin receptor,** which is a **G protein-linked receptor.**

III Insulin Receptor and Signal Transduction (Figure 19-2)

● **Figure 19-2 Diagram of the insulin receptor and signal transduction events.** A receptor (e.g., **insulin receptor**) that activates a chain of cellular events through the **autophosphorylation of tyrosine** is called a **receptor tyrosine kinase.** When insulin binds to the α-subunit of the insulin receptor, tyrosine kinase autophosphorylates tyrosine on the insulin receptor. The phosphorylated insulin receptor subsequently catalyzes the phosphorylation of **insulin receptor substrate-1** (*IRS-1*). The phosphorylated IRS-1 plays a role in (1) activation and deactivation of many metabolic enzymes; (2) activation of **phosphatidylinositol 3-kinase** (*PI 3 kinase*) to produce **inositol 3,4 phosphate** and **inositol 3,4,5 phosphate,** which causes translocation of glucose transporters (*GLUT4*) to the cell membrane; and (3) activation of **Ras protein, Raf protein kinase,** and **mitogen-activated protein** (*MAP*) **kinase,** which enters the nucleus where it activates gene regulatory proteins (e.g., jun) that promote gene transcription necessary for cell growth and differentiation.

Ⓘ Clinical Considerations

A. TYPE 1 DIABETES (POLYGENIC)

1. **Characteristics.** Type 1 diabetes is marked by **autoantibodies** and an **insulitis reaction** that results in the **destruction of pancreatic beta cells.** Clinical findings include: hyperglycemia, ketoacidosis, and exogenous insulin dependence. Long-term clinical effects include: neuropathy, retinopathy leading to blindness, and nephropathy leading to kidney failure.

2. **Genetic studies.** Type 1 diabetes is a **multifactorial inherited disease,** which means that many genes that have a small, equal, and additive effect (genetic component) and an environmental component are involved. If one considers only the genetic component of a multifactorial disease, the term **polygenic** is used. Type 1 diabetes shows an association with HLA (human leukocyte antigen complex) loci named **HLA-DR3** and **HLA-DR4,** located on the p arm of **chromosome 6 (p6).** It is hypothesized that genes closely linked to HLA-DR3 and HLA-DR4 loci somehow alter the immune response such that the individual has an immune response to an environmental antigen (e.g., virus). The immune response "spills over" and leads to the destruction of pancreatic beta cells, whereby **glutamic acid decarboxylase (GAD_{65}), insulin,** and **tyrosine phosphatases IA-2 and IA-2β autoantibodies** may play a role. The insulitis reaction is characterized mainly by infiltration of islets by **CD8$^+$ cytotoxic T lymphocytes.**

B. TYPE 2 DIABETES (POLYGENIC)

1. **Characteristics.** Type 2 diabetes is marked by **insulin resistance of peripheral tissues** and **abnormal beta cell function.** It is often detected during routine screening by detection of hyperglycemia or by patient complaints of polyuria. Before the onset of frank symptoms, individuals pass through phases that include the following: (1) hyperinsulinemia is present and euglycemia is maintained, (2) hyperinsulinemia is present but postprandial hyperglycemia is observed, and (3) insulin secretion declines in the face of persistent insulin resistance of peripheral tissues.

2. **Genetic studies.** Type 2 diabetes is a **multifactorial inherited disease.** At this time, genetic studies show no association with a major susceptibility gene. Instead, type 2 diabetes may involve multiple genes that convey limited degrees of susceptibility.

C. MONOGENIC FORMS OF TYPE 2 DIABETES. Genetic studies of family pedigrees prevalent with type 2 diabetes have identified mutations in a single gene. These are **rare** forms of type 2 diabetes.

1. **Mitochondrial type 2 diabetes** results from a mutation in the **mitochondrial tRNA^{Leu} gene.**

2. **Maturity onset diabetes of the young (MODY) 1** results from a mutation in the **hepatocyte nuclear factor 4α (HNF-4α) gene** located on chromosome 20 (20q). HNF-4α is a transcription factor that is a member of the steroid-thyroid superfamily of nuclear receptors.

3. **MODY 2** results from a mutation in the **glucokinase gene** located on chromosome 7. Glucokinase is an enzyme that catalyzes the conversion of glucose → glucose-6-phophate and plays a key role in generating the metabolic signal for insulin secretion.

4. **MODY 3** results from a mutation in the **HNF-1α gene** located on chromosome 12 (12q). HNF-1α is a homeodomain transcription factor.

5. **Leprechaunism** results from a mutation in the **insulin receptor gene.** Leprechaunism is characterized clinically by extreme insulin resistance, growth retardation, dysmorphic facies, and acanthosis nigricans.

D. DRUG TREATMENT OF DIABETES

1. **Injectable hypoglycemic agents** are used to treat type 1 diabetes.
   a. **Crystalline zinc insulin** (CZI; regular insulin; ultrashort acting) is a crystalline precipitate of insulin and zinc.
   b. **Prompt zinc insulin** (semilente insulin; ultrashort acting) is an amorphous insulin and zinc suspension.
   c. **Isophane insulin suspension** (neutral protamine Hagedorn; NPH; short acting) is a suspension of CZI and protamine.
   d. **Insulin zinc suspension** (lente insulin; short acting) is composed of 30% semilente and 70% ultralente insulins.
   e. **Protamine zinc insulin** (PZI; long acting) is a precipitate of CZI and protamine.
   f. **Extended insulin zinc suspension** (ultralente insulin; long acting) is a poorly soluble CZI.

2. **Oral hypoglycemic agents** are used to treat type 2 diabetes.
   a. **Tolbutamide (Orinase), acetohexamide (Dymelor), tolazamide (Tolinase), chlorpropamide (Diabinase), glyburide (Micronase), and glipizide (Glucotrol)** are sulfonylurea derivatives that block K^+ ion channels, causing depolarization of beta cells and triggering insulin secretion. The second-generation sulfonylureas (glyburide and glipizide) are more potent than their first-generation counterparts.
   b. **Metformin (Glucophage)** is a biguanide that **promotes** peripheral glucose utilization and reduces hepatic gluconeogenesis.
   c. **Troglitazone and Rezulin** are thiazolidinediones that improve insulin action by activating the peroxisome proliferator-activated receptor γ (PPAR γ), which modulates a number of genes involved in lipid metabolism.
   d. **Acarbose and miglitol** are α-glucosidase inhibitors that slow down carbohydrate absorption from the intestine.
   e. **Byetta** (which is GLP-1) increases insulin secretion in both normal physiology and type 2 diabetes. Byetta is the first in a new class of drugs called **incretin-mimetics** for the treatment of type 2 diabetes.
   f. **Januvia** and **Galvus** inhibit the enzyme dipeptidyl peptidase 4 (DPP. 4), which quickly inactivates both GIP and GLP-1.

E. ISLET CELL TUMORS

1. **Insulinoma.** An insulinoma (most common islet cell tumor) is a benign tumor consisting of islet ß cells and is generally associated with the MEN I syndrome. An insulinoma secretes **excess insulin and C peptide,** thereby producing a fasting hypoglycemia. Clinical findings include neuroglycopenia (brain without glucose); hypoglycemia; increased serum insulin levels; and increased serum C-peptide levels. The differential diagnosis is **factitious hypoglycemia** caused by surreptitious insulin injections. In factitious hypoglycemia, there is hypoglycemia; increased serum insulin levels; but decreased serum C-peptide levels caused by the suppression of endogenous insulin secretion by hypoglycemia.

2. **Glucagonoma.** A glucagonoma is a malignant tumor consisting of islet α cells. A glucagonoma secretes **excess glucagon,** thereby producing a fasting hyperglycemia (i.e., diabetes). Clinical findings include characteristic rash called necrolytic migratory erythema.

3. **Somatostatinoma.** A somatostinoma is a malignant tumor consisting of islet δ cells. A somatostatinoma secretes **excess somatostatin.** Clinical findings include: achlorhydria (lack of HCl production due to the inhibition of gastrin by somatostatin); cholelithiasis (formation of gallstones due to the inhibition of CCK by somatostatin); diabetes (increased blood glucose levels due to inhibition of GIP by somatostatin); steatorrhea (excessive amount of fat in the feces caused by inhibition of secretin and CCK by somatostatin).

V   Selected Photomicrographs

A. Normal exocrine pancreas and pancreatitis (Figure 19-3)

B. Islet of Langerhans in normal, type 1 diabetes, and type 2 diabetes (Figure 19-4)

● **Figure 19-3 Normal pancreas and pancreatitis. (A)** LM of normal exocrine pancreas. Acinar cells containing numerous granules (*gr*) are arranged in an acinus (*dotted lines*). A small capillary (*cap*) can be observed. **(B)** LM of pancreatitis. A large area of exocrine pancreas (*ex*) is shown surrounded by thick fibrous bands (*fib*) that are highly infiltrated with lymphocytes (inflammatory response). Acinar cells undergoing autolysis are shown (*arrows*). **(C)** Enzyme panel after acute pancreatitis.

● **Figure 19-4 Normal and diabetic islets. (A)** LM of a normal islet of Langerhans. A normal islet of Langerhans (*dotted circle*) is shown surrounded by exocrine pancreas (*ex*). **(B)** LM of an islet of Langerhans in type 1 diabetes. The islet (*dotted circle*) is shown with conspicuous lymphocytic infiltration (insulitis reaction; *arrow*), which probably leads to the destruction of the beta cells within the islet. **(C)** LM of an islet of Langerhans in type 2 diabetes. The islet (*dotted circle*) is shown with conspicuous amyloid deposition (*arrows*).

Case Study

A father brings his 10-year-old daughter into your office complaining that "she is always thirsty and drinks a heck of a lot of water." He also tells you that "she doesn't want to eat or drink today because she says she feels sick to her stomach and is vomiting. But, she is still urinating a lot." After some discussion, he informs you his daughter had a high fever about 2 weeks ago and he took her to the emergency room. The father is obviously concerned about his daughter but you sense a deeper level of worry and you ask him about it. He tells you "Doc, I lost my wife last year because of kidney failure and I am afraid my daughter has the same thing. I can't lose my daughter, too. She is all I got left." What is the most likely diagnosis?

Differentials

- Gastroenteritis, hypoglycemic coma, metabolic acidosis, nonketotic hyperglycemic hyperosmolar coma (NHHK)

Relevant Physical Exam Findings

- Breathing is rapid and deep (Kussmaul respirations)
- Sweet smell on her breath
- Dry skin and oral mucosa

Relevant Lab Findings

- Blood chemistry: Glucose = 490 mg/dL (High); Ketone bodies = High; Na^+ = 128 mEq/L (Low); K^+ = 6.2 mEq/L (High); HCO_3^- = 9.8 mEq/L (Low); pH = 7.1 (Low); Anion gap = 22 (High); Osmolarity = 330 mOsm/kg (High); BUN = 25 mg/dL (High); Creatinine = 1.0 mg/dL (Normal); Lactate = Normal
- Urinalysis: Ketones = >80 (High); Glucose = >1,000 mg/dL (High)

Diagnosis

Diabetic Ketoacidosis (DKA). DKA occurs secondary to infection or lack of insulin therapy in Type 1 diabetics (who lack endogenous circulating insulin). Therefore, the metabolic breakdown of fat stores in adipose tissue into fatty acids causes an increase in ketone body formation. Note: One of the functions of insulin is to inhibit the metabolic breakdown of fat stores in adipose tissue into fatty acids. The lack of insulin in Type 1 diabetics also results in a rise of counter-regulatory hormones (e.g., glucagons, epinephrine, cortisol, and growth hormone), which causes increased glycogen breakdown, increased gluconeogenesis in the liver, inhibition of glycolysis, and decreased peripheral utilization of glucose; all of which lead to hyperglycemia. The increased levels of glucose and ketone bodies in the glomerular filtrate (caused by exceeding the transport maximum T_M) results in an osmotic diuresis, which provokes hypovolemia, dehydration, and loss of electrolytes in the urine. The dehydration activates the renin-angiotensin system, which causes the release of aldosterone. Aldosterone acts on the principal cells of the cortical collecting duct and causes increased K^+ secretion (plasma $\rightarrow$ tubular fluid) and, thereby, increases K^+ excretion in the urine. The hyperkalemia results from the movement of K^+ out of the cells in exchange for H^+ that are prevalent in the serum because of the metabolic acidosis. Metabolic acidosis causes Kussmaul respirations in response to a $\downarrow$ serum pH. The elevated anion gap acidosis results from the production of excess organic acids (e.g., ketone bodies) and the body's inability to neutralize the excess acid. Gastroenteritis is a viral or bacterial infection of the stomach or small bowel. Clinical findings of gastroenteritis include a profuse vomiting that results in a metabolic alkalosis (i.e., loss of H^+ and Cl^- from the stomach). Clinical findings of hypoglycemic coma include low blood glucose levels, pallor, sweating, hunger, tremors, and increased heart rate owing to increased levels of epinephrine. Metabolic acidosis ($\downarrow$ serum pH and $HCO3^-$ levels) has several causes besides DKA. A normal-gap metabolic acidosis may be caused by diarrhea, renal tubular acidosis, or acetazolamide overdose. An elevated gap metabolic acidosis may be caused by chronic renal failure, uremia, lactic acidosis, DKA, salicylate overdose, methanol ingestion, and ethylene glycol ingestion. The normal creatinine levels rule out chronic renal failure. The normal lactate levels rule out lactic acidosis. NHHK is a condition that occurs in older adults with Type 2 diabetes and may be caused by infection, increased glucose consumption, or a cerebrovascular accident. Clinical findings of NHHK include hyperosmolarity without ketosis. The elevated ketone bodies in the blood and urine rule out NHHK.

Chapter 20

Respiratory System

① General Features (Figure 20-1). The respiratory system is divided into a **conduction portion** and a **respiratory portion.** The conduction portion **only conducts air into the lung;** no blood-air gas exchange occurs. Airflow through the conduction portion follows this route: **nasal cavities → nasopharynx → oropharynx → larynx → trachea → bronchi → bronchioles → terminal bronchioles.** The respiratory portion is where **blood-air gas exchange occurs.** Airflow through the respiratory portion follows this route: **respiratory bronchioles → alveolar ducts → alveoli.** The larger airways of the conduction portion (i.e., trachea and bronchi) are organized into a **mucosa (epithelium and lamina propria), muscular layer, submucosa,** and **adventitia.** As the airways get progressively smaller down to the alveoli, the components of the wall change significantly and this organization is lost.

⑪ Trachea

A. **MUCOSA.** The epithelium is a **respiratory epithelium** that is classically described as a **ciliated pseudostratified epithelium with goblet cells,** which contains the following cell types. **Ciliated cells** (≅30%) beat toward the pharynx thereby moving mucus and/or particulate matter to the mouth, where it can be swallowed or expectorated. **Goblet cells** (≅30%) secrete mucus. **Brush cells** contain microvilli and have been interpreted as either an intermediate stage in the differentiation to ciliated cells or a sensory cell, since it may be found in association with nerve terminals. **Endocrine cells (Kulchitsky cells)** secrete peptide hormones and catecholamines. **Basal cells** (≅30%) have mitotic capacity and thereby function as stem cells to regenerate the epithelium. The lamina propria consists of **collagen and elastic fibers.**

B. **MUSCULAR LAYER.** The muscular layer consists of smooth muscle that spans the dorsal ends of the cartilage rings called the **trachealis muscle.**

C. **SUBMUCOSA.** The submucosa consists of **seromucous glands** surrounded by **collagen and elastic fibers.**

D. **ADVENTITIA.** The adventitia consists of **C-shaped hyaline cartilage rings** surrounded by **collagen and elastic fibers.**

SUMMARY TABLE OF HISTOLOGY

	Mucosa	Smooth Musclular Layer	Submucosa	Adventitia
Trachea	Respiratory epithelium Collagen and elastic fibers	Trachealis muscle	Seromucous glands Collagen and elastic fibers	C-shaped hyaline cartilage rings Collagen and elastic fibers
Bronchi	Respiratory epithelium Collagen and elastic fibers	Prominent circular layer	Seromucous glands Collagen and elastic fibers	Irregular hyaline cartilage plates Collagen and elastic fibers
Bronchioles	Simple ciliated columnar with Goblet cells and Clara cells Collagen and elastic fibers	Prominent circular layer	Absent	Absent
Terminal bronchioles	Simple ciliated cuboidal with Clara cells Collagen and elastic fibers	Reduced, incomplete circular layer	Absent	Absent
Respiratory bronchioles	Simple ciliated cuboidal with Clara cells Collagen and elastic fibers	Prominent, incomplete circular layer	Absent	Absent
Alveolar ducts	Simple squamous epithelium Collagen and elastic fibers	Smooth muscle "knobs"	Absent	Absent
Alveoli	Type I pneumocytes Type II pneumocytes, Alveolar macrophages Collagen and elastic fibers	Absent	Absent	Absent

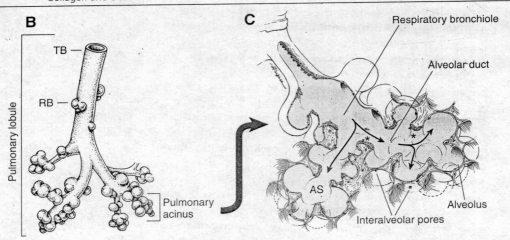

● **Figure 20-1 General features of the lung. (A)** Table illustrating changes in the respiratory tree from the trachea to alveoli. In the trachea and bronchi, collagen and elastic fibers span the cartilage rings and plates and also are found in the lamina propria beneath the epithelium. In the remaining portion of the respiratory tree, collagen and elastic fibers are found in the lamina propria, where the elastic fibers are arranged in longitudinal bands. Collagen and elastic fibers (minor component) along with surfactant (major component) contribute to the elastance of the lung (i.e., the collapsing force that develops in the lung as the lung expands). Note that cilia extend farther down the respiratory tree than mucous glands and goblet cells. **(B)** Diagram of a respiratory lobule consisting of a terminal bronchiole (TB), respiratory bronchioles (RB), alveolar ducts, and alveoli. **(C)** Diagram of a respiratory acinus. A respiratory acinus consists of a respiratory bronchiole, alveolar duct, and alveoli. Note the smooth muscle arranged in a circular layer in the respiratory bronchiole and as "knobs" (*) in the alveolar duct. The respiratory lobule-respiratory acinus concept is important pathologically in classifying types of emphysema: (1) centriacinar emphysema involves widening of air spaces within the respiratory bronchioles only at the apex of an acinus, whereas (2) panacinar emphysema involves widening of air spaces distal to the terminal bronchiole involving the entire acinus.

III Bronchi

A. **MUCOSA.** The epithelium is a **respiratory epithelium** as described above. The lamina propria consists of **collagen and elastic fibers.**

B. **MUSCULAR LAYER.** The muscular layer consists of a **prominent circular layer of smooth muscle.**

C. **SUBMUCOSA.** The submucosa consists of **seromucous glands** surrounded by **collagen and elastic fibers.**

D. **ADVENTITIA.** The adventitia consists of **irregular hyaline cartilage plates** surrounded by **collagen and elastic fibers.**

IV Bronchioles

A. **MUCOSA.** The epithelium is a **simple ciliated columnar epithelium** with **goblet cells** and **Clara cells.** The lamina propria consists of **collagen and elastic fibers.** Clara cells **secrete a component of surfactant, secrete Clara cell protein (CC16),** which is used as a marker of pulmonary function in bronchopulmonary lavage fluid and serum, **metabolize airborne toxins** using cytochrome P450, and **release Cl⁻ into the lumen** via a Cl⁻ ion channel regulated by cGMP-guanylate cyclase mechanism. Clara cells are nonciliated, have a dome-shaped protrusion extending into the lumen, and have the ultrastructural characteristics of a protein-secreting cell (rER, Golgi, secretory granules).

B. **MUSCULAR LAYER.** The muscular layer consists of a **prominent circular layer of smooth muscle.**

V Terminal Bronchioles

A. **MUCOSA.** The epithelium is a **simple ciliated cuboidal epithelium** with **Clara cells.** The lamina propria consists of **collagen and elastic fibers.**

B. **MUSCULAR LAYER.** The muscular layer consists of a **reduced, incomplete circular layer of smooth muscle.**

VI Respiratory Bronchioles

A. **MUCOSA.** The epithelium is a **simple ciliated cuboidal epithelium** with numerous **Clara cells.** The lamina propria consists of **collagen and elastic fibers.**

B. **MUSCULAR LAYER.** The muscular layer consists of a **prominent, incomplete circular layer of smooth muscle.** Note that respiratory bronchioles are distinguished histologically by the presence of alveoli that open into its wall.

VII Alveolar Ducts

A. **MUCOSA.** The epithelium is a **simple squamous epithelium.** The lamina propria consists of **collagen and elastic fibers.**

B. **MUSCULAR LAYER.** The muscular layer consists of **smooth muscle "knobs."**

VIII Alveoli contain the following:

A. **TYPE I PNEUMOCYTES** are a simple squamous epithelium joined by tight junctions (zonula occludens) that line alveoli and have no mitotic capacity.

B. **TYPE II PNEUMOCYTES** are cuboidal-shaped cells that are most commonly found at the junction of interalveolar septae and bulge into the air space. These cells secrete **surfactant** (which is stored as **lamellar bodies**) and have mitotic capacity thereby functioning as stem cells to regenerate the epithelium. Hyperplasia of Type II pneumocytes is an important marker of alveolar injury and repair of alveoli.

C. **ALVEOLAR MACROPHAGES** migrate over the surface of the alveoli and into the interalveolar septae to phagocytose inhaled dust, bacteria, and degraded surfactant.

D. **ALVEOLAR PORES (PORES OF KOHN)** are found within interalveolar septae and equalize pressure within alveoli. These pores play a significant role in obstructive lung disease by serving as a bypass to aerate alveoli distal to the blockage. The **interalveolar septae** of the alveoli contain **collagen and elastic fibers.**

IX Surfactant is composed of **cholesterol (50%), dipalmitoyl phosphatidylcholine (DPPC; 40%),** and **surfactant proteins (10%) SP-A, SP-B, and SP-C.** SP-A and SP-B combine with DPPC in the lamellar bodies within type II pneumocytes. SP-B and SP-C stabilize the surfactant coat. Surfactant lines the alveoli and reduces surface tension, preventing the collapse of small alveoli (atelectasis), cyanosis, and respiratory distress.

A. Surfactant is the major contributor to the elastance of the lung. **Elastance** is the collapsing force that develops in the lung as the lung expands. Elastance is described by the **Laplace Law** as shown below:

$$E = \frac{2T}{r}$$

where

E = collapsing force (elastance)

T = surface tension

r = radius of the alveolus

B. The Laplace law indicates that:
1. **Large alveoli** have a low collapsing force (elastance) and are easy to keep open.
2. **Small alveoli** have a high collapsing force (elastance) and are difficult to keep open.

X Blood-Air Barrier. The components of the blood-air barrier include the: **surfactant layer, type I pneumocyte, basement membrane,** and **capillary endothelial cell.** The rate of diffusion across the blood-air barrier is described by the Fick law as shown below:

$$RD = \frac{A}{T} \times D \times (P_1 - P_2)$$

where

RD = rate of diffusion

A = surface area of the alveoli

T = thickness of the blood-air barrier

D = solubility of the gas

$P_1 - P_2$ = pressure difference across the blood-air barrier

Note that increases in the thickness of the blood-air barrier will decrease the rate of diffusion of O_2 and CO_2 across the blood-air barrier.

XI **Air flow** through the lung from the bronchi to alveoli is inversely proportional to airway resistance.

A. AIRWAY RESISTANCE is described by the **Poiseuille law** as shown below:

$$R = \frac{8n\,l}{\pi r^4}$$

where

R = resistance

n = the viscosity of the inspired gas

l = length of the airway

r = radius of the airway

Note the strong relationship of r to R. If airway radius (r) is reduced by a factor of 2, then airway resistance (R) is increased by a factor of 16 (2^4). Therefore, airflow will be dramatically reduced.

B. The **medium-sized bronchi** are the **main site of airway resistance** through the contraction or relaxation of smooth muscle.
1. **Parasympathetic stimulation, leukotrienes (LTC$_4$, LTD$_4$), prostaglandin F$_{2\alpha}$ (PGF$_{2\alpha}$), and thromboxane (TXA$_2$)** constrict the airways (i.e., reduce r) and thereby increase airway resistance (R). These are bronchoconstrictors.
2. **Sympathetic stimulation, PGE$_2$, and β_2-adrenergic agonists (e.g., terbutaline, albuterol, metaproterenol, salmeterol)** dilate the airways (i.e., increase r) and thereby decrease airway resistance (R). These are bronchodilators.

XII **Clinical Considerations**

A. INFANT RESPIRATORY DISTRESS SYNDROME (RDS) is caused by a deficiency of surfactant that may be caused by prolonged intrauterine asphyxia or premature birth, or it may occur in infants of diabetic mothers. **Thyroxine and cortisol treatment** increase production of surfactant. RDS threatens the infant not only with immediate asphyxiation but also by triggering repeated gasping inhalations that can damage the alveolar lining, leading to **hyaline membrane disease.**

B. **BRONCHOGENIC CARCINOMA** begins as hyperplasia of the respiratory epithelium that lines the bronchi. Types of bronchogenic carcinoma include:

1. **Adenocarcinoma (AD)** is the most common type (35%). The lesions are peripherally located within the lung as they arise from distal airways and alveoli. AD forms well-circumscribed gray-white masses with obvious glandular elements that contain **mucin.** AD is less closely associated with a smoking history than squamous cell carcinoma.

2. **Squamous cell carcinoma (SQ)** is the second most common type (25%). The lesions are centrally located as they arise from larger bronchi. SQ begins as a small, red, granular plaque and progresses to a large intrabronchial mass that may produce **keratin** and secrete **parathyroid hormone (PTH),** causing hypercalcemia. SQ is closely associated with a **smoking history.**

3. **Small cell carcinoma (SC)** is the least common type (15%). The lesions are centrally located as they arise from larger bronchi. SC forms large, soft, gray-white masses and contains small, oval-shaped cells **(oat cells)** derived from **Kulchitsky cells** that may produce **adrenocorticotropic hormone (ACTH)** or **antidiuretic hormone (ADH),** causing Cushing syndrome or syndrome of inappropriate secretion of ADH (SIADH), respectively. SC is associated with a smoking history.

C. **CYSTIC FIBROSIS (CF)** is caused by production of abnormally thick mucus by epithelial cells lining the respiratory (and gastrointestinal tract). This results clinically in obstruction of airways and recurrent bacterial infections (e.g., *Staphylococcus aureus, Pseudomonas aeruginosa*). CF is caused by autosomal recessive mutations of the CF gene that is located on the long arm of chromosome 7 (q7). The CF gene encodes for a protein called **CFTR (c**ystic **f**ibrosis **t**ransporter) that functions as a **Cl⁻ ion channel.** In North America, 70% of CF cases are caused by a 3-base deletion that codes for the amino acid **phenylalanine at position 508** such that phenylalanine is missing from CFTR.

D. **LUNG INFECTIONS**

1. *Staphylococcus aureus* produces lung abscesses and is a common secondary infection in rubeola or influenza.

2. *Chlamydia trachomatis* produces pneumonia that is contracted as a newborn infant passes through the birth canal.

3. *Candida albicans* produces pneumonia that is associated with an indwelling catheter and immunodeficiency states.

4. *Coxiella burnetii* is a respiratory pathogen that is commonly found in individuals who have close association with cows, sheep, or goats.

5. *Histoplasma capsulatum* is a fungal infection characterized by multiple granulomas with calcification in the lung. It is acquired by inhalation of spores and is the most common systemic fungal in Midwest United States.

6. *Aspergillus fumigatus* is a fungal infection that resides in old tuberculous cavities.

7. *Coccidioides immitis* (valley fever) is a fungal infection. It is acquired by inhalation of spores and is most common in the Southwest United States (San Joaquin Valley).

8. *Pneumocystis carinii* is an opportunistic fungal infection that is a common initial presentation of AIDS.

E. **ALLERGIES, SEASONAL HAYFEVER, RHINITIS,** and **urticaria** can be treated with the following drugs:

1. **Diphenhydramine (Benadryl), dimenhydrinate (Dramamine), chlorpheniramine (Chlor-Trimeton),** and **meclizine (Antivert)** are first-generation H_1-receptor antagonists that block the effect of histamine released from mast cells on vascular permeability, vasodilation, and smooth muscle contraction of bronchi. The H_1-receptor is a G protein–linked receptor that increases inositol triphosphate (IP_3) and diacylglycerol (DAG) levels.

2. **Terfenadine (Seldane), loratadine (Claritin), and astemizole (Hismanal)** are second-generation H_1-receptor antagonists. These drugs do not cross the blood-brain barrier and therefore do not have a sedative effect like first-generation drugs above.

F. **EMPHYSEMA**
   1. **General features.** Patients are referred to as **"pink puffers"** with the following characteristics: a thin, barrel-shaped chest, increased breathing rate (tachypnea), a mildly decreased Pao_2 (mild hypoxemia), and a mildly decreased or normal $Paco_2$ (hypocapnia or normocapnia).
   2. **Pathology**
      a. **Panacinar emphysema** (related to α_1-**antitrypsin deficiency**). Pathologic findings include: a widening of the air spaces distal to the terminal bronchioles as a result of destruction of the alveolar walls by enzymes.
      b. **Centriacinar emphysema** (related to **smoking**). Pathologic findings include: a widening of the air spaces within the respiratory bronchioles only while the surrounding alveoli remain fairly well preserved.

G. **CHRONIC BRONCHITIS** (related to smoking)
   1. **General features.** Patients are referred to as **"blue bloaters"** with the following characteristics: a muscular, barrel-shaped chest, severely decreased Pao_2 (severe hypoxemia with cyanosis), increased $Paco_2$ (hypercapnia) leading to chronic respiratory acidosis, increased HCO_3^- reabsorption by the kidney to buffer the acidemia, right ventricular failure, and systemic edema.
   2. **Pathology.** Pathologic findings include: an excessive mucus production leading to copious, purulent sputum production, bronchi that demonstrate inflammatory cell infiltrates, and hypertrophy of mucous glands (increase in Reid index).

H. **ASTHMA** (Figure 20-2).

● **Figure 20-2** Diagram indicating the various factors that control bronchial smooth muscle relaxation and contraction.

1. **General features.** Asthma is associated with **smooth muscle hyperreactivity within bronchi and bronchioles, increased mucus production, and edema of the bronchial wall.**

2. **Pathology.** Pathologic findings include: inflammatory cell infiltrates containing numerous **eosinophils** within the bronchial wall, hyperplasia of bronchial smooth muscle cells, hyperplasia of mucous glands, **Curschmann spirals** (formed from shed epithelium), and **Charcot-Leyden crystals** (formed from eosinophil granules) within the mucous plugs.

3. **Pharmacology**
   a. **Terbutaline, albuterol, metaproterenol,** and **salmeterol** are β_2-adrenergic receptor agonists (i.e., β_2-agonist) that promote bronchodilation. The β_2-adrenergic receptor is a G protein-linked receptor that increases cAMP levels. **In asthma, the FEV_1 (the volume of air that can be expired in 1 second after a maximal inspiration) is reduced. After treatment with a β_2-agonist, the FEV_1 is increased.**
   b. **Atropine and ipratropium** are muscarinic acetylcholine receptor (mAChR) antagonists that inhibit bronchoconstriction. The mAChR is a G protein-linked receptor that increases IP_3 and DAG levels.
   c. **Cromolyn (NasalCrom)** inhibits the release of histamine from mast cells.
   d. **Beclomethasone, budesonide,** and **triamcinolone** are corticosteroids that have an anti-inflammatory effect by reducing the synthesis of arachidonic acid by phospholipase A_2 and inhibiting the expression of cyclooxygenase II (COX II).

XIII   Selected Photomicrographs

A. Blood-air barrier and type II pneumocyte (Figure 20-3)

B. Hyaline membrane disease, squamous cell carcinoma, cystic fibrosis (Figure 20-4)

C. Lung infections (Figure 20-5)

● Figure 20-3 Blood-air barrier and type II pneumocyte. (A) LM of an interalveolar septum. The junction of three alveoli (*alv*) is shown. The area within the box demonstrates the blood-air barrier, which separates the blood (RBC within the capillary) and air within the alveolus. **(B)** EM of boxed area in A shows the components of the blood-air barrier. The type I pneumocyte borders the air interface and the basal lamina, and the capillary endothelial cell borders the blood interface. The surfactant layer covering the type I pneumocyte is not shown. Note the histologic layers that air must traverse to get to the RBC. **(C)** EM of a type II pneumocyte with lamellar bodies (*LB*, and inset) that contain surfactant.

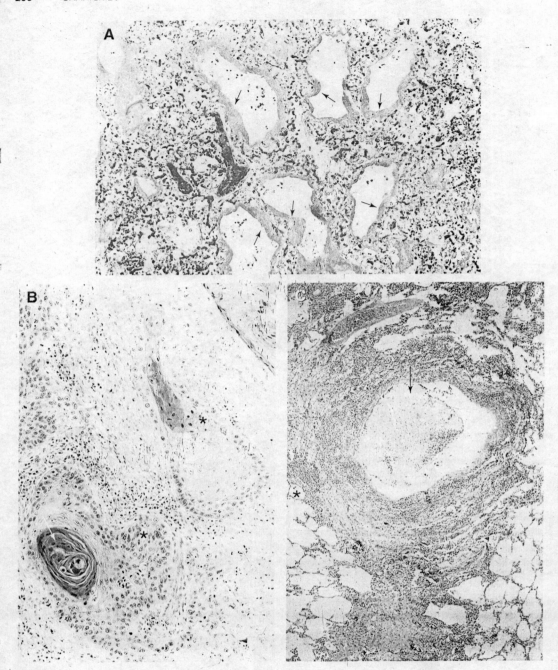

● **Figure 20-4 Lung pathology. (A)** LM of hyaline membrane disease as a result of respiratory distress syndrome (i.e., deficiency of surfactant). Note the air-filled bronchioles and alveolar ducts that are widely dilated. They are lined by a homogeneous hyaline material consisting of fibrin and necrotic cells (*arrows*). In addition, atelectasis or collapse of more distal alveoli is present. **(B)** LM of squamous cell carcinoma. Note the irregular nests (*) of squamous cell carcinoma. In some nests, keratinization is present (*arrow*). **(C)** LM of cystic fibrosis. A bronchus that is filled with thick mucus and inflammatory cells is shown (*arrow*). Smaller bronchi may be completely plugged by this material. In addition, surrounding the bronchus there is a heavy lymphocyte infiltration (*).

● **Figure 20-5 Lung infections. (A)** Aspergillosis. Fungal hyphae are impregnated with silver and appear as branching strands. **(B)** *Pneumocystis carinii*. The lung alveoli are filled with bubbly, protein-rich exudates. The cysts of *P. carinii* in the exudates are impregnated with silver and appear black. **(C)** Cytomegalovirus (CMV). Desquamated alveolar cells infected with CMV are markedly enlarged with large purple intranuclear inclusions surrounded by a clear halo. **(D)** Asbestosis. Asbestos bodies are beaded, dumbbell-shaped rods that stain with Prussian blue iron stain. **(E, F)** Tuberculosis. **(E)** Tuberculosis is characterized by caseating granulomas containing giant Langerhans' cells (*arrow*), which have a horseshoe-shaped pattern of nuclei. **(F)** *Mycobacterium tuberculosis* organisms are identified as red rods ("red snappers") by acid-fast Ziehl-Neelsen stain.

Case Study

A mother brings her 4-year-old son to your office complaining that "he coughs constantly and spits up a green mucus." After some discussion, she informs you that her son also has pungent, fatty stools; has had several bouts of severe coughing and fever within the past few months; and he had meconium ileus (obstruction of the bowel with a thick meconium) as a baby. Finally, she asks you this question, "Why is my son so small?" What is the most likely diagnosis?

Differentials

- Asthma, foreign body aspiration, pneumonia, selective IgA deficiency

Relevant Physical Exam Findings

- The boy is in the 10th percentile for height and 5th percentile for weight for children 4 years of age
- Fever = 101°F, tachypnea = 40 breaths/min, tachycardia = 155 bpm
- Auscultation of the lungs reveals diffuse, bilateral wheezing, rales, and coarse breath sounds.

Relevant Lab Findings

- Sweat test: Na^+ = High; Cl^- = High
- Stool sample showed steatorrhea
- Pulmonary function test: residual volume: total lung volume = High; FEV_1:FVC = Low
- Sputum culture: *Staphylococcus aureus* and *Pseudomonas aeruginosa* positive
- Radiograph: hyperinflation of lungs, early signs of bronchiectasis.

Diagnosis

Cystic Fibrosis (CF). CF is caused by production of abnormally thick mucus by epithelial cells lining the respiratory (and gastrointestinal tract). This results in obstruction of airways and recurrent bacterial infections (e.g., *Staphylococcus aureus*, *Pseudomonas aeruginosa*). CF is an autosomal recessive disease due to mutations of the CF gene, which is located on the long arm of chromosome 7 (q7). The CF gene encodes for a protein called CFTR (cystic fibrosis transporter), which functions as a Cl^- ion channel. In North America, 70% of CF cases are due to a three base deletion that codes for the amino acid phenylalanine at position #508 such that phenylalanine is missing from CFTR. CF is the most common lethal genetic disorder among whites. The primary manifestation of CF occur in the lungs and pancrease. In the lungs, the excessively viscous mucus leads to plugging of the lungs. In the pancreas, the release of pancreatic digestive enzymes is deficient leading to malabsorption and steatorrhea. One of the earliest signs of CF is failure to thrive in early childhood. Asthmatic patients have a low FEV_1: FVC and hyperinflation (similar to CF), but asthma is characterized by the reversibility of attacks and predisposes the patient to infections. Foreign body aspiration is usually unilateral and occurs most often on the right side. This 4-year-old boy has pneumonia but it is secondary to CF and the sputum culture is classic for pneumonia secondary to CF. Selective IgA deficiency is a congenital disorder in which class switching in the heavy chain fails to occur and is the most common congenital B cell defect. IgA is found in bodily secretions and plays an important role in preventing bacterial colonization of mucosal surfaces, which makes these patients susceptible to recurrent sinopulmonary infections.

Case Study

A 70-year-old man comes to your office complaining that "I'm starting to cough up blood. It's bright red and it scares me. I know I cough a lot because I'm a heavy smoker and when I get a cold in the winter it gets real bad. But it's always been a green mucus, never blood." He also tells you that "I'm short of breath and I've lost 15 pounds this past month because I have no appetite. I can't describe it, but this cough seems different." After some discussion, he informs you that he has smoked three packs of cigarettes a day for about 50 years and drinks a lot. "You know, Doc, when I smoke I like to drink and when I drink I like to smoke. It's a vicious cycle. But, like I tell my wife, I only have two bad habits in life. That's pretty good, isn't it?" What is the most likely diagnosis?

Differentials

- Bronchiectasis, Goodpasture syndrome, pneumonia, tuberculosis

Relevant Physical Exam Findings

- Tachypnea, positive end-expiratory wheezing, clubbing of the digits
- Lung auscultation: decreased breath sounds on the right side
- Patient appears frail.

Relevant Lab Findings

- Blood chemistry: WBCs = 8500/μL (Normal); Hct = 30% (Low); Mean corpuscular volume = 100 μm^3 (High); serum Ca^{2+} = 14.1 mg/dL (High)
- Sputum culture: normal respiratory flora; no acid-fast bacilli
- Urinalysis: ketones = none; leukocyte esterase = none; bacteria = none
- Chest radiograph: large mass in the lower right hilum; atelectasis in the right lower lobe
- Biopsy: keratin pearls and intercellular bridging are observed

Diagnosis

Squamous cell carcinoma (SQ). SQ has a 35% incidence and is most closely associated with smoking history. SQ is centrally located as it arises from larger bronchi owing to injury of the bronchial epithelium followed by regeneration from the basal layer in the from of squamous metaplasia. SQ begins as a small red granular plaque and progresses to a large intrabronchial mass. Cavitation of the lung may occur distal to the mass. SQ may secrete parathyroid hormone (PTH) causing hypercalcemia. SQ appears histologically as polygonal-shaped cells arranged in solid cell nests and bright eosinophilic aggregates of extracellular keratin ("pearls"). Intracellular keratinization may also be apparent such that the cytoplasm appears glassy and eosinophilic. In well-differentiated squamous cell carcinomas, intercellular bridges may be observed that are cytoplasmic extensions between adjacent cells. Another important histological characteristic of squamous cell carcinoma is the in *situ* replacement of the bronchial epithelium. As a rule, neither adenocarcinoma nor small cell carcinoma replaces the bronchial epithelium; instead, it tends to grow beneath the epithelium. Bronchiectasis is the abnormal, permanent dilatation of bronchi resulting from chronic necrotizing infection (e.g., *Staphylococcus, Streptococcus, Haemophilus influenzae*), bronchial obstruction (e.g., foreign body, mucous plugs, or tumors), or congenital conditions (e.g., Kartagener syndrome, cystic fibrosis, immunodeficiency disorders). The lower lobes of the lung are predominantly affected and the affected bronchi have a saccular appearance. Clinical findings of bronchiectasis include cough; fever; expectoration of large amounts of foul-smelling purulent sputum; crackles, rhonchi, and wheezing heard upon lung auscultation; chest radiograph shows prominent cystic spaces. Antiglomerular basement membrane glomerulonephritis (ABMG; Goodpasture syndrome) is caused by deposition of IgG immune complexes (i.e., autoantibodies to a globular noncollagenous domain of Type IV collagen) within the glomerular basement membrane. The autoantibodies generally cross, react with pulmonary basement membranes and therefore when both the lungs and kidneys are involved, the term Goodpasture syndrome is used. Pathologic findings of ABMG include glomerular crescents in >50% of glomeruli, which are formed by an inflammatory exudate containing macrophages and fibrin filling the urinary space and a proliferation of the simple squamous epithelium lining Bowman's capsule; immunofluorescence localizes IgG in a linear fashion along the GBM; electron microscopy shows focal breaks in the GBM but not immune dense deposits. Clinical findings of ABMG include patients present with a rapidly progressive renal failure; severe bloody cough (hemoptysis), dyspnea, hematuria, and nephritic syndrome. *Streptococcus pneumoniae* causes pneumococcal pneumonia. Pneumococcal pneumonia is the most common bacterial pneumonia in older adults (>65 years of age). Pneumococcal pneumonia is generally a consequence of altered immunity within the respiratory tract most frequently following a viral infection (e.g., influenza), which damages the mucociliary elevator, or chronic obstructive pulmonary disease (COPD), or alcoholism. Four stages of a classic bacteria pneumomia are described: 1) the initial stage features acute congestion, intra-alveolar fluid containing many bacteria, and few neutrophils. 2) the early consolidation or "red hepatization" (2–4 days) stage features consolidation with infiltration of a large number of neutrophils and intra-alveolar hemorrhage. The lung is red due to extravasated RBCs, firm, and airless with a liver-like consistency. 3) the late consolidation or "gray hepatization" (4–8 days) stage features large amounts of fibrin within the alveoli, lysis of the neutrophils, and appearance of macrophages which phagocytose the inflammatory debris. The lung has a gray-brown dry surface. 4) the resolution stage begins after 8 days. Clinical findings of pneumococcal pneumonia include: acute onset with fever, chills, chest pain secondary to pleural involvement, hemoptysis (rusty, blood-tinged sputum), chest radiograph shows lobar lung infiltrate. *Mycobacterium tuberculosis* causes tuberculosis (TB), which is the classic mycobacterial disease. Aerosolized infectious particles travel to terminal airways where *Mycobacterium tuberculosis* penetrates unactivated alveolar macrophages and inhibits acidification of endolysosomes so that alveolar macrophages can not kill the bacteria. However, replicating intracellular *Mycobacterium tuberculosis* stimulates CD8$^+$ cytotoxic T cells, which lyse infected cells and CD4$^+$ helper T cells, which release interferon-γ and other cytokines that activate macrophages to phagocytose and kill the bacteria. The Ghon complex is the first lesion of primary TB and consists of a parenchymal granuloma (location is subpleural and in lower lobes of the lung) and prominent, infected mediastinal lymph nodes. Most cases of primary TB are asymptomatic and resolve spontaneously. The genus *Mycobacterium* are Gram-positive bacilli that are poorly Gram-positive bacilli (rods), obligate aerobic, acid-fast (due to a waxy, hydrophobic, arabino-galactan-mycolate cell wall), endospore-negative, non-motile, and an intracellular pathogen. Clinical findings of TB include hemoptysis, weakness, night sweats, weight loss, chest radiograph shows localized consolidation, possibly with cavitation.

Chapter 21

Urinary System

I **General Features** (Figure 21-1). The kidneys are retroperitoneal organs that lie on the ventral surface of the quadratus lumborum muscle and lateral to the psoas muscle and vertebral column. They are covered by a fibrous capsule called the **renal capsule (or true capsule)**, which can be readily stripped from the surface of the kidney except in some pathologic conditions in which it is strongly adherent because of scarring. A *fresh* kidney that is hemisected in the sagittal plane shows a distinct outer **cortex** (a reddish-brown band 1–2 cm thick; its color is caused by its high degree of vascularization), inner **medulla** (lighter in color than the cortex), and **collecting system.** The functions of the kidney include regulation of the volume, osmolarity, mineral composition, and acidity (acid-base balance) of the body by excreting water and inorganic electrolytes (Na^+, Cl^-, K^+, Ca^{2+}, Mg^{2+}, SO_4^{2-}, PO_4^{2-}, H^+) in adequate amounts to achieve total-body balance and maintain their normal concentration in the extracellular fluid; excretion of metabolic waste products (urea, uric acid, creatinine, end products of hemoglobin breakdown, metabolites of various hormones, etc.); excretion of many foreign chemicals (drugs, pesticides, food additives, etc.); gluconeogenesis (during prolonged fasting, the kidneys synthesize glucose from amino acids and release glucose into the blood); secretion of the hormone **erythropoietin** by peritubular interstitial fibroblasts in the kidney cortex, which acts on the bone marrow to stimulate RBC formation (erythropoiesis); secretion of the enzyme **renin** by juxtaglomerular (JG) cells, which regulates blood pressure; hydroxylation of **25-(OH) vitamin D** to form 1,25-$(OH)_2$ vitamin D, which acts directly on osteoblasts to secrete IL-1, which stimulates osteoclasts to increase bone resorption and increases the absorption of Ca^{2+} from the intestinal lumen, thereby elevating blood Ca^{2+} levels.

A. **RENAL CAPSULE.** The kidney surface is covered by a connective tissue capsule that consists of fibroblasts, collagen, and myofibroblasts (with a contractile function). The capsule passes inward at the hilum, where it is continuous with the connective tissue of the renal sinus, renal pelvis, major calyces, and minor calyces.

B. **RENAL CORTEX.** The renal cortex lies under the capsule and also extends between the renal pyramids as the **renal columns of Bertin.** The renal cortex may be divided into the cortical labyrinth and the medullary rays.
1. **Cortical labyrinth.** The cortical labyrinth consists predominantly of: renal corpuscles [renal glomeruli plus the glomerular (Bowman's) capsule], proximal convoluted tubules, distal convoluted tubules, interlobular arteries, afferent and efferent arterioles, and a peritubular capillary bed.
2. **Medullar rays of Ferrein.** The medullary rays by light microscopy appear as striations perpendicular to the kidney surface that emanate from the renal medulla. The medullary rays consist predominantly of proximal straight tubules, distal straight tubules, cortical collecting ducts, and a peritubular capillary bed.

C. **RENAL MEDULLA.** The renal medulla is composed of **5–11 renal pyramids of Malpighi** whose tips terminate as 5–11 renal papille. The base of a renal pyramid abuts the renal cortex, whereas the tip of a renal pyramid (i.e., the renal papillae) abuts a minor calyx. The renal medulla may be divided into the outer medulla and inner medulla.

1. **Outer medulla.** The outer medulla consists predominantly of proximal straight tubules, descending thin limbs of the loop of Henle, ascending thin limbs of the loop of Henle, distal straight tubules, medullary collecting ducts, vasa recta, and a peritubular capillary bed.

2. **Inner medulla.** The inner medulla consists predominantly of descending thin limbs of the loop of Henle, ascending thin limbs of the loop of Henle, medullary collecting ducts, vasa recta, and a peritubular capillary bed. Vasa recta are absent near the tip of the renal papillae.

D. **RENAL LOBES.** A renal lobe consists of a renal pyramid and its associated cortical tissue at its base and sides (1/2 of each adjacent renal column). There are 5–11 renal lobes in the adult that corresponds to the number of renal pyramids. The renal lobes are conspicuous in the fetal kidney as a number of convexities on the surface, but these typically disappear in the adult kidney.

E. **RENAL LOBULE.** A renal lobule consists of a central medullary ray and its surrounding cortical labyrinth. Although the central medullary ray is conspicuous, the borders of a renal lobule within the cortical labyrinth are not distinct. The renal lobule extends into the medulla, although the borders of a renal lobule with the medullar are not distinct. A renal lobule is basically composed of all the nephrons that drain into the single collecting duct located in the medullary ray.

F. **COLLECTING SYSTEM.** The collecting system of the kidney includes the following:

1. **Collecting ducts.** The distal convoluted tubule is connected to the collecting ducts by **connecting tubules.** The collecting ducts located in the cortex are called **cortical collecting ducts.** As the cortical collecting ducts travel into the medulla, they are called **medullary collecting ducts.** As the medullary collecting ducts travel toward the renal papillae, they merge into larger collecting ducts called the **papillary ducts of Bellini.** The papillary ducts open onto the surface of the renal papillae at the **area cribrosa.** The collecting ducts are lined by a simple cuboidal epithelium that transitions into a simple columnar epithelium as the collecting ducts increases in size toward the renal papillae. The epithelium is composed of two cell types: **principal cells** and **intercalated cells (Type A and Type B).**

2. **5–11 Minor calyces.** The minor calyces are cup-shaped structures that abut the 5–11 renal papillae. The minor calyces consist of a transitional epithelium, a lamina propria rich in collagen and elastic fibers, and a smooth muscle layer that undergoes rhythmic peristaltic movements.

3. **2–3 Major calyces.** The major calyces are continuous with the minor calyces. The major calyces consist of a transitional epithelium, a lamina propria rich in collagen and elastic fibers, and a smooth muscle layer that undergoes rhythmic peristaltic movements.

4. **Renal pelvis.** The renal pelvis is continuous with the major calyces. The renal pelvis consists of a transitional epithelium, a lamina propria rich in collagen and elastic fibers, and a smooth muscle layer that undergoes rhythmic peristaltic movements.

G. **RENAL (URINIFEROUS) TUBULES** are classically considered the structural and functional units of the kidney and consist of the **nephron** and **collecting duct,** although this definition ignores the role of the renal vasculature (i.e., peritubular capillary bed, vasa recta).

H. **TYPES OF NEPHRONS.** Nephrons can be described based on their site of origin or the length of the loop of Henle.

1. **Site of origin.**
   a. **Cortical nephrons** originate in the outer region of the renal cortex.
   b. **Midcortical nephrons** originate in the middle region of the renal cortex.
   c. **Juxtamedullary nephrons** originate at the junction of the renal cortex and renal medulla (i.e., corticomedullary junction).

2. **Length of the loop of Henle**
   a. **Short-looped nephrons** have a loop of Henle that bends back in the outer medulla. Cortical nephrons and most midcortical nephrons are short-looped nephrons.
   b. **Long-looped nephrons** have a loop of Henle that bends back in the inner medulla. Some midcortical nephrons and all juxtamedullary nephrons are long-looped nephrons.

Ⅱ Renal Interstitium.

The renal interstitium is the connective tissue space between the uriniferous tubules and the blood vessels and is divided into the cortical interstitium and medullary interstitium.

A. **CORTICAL INTERSTITIUM.** The cortical interstitium makes up 7% of the total volume and contains the following components: predominantly fibroblasts, which synthesize an extracellular matrix (i.e., connective tissue), dendritic cells (antigen-presenting cells), macrophages, lymphocytes, and interstitial fluid (which plays an important physiologic role).

B. **MEDULLARY INTERSTITIUM.** The medullary interstitium makes up 20%–25% of the total volume and contains the following components: predominantly fibroblasts which synthesize an extracellular matrix (i.e., connective tissue), **interstitial cells,** which are oriented perpendicular to the long axis of the renal tubules and contain conspicuous lipid droplets, dendritic cells (antigen-presenting cells), macrophages, lymphocytes, and interstitial fluid (which plays an important physiologic role).

Ⅲ Nephrons

(Figure 21-1 and Table 21-1) consist of the following components:

A. **RENAL GLOMERULUS.** A renal glomerulus is a capillary bed (or tuft) that consists of a single layer of endothelial cells surrounded by a glomerular basement membrane. The capillaries within the renal glomerulus are **continuous, fenestrated capillaries without diaphragms.** A renal glomerulus receives blood from an **afferent arteriole** (a major site of autoregulation of renal blood flow) and is drained by an **efferent arteriole** (i.e., the **vascular pole**). A renal glomerulus is surrounded by a **glomerular (Bowman's) capsule.** A renal glomerulus is associated with a **glomerular mesangium,** which lies between the capillaries and consists of a **mesangial matrix** and **glomerular mesangial cells.** The mesangial matrix is an extracellular matrix of microfibrils and contains collagen (Types III, IV, V, and VI), microfibrillar proteins (fibrillin, MAGP, MP78, MP340), and fibronectin. The glomerular mesangial cells are irregular in shape, have many cell processes that extend toward the glomerular basement membrane, are attached to each other by desmosomes, and communicate with each other by gap junctions. The functions of mesangial cells include the following: synthesis of the mesangial matrix, which is frequently increased in glomerular disease; phagocytosis of colloids, macromolecules, protein aggregates, and immune complexes trapped by the glomerular basement membrane; contraction and relaxation in response to a number of vasoactive agents [e.g., angiotensin II and atrial natriuretic peptide (ANP)] produce cytokines and prostaglandins; and a target cell in many glomerular diseases and respond by injury, repair, and proliferation.

B. GLOMERULAR (BOWMAN'S) CAPSULE. The glomerular capsule is a double-layered capsule that consists of an outer **parietal layer** and an inner **visceral layer.** The parietal layer consists of a **simple squamous epithelium** that lines the outer wall of the glomerular capsule and becomes continuous with the simple cuboidal epithelium of the proximal convoluted tubule. The visceral layer consists of **podocytes** that extend cell processes to the glomerular basement membrane surrounding the capillaries of the renal glomerulus and is reflected to become continuous with the parietal layer. The space between the parietal and visceral layers of the glomerular capsule is called the **urinary (Bowman's) space.** The urinary space receives an ultrafiltrate of plasma produced by filtration through the glomerular filtration barrier and is continuous with the lumen of the proximal convoluted tubule (i.e., the **urinary pole**).

C. PROXIMAL CONVOLUTED TUBULE (PCT). The PCT consists of simple cuboidal epithelial cells with a distinctly acidophilic cytoplasm, brush border (i.e., microvilli), intercellular zonula occludens (tight junctions), apical endocytic vesicles, lateral interdigitations, and basal infoldings with numerous mitochondria. The physiological functions of the PCT include the following:

1. The PCT reabsorbs (tubular fluid → plasma) **100% of filtered organic nutrients** (e.g., glucose, amino acids, water-soluble vitamins (B complex and C), lactate, acetate, ketones (ß hydroxybutyrate, acetoacetate), Krebs cycle intermediates) using the carrier proteins: **Na^+-K^+ ATPase, Na^+-organic nutrient cotransporters,** and other **organic nutrient transporters.**

2. The PCT reabsorbs (tubular fluid → plasma) **100% of filtered proteins, 100% of filtered polypeptides, and 50% of filtered urea** using **specific protein receptors** and **peptidases.**

3. The PCT secretes (plasma → tubular fluid) **100% of non-filtered organic anions** (e.g., para-aminohippuric acid, urate, bile salts, fatty acids, hydroxybenzoates, acetazolamide, chlorothiazide, penicillin, salicylates, sulfonamides) using the carrier proteins: **Na^+-K^+ ATPase, Na^+-dicarboxylate/tricarboxylate cotransporter, organic anion-dicarboxylate/tricarboxylate exchanger,** and **organic anion-X exchanger.**

4. The PCT secretes (plasma → tubular fluid) **100% of the non-filtered organic cations** (e.g., acetylcholine, creatinine, dopamine, epinephrine, norepinephrine, histamine, serotonin, atropine, isoproterenol, cimetidine, morphine, etc.) using the carrier proteins: **Na^+-K^+ ATPase, organic cation-? exchanger,** and **organic cation-X^+ exchanger.**

5. The PCT reabsorbs (tubular fluid → plasma) **65% of the filtered Na^+** isosmotically using the carrier proteins: **Na^+-K^+ ATPase, Na^+-organic nutrient cotransporters, Na^+-H^+ exchanger,** and **Na^+-HCO_3^- cotransporer.**

6. The PCT reabsorbs (tubular fluid → plasma) **65% of filtered Cl^-** using the carrier proteins: **Na^+-K^+ ATPase, Na^+-H^+ exchanger, Cl^- base exchanger,** and **K^+-Cl^- cotransporter.**

7. The PCT reabsorbs (tubular fluid → plasma) **65% of the filtered H_2O** using **aquaporin H_2O channels** and the paracellular route.

8. The PCT reabsorbs (tubular fluid → plasma) **55% of the filtered K^+** using the paracellular route.

9. The PCT reabsorbs (tubular fluid → plasma) **80% of the filtered Ca^{2+} using the paracellular route.**

10. The PCT reabsorbs (tubular fluid → plasma) **85% of the filtered PO$_4$$^{2-}$ using the carrier proteins: Na$^+$-K$^+$ ATPase, Na$^+$- PO$_4$$^{2-}$ cotransporter, and PO$_4$$^{2-}$-anion exchanger.**

11. The PCT reabsorbs (tubular fluid → plasma) **80% of the filtered HCO$_3$$^-$ using the carrier proteins: H$^+$ ATPase, Na$^+$-H$^+$ exchanger, and Na$^+$-HCO$_3$$^-$ cotransporter.**

12. The PCT **secretes H$^+$ and NH$^+$$_4$ using the carrier proteins: H$^+$ ATPase, Na$^+$-H$^+$ exchanger, and Na$^+$-NH$_4$$^+$ exchanger.**

D. LOOP OF HENLE

1. **Proximal straight tubule (PST).** The PST is similar in morphology to the PCT. The physiologic functions of the PST include the following:
    a. The PST reabsorbs (tubular fluid → plasma) **5% of the filtered H$_2$O using aquaporin H$_2$O channels** and the paracellular route.
    b. The PST is **permeable to H$_2$O.**

2. **Descending thin limb (DTL).** The DTL consists of simple squamous epithelial cells with deep intercellular zonula occludens (tight junctions), no lateral interdigitations, and a few microvilli. The physiologic functions of the DTL include the following:
    a. The DTL reabsorbs (tubular fluid → plasma) **5% of the filtered H$_2$O using aquaporin H$_2$O channels** and the paracellular route.
    b. The DTL is **permeable to H$_2$O.**

3. **Ascending thin limb (ATL).** The ATL consists of simple squamous epithelial cells with shallow intercellular zonula occludens (tight junctions) and extensive lateral interdigitations. The physiologic functions of the ATL include the following:
    a. The ATL reabsorbs (tubular fluid → plasma) **10% of the filtered Na$^+$ by passive transport ("downhill"),** the mechanism of which is poorly understood.
    b. The ATL reabsorbs (tubular fluid → plasma) **10% of the filtered Cl$^-$ by passive transport ("downhill"),** the mechanism of which is poorly understood.
    c. The ATL is **impermeable to H$_2$O.**

4. **Distal straight tubule (DST).** The DST consists of simple cuboidal epithelial cells with intercellular zonula occludens (tight junctions), lateral interdigitations, and basal infoldings with numerous mitochondria. The DST has no conspicuous brush border (i.e., microvilli). In the region of the afferent and efferent arterioles, the DST contains specialized cells called **macula densa cells.** The DST synthesizes the **Tamm-Horsfall glycoprotein,** which is the most abundant constituent of renal tubule casts found in many diseases. The physiologic functions of the DST include the following:
    a. The DST reabsorbs (tubular fluid → plasma) **15% of the filtered Na$^+$** by the paracellular route and using the carrier proteins: **Na$^+$-K$^+$ ATPase, Na$^+$-K$^+$-2Cl$^-$ cotransporter, Na$^+$-H$^+$ exchanger, and Na$^+$-HCO$_3$$^-$ cotransporter.**
    b. The DST reabsorbs (tubular fluid → plasma) **15% of the filtered Cl$^-$ using** the carrier proteins and ion channel proteins: **Na$^+$-K$^+$ ATPase, Na$^+$-K$^+$-2Cl$^-$ cotransporter, K$^+$-Cl$^-$ cotransporter, and Cl$^-$ ion channel protein.**
    c. The DST reabsorbs (tubular fluid → plasma) **30% of the filtered K$^+$** by the paracellular route and using the carrier proteins: **Na$^+$-K$^+$ ATPase and Na$^+$-K$^+$-2Cl$^-$ cotransporter.**
    d. The DST reabsorbs (tubular fluid → plasma) **10% of the filtered Ca^{2+}** by the paracellular route.
    e. The DST reabsorbs (tubular fluid → plasma) **10% of the filtered HCO$_3$$^-$ using the** carrier proteins: **H$^+$ ATPase, Na$^+$-H$^+$ exchanger, and Na$^+$-HCO$_3$$^-$ cotransporter.**

f. The DST secretes (plasma → tubular fluid) H^+ using the carrier proteins: **H^+ ATPase** and **Na^+-H^+ Exchanger.**

g. The DST is **impermeable to H_2O.**

E. **DISTAL CONVOLUTED TUBULE (DCT).** The DCT consists of simple cuboidal epithelial cells with intercellular zonula occludens (tight junctions), lateral interdigitations, and basal infoldings with numerous mitochondria. The DCT has no conspicuous brush border (i.e., microvilli). The physiologic functions of the DCT include the following:

1. The DCT reabsorbs (tubular fluid → plasma) **5% of the filtered Na^+** using the carrier proteins and ion channel proteins: **Na^+-K^+ ATPase, Na^+-Cl^- cotransporter,** and **Na^+ ion channel protein.**

2. The DCT reabsorbs (tubular fluid → plasma) **5% of the filtered Cl^-** using the carrier proteins and ion channel proteins: **Na^+-K^+ ATPase, Na^+-Cl^- cotransporter,** and **Cl^- ion channel protein.**

3. The DCT is **impermeable to H_2O.**

4. The DCT reabsorbs (tubular fluid → plasma) **filtered K^+** by the paracellular route when a person is on a low K^+ diet (K^+ depleted).

5. The DCT reabsorbs (tubular fluid → plasma) **5% of the filtered Ca^{2+}** using the carrier proteins and ion channel proteins: **Ca^{2+} ATPase, Na^+-Ca^{2+} exchanger, Na^+-K^+ ATPase,** and **Ca^{2+} ion channel protein.**

IV Collecting Duct (CD). The CD consists basically of a simple cuboidal → simple columnar epithelium composed of two cell types: **principal cells** and **intercalated cells (Type A and Type B).** Principal cells are found in both cortical and medullary collecting ducts and change in size from simple cuboidal → simple columnar. Intercalated cells are found predominantly in the cortical collecting ducts and their number gradually decreases in the medullary collecting ducts until they are completely absent in the largest papillary ducts. **Principal cells** have the following characteristics: simple cuboidal → simple columnar, a few short microvilli and one cilium, intercellular zonula occludens (tight junctions), apical endocytic profiles, no lateral infoldings, basal infoldings with numerous mitochondria, and they possess antidiuretic hormone (ADH) receptors. **Type A intercalated cells** have the following characteristics: polygonal-shaped, distinctive microfolds on the luminal membrane, intercellular zonula occludens (tight junctions), apical endocytic profiles, no lateral infoldings, no basal infoldings, and H^+ ATPase located on the luminal membrane. **Type B intercalated cells** have the following characteristics: polygonal-shaped, no distinctive microfolds on the luminal membrane, intercellular zonula occludens (tight junctions), apical endocytic profiles, no lateral infoldings, no basal infoldings, and H^+ ATPase located on the basolateral membrane. The CD is divided into the **cortical CD** (that portion of the CD found in the kidney cortex) and the **medullary CD** (that portion of the CD found in the kidney medulla). The physiologic functions of the various cell types of the CD include the following:

A. **PRINCIPAL CELLS**

1. The principal cells of the CD reabsorb (tubular fluid → plasma) **5% of the filtered Na^+** using the carrier proteins and ion channel proteins: **Na^+-K^+ ATPase** and **Na^+ ion channel protein.**

2. The principal cells of the CD reabsorb (tubular fluid → plasma) **5%–25% of the filtered H_2O** depending on the H_2O balance of the person by the paracellular route and using the **aquaporin H_2O channel.**

3. The principal cells of the CD reabsorb (tubular fluid → plasma) **5% of the filtered Ca^{2+}** using the carrier proteins and ion channel proteins: Ca^{2+} **ATPase, Na^+-Ca^{2+} exchanger, Na^+-K^+ ATPase and Ca^{2+} ion channel protein.**

4. The principal cells of the CD reabsorb (tubular fluid → plasma) **10% of the filtered urea** using the carrier protein: **urea transporter.**

5. The principal cells of the CD secrete (plasma → tubular fluid) **plasma K^+** when a person is on a high/normal K^+ diet using the carrier proteins and ion channel proteins: Na^+-K^+ **ATPase and K^+ ion channel protein.**

⊕ **Figure 21-1 Diagram of the kidney and renal tubules.** The renal tubules consist of a nephron and collecting duct. The nephron (shaded area) consists of the renal glomerulus formed by the afferent arteriole (aa) and efferent arteriole (ea), Bowman's capsule (BC), proximal convoluted tubule (PCT), proximal straight tubule (PST), descending thin limb (DTL), ascending thin limb (ATL), distal straight tubule (DST), and distal convoluted tubule (DCT). Note the histologic appearance of each of the tubules.

TABLE 21-1	PHYSIOLOGIC FUNCTIONS OF RENAL TUBULES

Tubules	Functions
PCT	**Reabsorption from tubular fluid → plasma:** 100% of organic nutrients (glucose, amino acids, water-soluble vitamins [B complex and C], lactate, acetate, ketones [β-hydroxybutyrate, acetoacetate], and Krebs cycle intermediates) 100% of proteins and polypeptides and 50% of urea, 65% of Na^+, 65% of Cl^-, 65% of H_2O, 55% of K^+, 80% of Ca^{2+}, 85% of PO_4^{2-}, and 80% of HCO_3^- **Secretion from plasma → tubular fluid:** 100% of organic anions (*para*-aminohippuric acid, urate, bile salts, fatty acids, hydroxybenzoates, acetazolamide, chlorothiazide, penicillin, salicylates, and sulfonamides) 100% of organic cations (acetylcholine, creatinine, dopamine, epinephrine, norepinephrine, histamine, serotonin, atropine, isoproterenol, cimetidine, and morphine) H^+ and NH_4^+
Loop of Henle	
PST	**Reabsorption from tubular fluid → plasma:** 5% of H_2O; (permeable to H_2O)
DTL	**Reabsorption from tubular fluid → plasma:** 5% of H_2O; (permeable to H_2O)
ATL	**Reabsorption from tubular fluid → plasma:** 10% of Na^+, 10% of Cl^-; (impermeable to H_2O)
DST	**Reabsorption from tubular fluid → plasma:** 15% of Na^+, 15% of Cl^-, 30% of K^+, 10% of Ca^{2+}, 10% of HCO_3^- (impermeable to H_2O) **Secretion from plasma → tubular fluid:** H^+
DCT	**Reabsorption from tubular fluid → plasma:** 5% of Na^+, 5% of Cl^-, K^+ (low K^+ diet), 5% of Ca^{2+}; (impermeable to H_2O)
CD (principal cells)	**Reabsorption from tubular fluid → plasma:** 5% of Na^+, 5%–25% of H_2O (depending on water balance), 5% of Ca^{2+}, 10% of urea **Secretion from plasma → tubular fluid:** K^+ (high/normal diet)
CD (Type A cells)	**Reabsorption from tubular fluid → plasma:** 10% of HCO_3^-, K^+ (low-K^+ diet) **Secretion from plasma → tubular fluid:** H^+
CD (Type B Cells)	**Reabsorption from tubular fluid → plasma:** 5% of Cl^- **Secretion from Plasma → tubular fluid:** HCO_3^-

PCT—proximal convoluted tubule; PST—proximal straight tubule; DTL—descending thin limb; ATL—ascending thin limb; DST—distal straight tubule; DCT—distal convoluted tubule; CD—collecting duct.

B. TYPE A INTERCALATED CELLS

1. The Type A cells of the CD reabsorb (tubular fluid → plasma) **10% of the filtered HCO_3^-** using the carrier proteins and ion channel proteins: **H^+ ATPase, H^+-K^+ ATPase, Cl^- -HCO_3^- exchanger, Cl^- ion channel protein**, and **K^+ ion channel protein**.

2. The Type A cells of the CD reabsorb (tubular fluid → plasma) **filtered K^+** when a person is on a low K^+ diet (K^+ depleted) using the carrier proteins and ion channel proteins: **H^+-K^+ ATPase** and **K^+ ion channel protein**.

3. The Type A cells of the CD secrete (plasma → tubular fluid) **H^+** using the carrier proteins and ion channel proteins: **H^+ ATPase, H^+-K^+ ATPase,** and **K^+ ion channel protein**.

C. TYPE B INTERCALATED CELLS

1. The Type B cells of the CD reabsorb (tubular fluid → plasma) **5% of the filtered Cl^-** using the carrier proteins and ion channel proteins: **H^+ ATPase, Cl^- -HCO_3^- exchanger, Cl^- ion channel protein**.

2. The Type B cells of the CD **secrete HCO_3^-** during alkalosis using the carrier proteins: **H^+ ATPase** and **Cl^--HCO_3^- exchanger**. Normally, HCO_3^- is minimal.

Renal Vasculature (Figure 21-2)

A. **ARTERIAL SUPPLY.** The **renal artery** branches into **five segmental arteries.** The segmental arteries branch into **5–11 interlobar arteries.** The interlobar arteries branch into the **arcuate arteries,** which travel along the base of the renal pyramids at the corticomedullary junction. The arcuate arteries branch into the **interlobular arteries,** which travel through the cortex toward the capsule and branch into numerous **afferent arterioles.** Each afferent arteriole forms a capillary bed (or tuft) called the **renal glomerulus,** which is drained by an **efferent arteriole.** The efferent arteriole has two fates:

1. **Formation of the cortical peritubular capillary bed.** The efferent arteriole of renal glomeruli from cortical and midcortical nephrons branches into a **cortical peritubular capillary bed** that is intimately associated with renal tubules in the cortex. Note that the renal glomerulus and cortical peritubular capillary bed are two capillary beds connected in series by the efferent arteriole.

2. **Formation of the vasa recta (hairpin loop).** The efferent arteriole of renal glomeruli from juxtamedullary nephrons branches into **12–25 descending vasa recta** which are long, straight capillaries that run to varying depths of the medulla. The ends of the descending vasa recta give rise to a **medullary peritubular capillary bed** that is intimately associated with renal tubules in the medulla. The venous ends of the capillaries converge to form **ascending vasa recta,** which then completes the hairpin loop. The vasa recta are part of the **countercurrent exchanger system,** which maintains the hyperosmolarity gradient of the interstitial fluid in the medulla that is crucial for urine concentration. Note that the renal glomerulus and the vasa recta/medullary peritubular capillary bed are two capillary beds connected in series by the efferent arteriole.

B. **VENOUS DRAINAGE.**

1. **Kidney surface and capsule.** The venous ends of a capillary bed near the kidney surface and capillaries of the kidney capsule drain into **stellate veins.** Stellate veins drain into **interlobular veins.** The interlobular veins drain into **arcuate veins.** The arcuate veins drain into **interlobar veins,** which anastomose and converge to form the **renal vein.**

2. **Cortical venous drainage.** The venous ends of the cortical peritubular capillary bed converge to drain into **interlobular veins.** The interlobular veins drain into **arcuate veins.** The arcuate veins drain into **interlobar veins,** which anastomose and converge to form the **renal vein.**

3. **Medullary venous drainage.** The venous ends of the medullary capillary bed converge to form **ascending vasa recta** which completes the hairpin loop. The ascending vasa recta drain into both **the interlobular veins** and **arcuate veins.** The arcuate veins drain into **interlobar veins,** which anastomose and converge to form the **renal vein.**

Hormonal Control of the Kidney (Figure 21-3)

A. **ANGIOTENSIN II.** Angiotensin II is produced by the conversion of angiotensin I by **angiotensin-converting enzyme (ACE)** primarily by the endothelium of lung capillaries. Angiotensin II has many widespread actions that include actions on the kidney.

1. Angiotensin II acts on the **epithelial cells of the proximal convoluted tubule** and causes **increased Na^+ reabsorption** (tubular fluid $\rightarrow$ plasma) and therefore **decreased Na^+ excretion in the urine.**

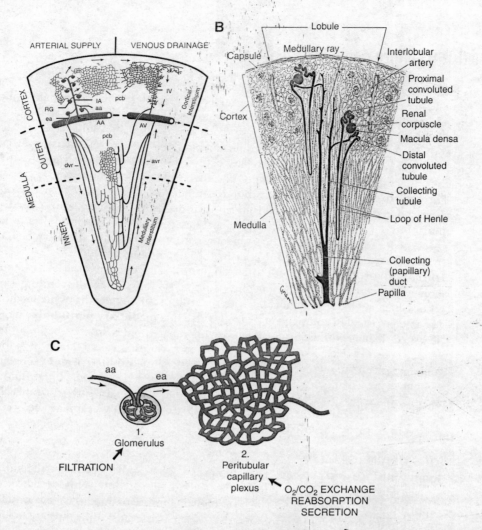

● **Figure 21-2 (A) Diagram of the arterial supply and venous drainage of the kidney.** The boundary between the renal cortex and renal medulla *(dashed line)* is shown. The renal medulla can be further subdivided into the outer medulla and inner medulla. The boundary between the outer medulla and inner medulla *(dotted line)* is shown. Note the various segments of the renal vasculature that are present in the cortex, outer medulla, and inner medulla. The arcuate arteries (AA) branch into interlobular arteries (IA). The interlobular arteries give off numerous afferent arterioles. The afferent arteriole forms a capillary bed (or tuft) called the renal glomerulus (RG). The renal glomerulus is drained by the efferent arteriole (ea). Note the two fates of the efferent arteriole (ea). **Fate One:** The efferent arteriole from renal glomeruli from cortical or midcortical nephrons branches into a cortical peritubular capillary bed (pcb). The venous ends of the cortical peritubular capillary bed converge to drain into the interlobular veins (IV). The interlobular veins drain into the arcuate veins (AV). **Fate Two:** The efferent arteriole of renal glomeruli from juxtamedullary nephrons branches into 12–25 descending vasa recta (dvr), which are long, straight capillaries that run to varying depths of the medulla. The ends of the descending vasa recta give rise to a medullary peritubular capillary bed (pcb). The venous ends of the medullary peritubular capillary bed converge to form the ascending vasa recta (avr). The ascending vasa recta drain into both the interlobular vein (IV) and the arcuate vein (AV). Arrows indicate the direction of blood flow. The renal interstitium is indicated by gray shading. **(B)** Diagram indicating the renal tubules (black) in the cortex and medulla of the kidney. The difficulty in understanding the histology of the kidney involves the superimposition of the renal vasculature network on the renal tubule system. Figure A and B will help the student in this superimposition. **(C)** A diagram to indicate that in the kidney there are two capillary networks **arranged in series.** The afferent arteriole forms a capillary network called the renal glomerulus, which is involved in filtration of the blood. The efferent arteriole forms the peritubular capillary plexus, which is involved in O_2/CO_2 exchange for the renal tubules, reabsorption of substances from the tubular fluid into the blood (tubular fluid → plasma), and secretion of substances from the blood into the tubular fluid (plasma → tubular fluid).

2. Angiotensin II acts on the **smooth muscle cells of the afferent and efferent arterioles** and causes **vasoconstriction** of the afferent and efferent arterioles and therefore **decreases the glomerular filtration rate (GFR).**

3. Angiotensin II also plays a role in ADH and ALD secretion.

B. **ANTIDIURETIC HORMONE (ADH).** ADH is secreted by axon terminal within the **neurohypophysis** whose cell bodies are located in the **supraoptic nucleus** and **paraventricular nucleus** of the hypothalamus. The most important inputs to these neurons are from baroceptors and osmoreceptors. **Baroreceptors** in the walls of the common carotid arteries (carotid sinus), great veins, atria, and aortic arch respond to decreased blood pressure and stimulate ADH secretion. **Osmoreceptors** in the hypothalamus respond to increased plasma osmolarity and stimulate ADH secretion. **Angiotensin II** also stimulates ADH secretion.

1. ADH acts on the **principal cells of the cortical and medullary collecting ducts** and causes **increased H_2O reabsorption** (tubular fluid → plasma) and therefore **decreased H_2O excretion in the urine.**

2. **Clinical consideration. Syndrome of inappropriate ADH secretion (SIADH)** is caused by pulmonary disorders (e.g., small cell carcinoma with ectopic secretion of ADH, tuberculosis), drugs (e.g., chlorpropamide, cyclophosphamide, morphine, carbamazepine, oxytocin), and central nervous system disorders (e.g., tumor, infection, hypopituitarism) cause the loss of the inhibitory effect of cortisol on ADH. SIADH is characterized by **excessively increased H_2O reabsorption** (tubular fluid → plasma) and, therefore, **excessively decreased H_2O excretion** in the urine. This results in a dilutional hyponatremia (low serum Na^+) and a great increase in total body water. Eventually, the effective arterial blood volume is increased, leading to an inhibition of the rennin-angiotensin system; hence, no aldosterone is secreted. This leads to decreased Na^+ reabsorption, increased loss of urea, and increased loss of uric acid. The trial of **hyponatremia, low serum BUN (blood urea nitrogen)**, and **hypouricemia** is virtually pathognomonic for SIADH.

C. **ALDOSTERONE (ALD).** ALD is secreted by the **zona glomerulosa cells of the adrenal cortex.** The secretion of ALD is controlled by **angiotensin II** of the renin-angiotensin system.

1. ALD acts on the **principal cells of the cortical collecting duct** and causes **increased Na^+ reabsorption** (tubular fluid → plasma) and therefore **decreased Na^+ excretion in the urine.** ALD is the most important controller of Na^+ reabsorption.

2. ALD acts on the **principal cells of the cortical collecting duct** and causes **increased K^+ secretion** (plasma → tubular fluid) and thereby **increases K^+ excretion in the urine.**

3. ALD acts on the **Type A intercalated cells of the cortical collecting duct** and causes **increased H^+ secretion** (plasma → tubular fluid).

D. **A-TYPE NATRIURETIC PEPTIDE (ANP).** ANP is secreted by **myocardial endocrine cells** located within the right and left atria of the heart. ANP is secreted in response to increased blood volume (pressure) or increased venous pressure with the atria of the heart. ANP binds to the NPR-A and NPR-C receptors. The NPR-A receptor is a G protein–linked receptor. The NPR-C receptor is believed to be a "decoy receptor," because it lacks an intracellular domain.

1. ANP acts on the **principal cells of the medullary collecting ducts** and causes **decreased Na^+ reabsorption** (tubular fluid → plasma) and therefore **increased Na^+ secretion in the urine.**

2. ANP acts on the **smooth muscle cells of the efferent arteriole** and causes **vaso-constriction** of the efferent arteriole and therefore **increases glomerular filtration rate (GFR).**

E. B-TYPE NATRIURETIC PEPTIDE (BNP). BNP is secreted by myocardial endocrine cells located within the right and left ventricles of the heart. BNP binds to the NPR-A and NPR-C receptors. BNP is secreted in congestive heart failure and has a diuretic effect on the kidney (similar to that of ANP). **Natrecor (nesiritide)** is a relatively new recombinant DNA human sequence of BNP and has been approved for short-term management of decompensated congestive heart failure.

● **Figure 21-3 Diagram of hormonal control of the kidney.** *BG* = Bowman's or glomerular capsule; *PCT* = proximal convoluted tubule; *PST* = proximal straight tubule of the loop of Henle; *DTL* = descending thin limb of the loop of Henle; *ATL* = ascending thin limb of the loop of Henle; *DST* = distal straight tubule of the loop of Henle; *DCT* = distal convoluted tubule; *corCD* = cortical collecting duct medCD; *CT* = connecting tubule; *aa* = afferent arteriole; *ea* = efferent arteriole; *ANGI II* = angiotensin II; *ADH* = antidiuretic hormone; *ALD* = aldosterone; *ANP* = atrial natriuretic peptide.

VII Glomerular Filtration Barrier (GFB) (Figure 21-4) Urine formation begins with filtration, which occurs where the renal glomerulus and the glomerular (Bowman's) capsule interact to form the GFB. Filtration is the bulk flow of fluid from the glomerular capillaries into the urinary (Bowman's) space to form tubular fluid.

A. THE COMPONENTS OF GFB include:

1. **Glomerular capillary endothelium.** The glomerular capillary endothelium is a **continuous, fenestrated (without diaphragms) endothelium.** The fenestrae are 70- to 90-nm diameter pores that are not bridged by diaphragms, as usually occurs in other capillaries. The endothelial cells possess **aquaporin H_2O channels** that allow fast movement of H_2O through the endothelium, **cell surface polyanionic glycoproteins** (e.g., podocalyxin) that impart a negative surface charge to the endothelial cells and **integrins** that bind to fibronectin in the glomerular basement membrane.

2. **Glomerular basement membrane (GBM).** The GBM is a 300- to 350-nm thick basement membrane that is synthesized jointly by the glomerular capillary endothelium and podocytes. The GBM consists of **Type IV collagen ($\alpha_1 - \alpha_6$) chains), heparan sulfate proteoglycan (also called perlecan),** which is important in imparting a negative charge, **laminin (glycoprotein), fibronectin (glycoprotein),** and **entactin (glycoprotein).** By electron microscopy three layers of the GBM have been described:

   a. **Lamina rara interna.** The lamina rara interna is an electron-lucent layer of the GBM located adjacent to the glomerular capillary endothelium. This layer is characterized by the α_1 and α_2 chains of Type IV collagen [α_1 (IV) and α_2 (IV)] and a large amount of **heparan sulfate,** which imparts a high negative charge to this layer.

   b. **Lamina densa.** The lamina densa is an electron-dense layer of the GBM located between the lamina rara interna and lamina rara externa. This layer is characterized by a fairly dense network of the α_3 and α_4 chains of Type IV collagen [α_3 (IV) and α_4 (IV)].

   c. **Lamina rara externa.** The lamina rara externa is an electron-lucent layer of the GBM located adjacent to the podocytes. This layer is characterized by a large amount of **heparin sulfate,** which imparts a high negative charge to this layer.

3. **Slit diaphragms of podocytes.** The podocytes have voluminous cell bodies that bulge into the urinary space and make up the visceral layer of the glomerular (Bowman's) capsule. The cell bodies give rise to **foot processes** that extend toward and make contact with the GBM. The foot processes from neighboring podocytes regularly interdigitate with one another, thereby forming elongated 25-nm wide spaces called **filtration slits.** The filtration slits are bridged by **slit diaphragms,** which by electron microscopy appear as rows of "pores" on either side of a central, electron dense bar through which filtration occurs. The podocytes possess **cell surface polyanionic glycoproteins** (e.g., podocalyxin) that impart a negative surface charge to the foot processes and slit diaphragms and **integrins** that bind to fibronectin in the glomerular basement membrane.

B. THE FUNCTIONS OF THE GFB include:

1. Prevents passage of red blood cells, leukocytes, and platelets

2. Restricts passage of proteins >70,000d (**"size filter"**) and negatively charged substances (**"charge filter"**). The GFB provides no hindrance to molecules <7,000d and almost total hindrance to plasma albumin (**70,000d**). For molecules between **7,000d** ⇔ **70,000d,** the amount filtered becomes progressively smaller as the molecule becomes larger. For any given molecular size, negatively charged molecules are

filtered to a lesser extent and positively charged molecules to a greater extent versus neutral molecules. The reason is that the GFB is negatively charged (due to heparan sulfate), which repels negatively charged molecules. Since almost all plasma proteins are negatively charged, the charge hindrance of the GFB plays an important role of enhancing the size hindrance. Note that the "charge filter" does not a affect ions.

3. Permits passage of water, cations, anions, and other small molecules.

4. Forms an ultrafiltrate of blood

● **Figure 21-4 (A) Diagram of the renal glomerulus and the glomerular (Bowman's) capsule.** Note that the renal glomerulus is actually part of the renal vasculature but there is an intimate histologic relationship between the glomerular capillaries and the glomerular capsule. Hence, the glomerular capillaries and the glomerular capsule are sometimes called the renal corpuscle. The glomerular capillaries are covered by podocytes and their foot processes called the visceral layer of glomerular capsule. The podocytes reflect to become continuous with the simple squamous epithelium of the parietal layer of the glomerular capsule. The parietal layer of the glomerular capsule becomes continuous with the simple cuboidal epithelium of the proximal convoluted tubule at the urinary pole (UP). The renal glomerulus receives blood from the afferent arteriole (aa) and is drained by the efferent arteriole (ea) at the vascular pole (VP). JG = juxtaglomerular cells; MD = macula densa cells; DST = distal straight tubule; EGM = extraglomerular mesangial cells; SM = smooth muscle; Pod = podocyte; FP = foot process; PCT = proximal convoluted tubule; BS = blood space; US = urinary space; GBM = glomerular basement membrane **(B)** LM of the glomerulus and Bowman's capsule. Podocytes (P), which comprise the visceral layer of Bowman's capsule are indicated. Simple squamous epithelium (single arrows), which comprise the parietal layer of Bowman's capsule are also indicated. Filtration from the blood space (BS) to the urinary space (US) is also indicated (see arrow). **(C)** EM of the glomerular filtration barrier. A podocyte (P) with its foot processes and filtration slits is adjacent to the basement lamina. The glomerular capillary consists of an endothelium that is fenestrated (pore) with no diaphragms. Filtration from the blood space (BS) to the urinary space (US) is indicated (see arrow). **(D)** Scanning electron micrograph of the renal glomerulus. A podocyte cell body (PCB) and foot processes (FP; arrows) are shown covering a capillary.

VIII **Juxtaglomerular (JG) Complex** (Figure 21.5). The JG complex is a composite specialized structure located where the distal straight tubule (DST) of the nephron makes contact with the vascular pole of the glomerulus (i.e. the afferent and efferent arterioles).

A. **THE COMPONENTS OF THE JG COMPLEX include:**
1. **Macula densa (MD) cells.** The MD cells are **modified epithelial cells of the DST** that are located where the DST makes contact with the vascular pole of the glomerulus. MD cells have the following characteristics: columnar-shaped, crowded nuclei that appear to be superimposed on each other, microvilli, and connected by desmosomes. **MD cells monitor changes in Na⁺ levels in the DST fluid and stimulate the release of renin from JG cells.**

2. **JG cells.** The JG cells are **modified smooth muscle cells** that are located in clusters of four to five cells in the tunica media of the afferent arteriole and early portion of the efferent arteriole. JG cells have the following characteristics: a spherical nucleus, many cell processes, communication with neighboring cells through gap junctions, and have distinct granules that contain **renin** (a proteolytic enzyme). **JG cells secrete renin, monitor changes in blood pressure** (i.e., act as intrarenal baroreceptors), and are **innervated by postganglionic sympathetic nerves.**

3. **Extraglomerular mesangium.** The extraglomerular mesangium is located at the vascular pole of the renal glomerulus and is continuous with the glomerular mesangium. The extraglomerular mesangium consists of a **mesangial matrix and extraglomerular mesangial cells (also called Lacis cells or Goormaghtigh cells).** The mesangial matrix is an extracellular matrix of microfibrils and contains collagen (Types III, IV, V, and VI), microfibrillar proteins (fibrillin, MAGP, MP78, MP340), and fibronectin. The extraglomerular mesangial cells are irregular in shape, have many cell processes, are attached to each other by desmosomes, and communicate with each other and neighboring cells through gap junctions. Although the function of the extraglomerular mesangial cells is not quite clear, it appears that **extraglomerular mesangial cells mediate signals received from MD cells for transmission to JG cells and glomerular mesangial cells.**

B. **THE FUNCTION OF THE JG COMPLEX** (Figure 21-5). The JG complex is one of the most important regulators of **arterial blood pressure.** In most people, the daily average mean arterial blood pressure is strictly regulated at about **100 mm Hg** with fluctuations of **±20 mm Hg.** This strict regulation provides organs with a blood flow at a constant perfusion pressure and minimizes cardiac, vascular, and renal damage. There are two main mechanisms that regulate arterial blood pressure as indicated below.
1. **Baroreceptor mechanism** involves the **autonomic nervous system** and regulates blood pressure in a **fast, moment-to-moment, neurotransmitter fashion.** The baroreceptors are stretch receptors that monitor **changes in blood pressure** and are located in the walls of the common carotid arteries (i.e., **carotid sinus**), great veins, atria, and aortic arch. Afferent (sensory) neurons of **CN IX** (also called **Hering nerve** or **carotid sinus nerve**) whose cell bodies are located in the petrosal ganglion innervate the carotid sinus and relay information to the **solitary nucleus (SN)** within the CNS. Afferent (sensory) neurons of **CN X** whose cell bodies are located in the nodose ganglion innervate the baroceptors in the great veins, atria, and aortic arch and relay information to the **solitary nucleus** within the CNS. The SN controls the activity of other CNS nuclei involved in the parasympathetic and sympathetic nervous system as indicated below.

DECREASED BLOOD PRESSURE (HEMORRHAGE)

● **Figure 21-5 Flow chart of physiologic responses to decreased blood pressure (e.g., hemorrhagic or hypovolemic shock).** The physiologic response to hemorrhage involves both the baroreceptor mechanism and the renin-angiotensin II mechanism. First, we will discuss the baroreceptor mechanism. A decreased stretch on the baroreceptors is relayed via CN IX and X to the SN in the CNS. First, the SN inhibits the DVM and NA, which in turn inhibits the parasympathetic nervous system. This elicits the following actions: increases heart rate (positive chronotropism), increases conduction velocity (positive dromotropism), increases contractility (positive inotropism). Second, the SN stimulates the rostral ventrolateral medulla (RVLM), which in turn stimulates the intermediolateral cell column, which in turn stimulates the sympathetic nervous system. This elicits the following actions: increases heart rate (positive chronotropism), increases conduction velocity (positive dromotropism), increases contractility (positive inotropism), and increases vasoconstriction of arterioles and veins. These actions will increase arterial blood pressure. Second, we will discuss the renin-angiotensin mechanism. The MD cells sense a decreased Na^+ in the DST fluid, whereas the JG cells and sympathetic nerves sense a decreased blood pressure. This causes an increased renin release and increased angiotensin II. Increased angiotensin II elicits the following actions: affects vascular smooth muscle to contract, which increases arteriolar and venous constriction and leads to increased peripheral resistance; affects the CNS and PNS to increase sympathetic activity, which increases arteriolar and venous constriction and leads to increased peripheral resistance and to increased cardiac output; affects the adrenal cortex to increase aldosterone (ALD) secretion, which increases Na^+ reabsorption and leads to decreased Na^+ and H_2O excretion in the urine; affects the kidneys to increase Na^+ reabsorption by the proximal convoluted tubule (PCT) and decreases glomerular filtration rate (GFR) by vasoconstriction of the afferent and efferent arterioles, both of which lead to decreased Na^+ and H_2O excretion in the urine; affects the CNS (i.e., neurohypophysis) to increase anti-diuretic hormone (ADH) secretion, which works synergistically with ALD and increases H_2O reabsorption, both of which lead to decreased Na^+ and H_2O excretion in the urine; affects the CNS to increase the sensation of thirst, which increases H_2O ingestion and leads to decreased Na^+ and H_2O excretion in the urine. Increased peripheral resistance, increased cardiac output, and decreased Na^+ and H_2O excretion in the urine are physiologic actions that increase arterial blood pressure. + = stimulation, − = inhibition; ↑ = increases; ↓ = decreases; SN = solitary nucleus; RVLM = rostral ventrolateral medulla; DVN = dorsal vagal nucleus; NA = nucleus ambiguous; Ach = acetylcholine; NE = norepinephrine; DST = distal straight tubule; ea = efferent arteriole; aa = afferent arteriole; JG = juxtaglomerular; ACE = angiotensin converting enzyme; PCT = proximal convoluted tubule; ALD = aldosterone; ADH = anti-diuretic hormone; GFR = glomerular filtration rate; BP = blood pressure; CNS = central nervous system; PNS = peripheral nervous system; MD = macula densa cells.

a. **Parasympathetic control.** The SN controls the activity of the **dorsal vagal nucleus (DVN)** and **nucleus ambiguous (NA).** The DVN and NA are the source of preganglionic parasympathetic neurons of CN X. The preganglionic parasympathetic neurons synapse with postganglionic parasympathetic neurons that elicit the following actions in the heart.

   (1) Decreases heart rate (negative chronotropism), decreases conduction velocity (negative dromotropism), and decreases contractility (negative inotropism).

b. **Sympathetic control.** The SN controls the activity of the **rostral ventrolateral medulla (RVLM).** The RVLM controls the activity of preganglionic sympathetic neurons within the **intermediolateral cell column** of the spinal cord. The preganglionic sympathetic neurons synapse with postganglionic sympathetic neurons within the paravertebral chain ganglia. The postganglionic sympathetic neurons elicit the following actions in the heart, arterioles, and veins.

   (1) Increases heart rate (positive chronotropism), increases conduction velocity (positive dromotropism), and increases contractility (positive inotropism)

   (2) Increases vasoconstriction of arterioles and veins

2. **Renin-angiotensin II mechanism** involves the **juxtaglomerular (JG) complex** of the kidney and regulates blood pressure in a **slow, long-term, hormonal fashion.** The JG complex regulates blood pressure in three different ways all of which affect **renin** release from JG cells (modified smooth muscle cells of the afferent arteriole).

   a. The JG complex contains **macula densa (MD) cells** that monitor **changes in Na^+** within the fluid of the distal straight tubule (DST) and affect **renin** release.

   b. The JG complex contains **JG cells** (which act as intrarenal baroreceptors) that monitor **changes in blood pressure** and affect **renin** release.

   c. JG cells are innervated by sympathetic nerves under the control of peripheral baroreceptors (e.g., carotid sinus) that monitor **changes in blood pressure** and affect **renin** release. The preganglionic sympathetic neurons travel in the lesser and least splanchnic nerves and synapse in the aorticorenal ganglia. Postganglionic sympathetic neurons terminate on JG cells.

d. **Renin** is an enzyme that converts **angiotensinogen** (produced by the liver) to **angiotensin I**. Angiotensin I is converted to **angiotensin II** (primarily by endothelium of lung capillaries) by **angiotensin converting enzyme (ACE)**. Angiotensin II has widespread actions as indicated below.

(1) Affects vascular smooth muscle

(2) Affects CNS and PNS to modulate sympathetic activity

(3) Affects the adrenal cortex to modulate aldosterone

(4) Affects the kidneys to modulate Na^+ reabsorption and glomerular filtration rate (GFR)

(5) Affects the CNS to modulate antidiuretic hormone (ADH)

(6) Affects the CNS to modulate thirst.

IX Histophysiology

A. A sophisticated understanding of the kidney entails knowing the function of each renal tubule as indicated in Table 21-1, which is a comprehensive summary table. However, there are some noteworthy generalizations. In order to excrete waste products adequately, the glomerular filtration rate (GFR) must be very large (180 L/day!!). This means that filtered loads of all low molecular weight blood solutes is also very large. These must be put back into the blood. The **PCT** has the primary role of recovering these filtered loads by tubular reabsorption and has been called the **"mass reabsorber."** In addition (with the exception of K^+), the PCT is a major site of tubular secretion; a **"mass secretor."** The loop of Henle also reabsorbs relatively large loads of H_2O and ions. The extensive reabsorption of the PCT and loop of Henle ensure that the load of solutes and volume of H_2O entering the DCT, cortical CD, and medullary CD are relatively small. The DCT, cortical CD, and medullary CD then do the fine tuning and determine the final amounts of substances excreted into the urine by adjusting tubular reabsorption and tubular secretion. Therefore, most (but not all) homeostatic controls (e.g., hormone sensitivity) are exerted on the DCT, cortical CD, and medullary CD.

B. The three basic physiologic processes that occur in the kidney include:

1. **Glomerular filtration.** The formation of urine begins with filtration, which occurs where the glomerulus and Bowman's capsule interact to form a **glomerular filtration barrier (GFB)**. The formation of urine involves the process of glomerular filtration which is the bulk-flow of fluid from the glomerular capillaries → Bowman's space forming a **glomerular filtrate (or tubular fluid)**. The glomerular filtration rate (GFR) equals the amount of glomerular filtrate formed per unit time. The GFR in a typical normal adult is **0.125 L/min** (or an incredible **180 L/day**). GFR is measured by the **clearance of inulin.** Inulin is excreted by glomerular filtration only (no tubular reabsorption or tubular secretion is involved).

2. **Tubular reabsorption.** After filtration, the composition of the tubular fluid is altered by tubular reabsorption where transfer occurs from the tubular fluid to the plasma (**tubular fluid → plasma**). Tubular reabsorption may occur by two routes:

a. **Paracellular route.** Tubular reabsorption via the paracellular route occurs **between** renal tubular epithelial cells at the zonula occludens. Tubular reabsorption via the paracellular route occurs by **diffusion** ("downhill") or **solvent drag** (movement of water drags dissolved solutes with it). This diffusion requires that an electrochemical gradient exist for the substance and that the zonula occludens is permeable to the substance.

b. **Transcellular route.** Tubular reabsorption via the transcellular route occurs **across** renal tubular epithelial cells and therefore the substance must cross the luminal cell membrane → cytoplasm of the cell → basolateral cell membrane. Tubular reabsorption via the transcelluar route occurs by **diffusion** ("downhill") for lipid-soluble substances or by **active transport** ("uphill") for lipid-insoluble substances.

3. **Tubular secretion.** After filtration, the composition of the tubular fluid is altered by tubular secretion in which transfer occurs from the plasma to the tubular fluid (**plasma → tubular fluid**). Tubular secretion may occur by two routes:

a. **Paracellular route.** Tubular secretion via the paracellular route occurs **between** renal tubular epithelial cells at the zonula occludens. Tubular secretion via the paracellular route occurs by **diffusion** ("downhill"). This diffusion requires that an electrochemical gradient exist for the substance and that the zonula occludens is permeable to the substance.

b. **Transcellular route.** Tubular secretion via the transcellular route occurs across renal tubular epithelial cells and therefore the substance must cross the basolateral cell membrane → cytoplasm of the cell → luminal cell membrane. Tubular secretion via the transcellular route occurs by **diffusion** ("downhill") for lipid-soluble substances or by **active transport** ("uphill") for lipid-insoluble substances.

C. **RENAL CLEARANCE.** Renal clearance is the volume of plasma from which a substance is completely cleared by the kidneys per unit time. The clearance of inulin (C_{inulin}) is used as a benchmark because inulin is freely filterable at the glomerulus and does not undergo tubular secretion or tubular reabsorption. Note that C_{inulin} = GFR = 0.125 L/min. If substance A is present in the plasma but is not excreted in the urine, then **C_A = 0.** If substance B (like inulin) is freely filterable at the glomerulus and does not undergo tubular secretion or tubular reabsorption, then the clearance of inulin can be used to measure GFR. **C_{inulin} = GFR = 0.125 L/min.** If substance C is freely filterable at the glomerulus and undergoes tubular secretion, then **$C_C > C_{inulin} > 0.125$ L/min.** If substance D is freely filterable at the glomerulus and undergoes tubular reabsorption, then **$C_D < C_{inulin} < 0.125$ L/min.** Creatinine is freely filterable at the glomerulus and undergoes a small amount of tubular secretion but no tubular reabsorption. If the small amount of tubular secretion is ignored, then **$C_{CR} \sim C_{inulin} \sim$ GFR ~ 0.125 L/min.** In clinical practice, it is more common to measure plasma creatinine levels (P_{CR}) as an indicator of GFR because there is an excellent inverse relationship between P_{CR} and GFR.

D. **THE COUNTERCURRENT MULTIPLIER SYSTEM.** The countercurrent multiplier system **creates the hyperosmolarity gradient** within the interstitial fluid in the kidney medulla, which is crucial for urine concentration. The countercurrent multiplier system involves the **loops of Henle** from juxtamedullary nephrons, which extend very long loops of Henle deep into the medulla. In the loops of Henle, tubular fluid flows down the descending limb (PST and DTL) and then back up the ascending limb (ATL and DST); hence, the term **countercurrent.** The differences in permeability of the descending limb and ascending limb establish a small osmolarity difference at the higher levels of the loop of Henle so that the tubular fluid entering the next lower level of the loop of Henle is more concentrated. This process is repeated over and over as tubular fluid flows to lower levels of the loop of Henle. Consequently, the countercurrent flow multiplies a small osmolarity difference such that a hyperosmotic gradient of **300–1400 mOsm** is created within the medullary interstitial fluid; hence the term **multiplier.** The permeability differences of the descending limb and ascending limb of the loop of Henle are indicated below.

1. **Descending limb of the loop of Henle (PST and DTL)** is impermeable to Na^+ and Cl^- but permeable to H_2O.

2. **Ascending limb of the loop of Henle (ATL and DST)** is permeable to Na^+ and Cl^- but impermeable to H_2O.

E. **THE COUNTERCURRENT EXCHANGER SYSTEM MAINTAINS THE HYPEROSMOLARITY GRADIENT** of the interstitial fluid in the kidney medulla, which is crucial for urine concentration. The countercurrent exchanger system involves the **vasa recta** (capillaries) that arise from the efferent arteriole of juxtamedullary nephrons, which extend very long capillaries deep into the medulla. The vasa recta form a hairpin loop in which blood flows down the descending side and then back up the ascending side; hence, the term **countercurrent.** If the kidneys were supplied by an ordinary capillary bed (i.e., no hairpin loop) containing blood of 300 mOsm/L, H_2O would diffuse out of the capillaries and Na^+ and Cl^- ions would diffuse into the capillaries, thereby destroying the hyperosmolarity gradient. This is exactly what happens as blood flows down the descending side, but then the process is reversed or exchanged as blood flows up the ascending side; hence the term **exchanger.** This unique, hairpin loop arrangement of the vasa recta maintains the hyperosmolarity gradient of the medullary interstitial fluid.

Ⓧ Pharmacology of Diuretics (Figure 21-6). Diuretics cause an increase in the volume of urine. Many diuretics have been developed that elicit their action on a specific renal tubule. Most diuretics act on the luminal side of the renal tubule and therefore must be present in the tubular fluid for action to occur. Diuretics in conjunction with other drugs are frequently used in the management of congestive heart failure and hypertension.

A. **ACETAZOLAMIDE (DIAMOX)** inhibits **carbonic anhydrase** by acting primarily on the **PCT** resulting in decreased reabsorption of Na^+ (H_2O) and HCO_3^-. It is used clinically to treat glaucoma and altitude sickness.

B. **MANNITOL (OSMITROL)** promotes osmotic diuresis by acting primarily on the **PCT, and PST, DTL of the loop of Henle.** Mannitol is filtered at the glomerulus but is poorly reabsorbed so that mannitol "holds" H_2O within the lumen by virtue of its osmotic effect. It is used clinically to treat cerebral edema, increased intracranial pressure, or increased intraocular pressure.

C. **LOOP DIURETICS (SULFONAMIDE DERIVATIVES). Furosemide (Lasix; "lasts six" hours), bumetanide (Bumex), and torsemide (Demadex)** are Na^+-K^+-$2Cl^-$ **symporter inhibitors** that act on the **distal straight tubule (DST) of the loop of Henle** and cause a decreased NaCl reabsorption (tubular fluid → plasma). This results in **NaCl diuresis; hypokalemic alkalosis** due to the delivery of large amounts of Na^+ to the cortical collecting duct causing K^+ secretion (plasmsa → tubular fluid; K^+ wasting) and H^+ secretion (plasma → tubular fluid). Clinical uses include edema associated with congestive heart failure, liver disease, renal disease, and pulmonary disease; hypertension (due to decreased blood volume).

D. **THIAZIDES DIURETICS (SULFONAMIDE DERIVATIVES). Hydrochlorothiazide (HydroDIURIL), chlorthalidone (Hygroton), indapamide (Lozol), and metolazone (Mykrox)** are Na^+-Cl^- **symporter inhibitors** that act on the early **distal convoluted tubule (DCT)** and cause a decreased NaCl reabsorption (tubular fluid → plasma). This results in **NaCl diuresis; hypokalemic alkalosis** caused by the delivery of large amounts of Na^+ to the cortical collecting duct causing K^+ secretion (plasma → tubular fluid; K^+ wasting) and H^+ secretion (plasma → tubular fluid). Clinical uses include edema associated with congestive heart failure, liver disease, renal disease, and corticosteroid therapy; hypertension (owing to decrease in blood volume).

E. K⁺-SPARING DIURETICS

1. **Spironolactone (Aldactone)** is an **aldosterone antagonist** that acts by reducing gene expression of Na^+ ion channels and Na^+-K^+ ATPase in the cortical collecting ducts. This causes decreased NaCl reabsorption (tubular fluid → plasma), decreased K^+ secretion (plasma → tubular fluid; **K^+ sparing**), and decreased H^+ secretion (plasma → tubular fluid). This results in **NaCl diuresis with K^+-sparing.** Clinical uses include hypertension, edematous states, primary hyperaldosteronism (Conn syndrome).

2. **Amiloride (Midamor) and triamterene (Dyrenium)** are **Na^+ ion channel antagonists** that block Na^+ ion channels in the late distal convoluted tubule (DCT) and collecting ducts (CD). This causes a decreased NaCl reabsorption (tubular fluid →

● **Figure 21-6 Pharmacologic site of action of diuretics.** ea = efferent arteriole; aa = afferent arteriole; PCT = proximal convoluted tubule; BC = Bowman capsule; PST = proximal straight tubule; DTL = descending thin limb of the loop of Henle; ATL = ascending thin limb of the loop of Henle; DCT = distal convoluted tubule; CD = collecting duct.

plasma), decreased K^+ secretion (plasma $\rightarrow$ **tubular fluid; K^+ sparing**), and decreased H^+ secretion (plasma $\rightarrow$ tubular fluid). This results in: **NaCl diuresis with K^+-sparing.** Clinical uses include hypertension and edematous states.

XI Clinical Considerations (Figure 21-7)

A. **WILMS' TUMOR (WT).** WT is the **most common renal malignancy of childhood**, which usually presents between 1–3 years of age. WT presents as a large, solitary, well-circumscribed mass that on cut section is soft, homogeneous, and tan-gray in color. WT is interesting histologically in that this tumor tends to recapitulate different stages of embryologic formation of the kidney so that three classic histologic areas are described: a stromal area; a blastemal area of tightly packed embryonic cells; and a tubular area. In 95% of cases, the WT tumor is sporadic and unilateral. In 5% of cases, the WT tumor arises in association with the WAGR syndrome, Denys-Drash syndrome, or Beckwith-Wiedemann syndrome. WT is a neoplasm involving the **WT1 gene** and **WT2 gene** both located on the short arm of chromosome 11 (11p13). The WT1 gene and WT2 gene are anti-oncogenes (or tumor-suppressor genes) that encode proteins that suppress the cell cycle.

B. **AUTOSOMAL DOMINANT POLYCYSTIC KIDNEY DISEASE (ADPKD; ALSO CALLED ADULT POLYCYSTIC KIDNEY DISEASE).**
   1. **General features.** ADPKD is most commonly caused (85% of cases) by an **autosomal dominant** mutation of the ADPKD-1 gene, which is located on the **short arm (p arm) of chromosome 16 (16p)** and encodes for the protein **polycystin** (an integral membrane protein involved in cell-to-cell and cell-to-matrix interactions).
   2. **Pathologic findings** include bilaterally enlarged palpable kidneys; numerous cysts filled with a straw-colored fluid distort the external contours of the kidney; cysts are lined by simple cuboidal or columnar epithelium; cysts arise from any point along the nephron; associated with cystic disease in other organs (especially the liver); associated with berry aneurysms within the circle of Willis.
   3. **Clinical findings.** Symptoms become apparent around 40 years of age; heaviness in the loins; bilateral flank and abdominal masses; hematuria; hypertension; azotemia; uremia; leads to end-stage renal disease.

C. **AUTOSOMAL RECESSIVE POLYCYSTIC KIDNEY DISEASE (ARPKD; ALSO CALLED CHILDHOOD POLYCYSTIC KIDNEY DISEASE).**
   1. **General features.** ARPKD is caused by an **autosomal recessive** mutation of a gene linked to the **short arm (p arm) of chromosome 6 (6p)** and encodes for an as-yet-unidentified protein.
   2. **Pathologic findings** include bilaterally enlarged spongy kidneys that may impede delivery of the infant; numerous cysts are present but do not distort the external contours of the kidney; cysts arise from collecting ducts and tubules; cysts are arranged in a radial pattern perpendicular to the kidney surface; associated with congenital hepatic fibrosis.
   3. **Clinical findings** include leads to end-stage renal disease, in which 75% of these infants die in the perinatal period.

D. **GLOMERULONEPHRITIS.** Glomerulonephritis is a general term applied to kidney diseases in which inflammation is prominent due to the deposition of immune complexes within the glomeruli, *in situ* formation of immune complexes, or antineutrophil cytoplasmic autoantibodies. The inflammation may cause proliferation of endothelial cells lining the glomerular capillaries, mesangial cells, or epithelial cells (both simple squamous epithelium lining Bowman's capsule and podocytes). In severe cases, glomerular necrosis occurs. Glomerulonephritis causes **nephritic syndrome** whose clinical findings include **hematuria (hallmark finding), proteinuria, edema, hypoalbuminemia, and hypertension.** The various types of glomerulonephritis are indicated below:

1. **IgA nephropathy (Berger disease).**
    a. **General features.** IgA nephropathy is caused by the deposition of IgA immune complexes within the mesangium whose etiology is unknown but usually follows infection of the respiratory or gastrointestinal tracts. IgA nephropathy is the most common type of glomerulonephritis.
    b. **Pathologic findings** include mesangial cell proliferation; immunofluorescence localizes IgA to the mesangium; electron microscopy shows dense deposits within the mesangium.
    c. **Clinical presentation** is highly variable, ranging from asymptomatic microscopic hematuria → gross hematuria → end-stage renal disease; symptoms usually follow an episodic pattern exacerbated by respiratory and gastrointestinal infections.

2. **Acute poststreptococcal glomerulonephritis (APG).**
    a. **General features.** APG is caused by the deposition of IgG immune complexes within the GBM and complement (C3) activation most commonly as a result of infection with **Group A (ß-hemolytic) streptococci** (e.g., poststreptococcal pharyngitis, "strep throat," impetigo).
    b. **Pathologic findings** include increased size of glomeruli; glomerular hypercellularity resulting from proliferation of endothelial cells, mesangial cells, neutrophils, and monocytes; immunofluorescence localizes IgG and C3 to **"lumpy-bumpy"** areas; electron microscopy shows "lumpy-bumpy" subepithelial (beneath the podocytes) dense deposits.
    c. **Clinical findings** include most commonly seen in children with a primary infection of the pharynx; diagnosis relies on a rise of antibody titers to streptococcal products; hematuria; oliguria; proteinuria; facial edema; hypertension; a short-lived nephritic syndrome in which most children recover spontaneously.

3. **Type I membranoproliferative glomerulonephritis (MPG)**
    a. **General features.** Type I MPG is caused by the deposition of immune complexes within the mesangium and subendothelial (i.e., beneath the endothelium of the glomerular capillaries) as a result of persistent, indolent infections causing chronic antigenemia.
    b. **Pathologic findings** include increased size of glomeruli; capillary wall thickening; lobular distortion of glomeruli (hypersegmentation); mesangial cell proliferation; immunofluorescence localizes IgG and C3 to the mesangium and subendothelial areas; electron microscopy shows a focal loss of podocytic foot processes and a **"train track"** GBM, which appears as two layers.
    c. **Clinical findings** may present as either a nephritic syndrome, nephritic syndrome, or a combination of both.

4. **Type II membranoproliferative glomerulonephritis (MPG) or dense deposit disease.**
    a. **General features.** Type II MPG is caused by deposition of complement within the GBM and mesangium, the basis of which is unknown. In most patients, **C3 nephritic factor** (a circulating IgG autoantibody that stabilizes the activated C3 convertase enzyme and causes increased C3 cleaving activity) is present.

    b. **Pathologic findings** are similar to Type I MPG with capillary wall thickening; lobular distortion of glomeruli (hypersegmentation); but mesangial cell proliferation may be reduced or absent; immunofluorescence localizes C3 within the GBM and mesangium; electron microscopy shows **ribbon-like dense deposits** with the GBM.

    c. **Clinical findings** may present as a nephritic syndrome, nephritic syndrome, or a combination of both.

5. **Lupus glomerulonephritis (LG).**

    a. **General features.** LG is caused by the deposition of immune complexes (IgG, IgM, IgA) within the mesangium, subendothelial (i.e., beneath the endothelium of the glomerular capillaries), and subepithelia (i.e., beneath the podocytes) and complement activation as a complication of **systemic lupus erythematosus (SLE)**. SLE is an autoimmune disease characterized by the hyperactivity of B lymphocytes with the production of a wide variety of autoantibodies including those against DNA **(anti ds-DNA).**

    b. **Pathologic findings.** Pathologic findings are highly variable and include: **Class I** SLE patient with no glomerular lesion, no immune complexes, and no glomerular dysfunction; **Class II.** Mesangial proliferation, immune complexes located in the mesangium, mild hematuria and proteinuria; **Class III.** Focal proliferative (<50% of glomeruli affected), immune complexes located in the mesangium and subendothelial, moderate nephritis (poor prognosis); **Class IV.** Diffuse proliferative (>50% of glomeruli affected), immune complexes located in the mesangium and subendothelial ("wire loop lesion"), severe nephritis (worst prognosis); **Class V.** Membranous glomerulonephritis, immune complexes located subepithelial (i.e., beneath the podocytes), nephritic syndrome.

    c. **Clinical findings** include 70% of all SLE patients develop kidney disease, the clinical manifestations of which are varied as indicated by the different classes; renal biopsies of SLE patients are taken to evaluate the class, activity, and chronicity of the SLE rather than to diagnose LG; with current immunosuppressive therapy, 25% of Class IV SLE patients reach end-stage renal disease within 5 years.

6. **Antiglomerular basement membrane glomerulonephritis (ABMG; Goodpasture syndrome).**

    a. **General features.** ABMG is caused by deposition of IgG immune complexes (i.e., autoantibodies to a globular noncollagenous domain of Type IV collagen) within the GBM. The autoantibodies generally cross react with pulmonary basement membranes; therefore, when both the lungs and kidneys are involved the term **Goodpasture syndrome** is used.

    b. **Pathologic findings** include glomerular crescents in >50% of glomeruli, which are formed by an inflammatory exudate containing macrophages and fibrin filling the urinary space and a proliferation of the simple squamous epithelium lining Bowman's capsule; immunofluorescence localizes IgG in a linear fashion along the GBM; electron microscopy shows focal breaks in the GBM but not immune-dense deposits.

    c. **Clinical findings.** Patients present with rapidly progressive renal failure; nephritic syndrome.

7. **Antineutrophil cytoplasmic autoantibody glomerulonephritis (ANCAG).**

    a. **General features.** ANCAG is not caused by immune complexes within the GBM, but instead is an aggressive, neutrophil-mediated disease causing glomerular necrosis and crescents. However, 90% of ANCAG patients have circulating **antineutrophil cytoplasmic autoantibodies (ANCA)** directed against myeloperoxidase and proteinase 3. ANCAG also may affect the lungs; therefore, when both the lungs and kidney are involved the term **Wegener granulomatosis** is used.

b. **Pathologic findings** include focal glomerular necrosis; glomerular crescents in >50% of glomeruli, which are formed by an inflammatory exudates containing macrophages and fibrin filling the urinary space and a proliferation of the simple squamous epithelium lining Bowman's capsule; immunofluorescence does not localize immune complexes along the GBM; electron microscopy shows no immune dense deposits.

c. **Clinical findings** include patients present with a rapidly progressive renal failure; nephritic syndrome; 75% of ANCAG patients have systemic small vessel vasculitis; 80% of ANCAG patients develop end-stage renal disease within 5 years.

8. **Hereditary nephritis (Alport syndrome).**

a. **General features.** Hereditary nephritis is caused by a X-linked mutation in the COL4A5 gene that encodes for the a5 chain of **Type IV collagen,** which is a key component of the glomerular basement membrane (GBM) and leads to a leaky GBM. Hereditary nephritis is a proliferative and sclerosing glomerular disease that is accompanied by defects of the ears and eyes.

b. **Pathologic findings** include mild mesangial matrix expansion; mesangial hypercellularity; focal and diffuse glomerular sclerosis; interstitial foam cells; immunofluorescence does not localize the a5 chain of Type IV collagen to the GBM; electron microscopy shows an **irregularly thickened GBM with interlacing lamellae** surrounding electron lucent areas.

c. **Clinical findings** include disease is more severe in males; hematuria; proteinuria; hypertension; progressive renal failure; nearly all males and 20% of females develop endstage renal disease by 40–50 years of age.

E. **GLOMERULOPATHY.** Glomerulopathy is a general term applied to kidney diseases in which glomerular pathology can be observed but no inflammation is present. Glomerulopathy causes **nephritic syndrome** whose clinical findings include **proteinuria >3.5–4.0 g of protein/day (hallmark finding), edema, hypoalbuminemia,** and **hyperlipidemia.** The various types of glomerulopathy are indicated below:

1. **Membranous glomerulopathy.**

a. **General features.** Membranous glomerulopathy is caused by the deposition of IgG and C3 immune complexes in a subepithelial (beneath the podocytes) location within the glomerulus whose etiology is unknown but may be secondary to systemic lupus erythematosus (SLE), hepatitis B, cancer, or penicillamine. Membranous glomerulopathy is the most common primary renal cause of nephritic syndrome in young adults.

b. **Pathologic findings** include slightly increased size of glomeruli; no hypercellularity of glomeruli; silver staining shows spikes of basement membrane; glomerular sclerosis in advanced stages; immunofluorescence localizes IgG and C3 to subepithelial domes that lie between the spikes of basement membrane; electron microscopy shows spikes of basement membrane and dome-like subepithelial dense deposits. (**"spike and dome"** appearance).

c. **Clinical findings** include the clinical course is highly variable; 25% of patients shows spontaneous remission; 50% of patients have persistent proteinuria and only partial loss of kidney function; 25% of patients develop end-stage renal disease.

2. **Minimal change disease (lipoid nephrosis).**

a. **General features.** Minimal change disease is caused by immune system irregularities whose etiology is unknown. Minimal change disease is the most common cause of nephritic syndrome in children under 5 years of age.

b. **Pathologic findings** include glomeruli appear normal or "minimally changed." lipid droplets found in the renal cortex (i.e., lipoid nephrosis);

immunofluorescence does not localize immune complexes; electron microscopy shows fusion of podocyte foot processes, which leads to a disruption of the negative charge of the glomerular filtration barrier.

c. **Clinical findings include** proteinuria is caused by large amounts of albumin in the urine (although this is not diagnostic); 90% of patients show complete remission within 8 weeks of the start of corticosteroid therapy.

3. **Focal segmental glomerulosclerosis**

a. **General features.** Focal segmental glomerulosclerosis is caused by many factors, both idiopathic (primary) or secondary to obesity, renal mass reduction, sickle cell disease, cyanotic heart disease, AIDS, and intravenous drug abuse.

b. **Pathologic findings** include a variable number of glomeruli (focal) and only a portion of the glomerulus (segmental) show scarring (sclerosis) of the capillary loops; scarring involves collagen deposition along with lipid and proteinaceous material (e.g., plasma proteins; hyalinosis) accumulation; the remainder of the glomeruli appear normal; immunofluorescence localizes IgM and C3; electron microscopy shows fusion and focal detachment of podocyte foot processes along with dense deposits within the sclerotic areas which correspond to the hyalinosis seen in light microscopy.

c. **Clinical findings** include insidious onset with asymptomatic proteinuria; frequently progresses to nephritic syndrome; progressive decline in renal function leading to end-stage renal disease in 5–20 years.

4. **Diabetic glomerulosclerosis**

a. **General features.** Diabetic glomerulosclerosis is caused by Type 1 or Type 2 diabetes.

b. **Pathologic findings** include glomerular basement membrane (GBM) thickening; diffuse mesangial matrix expansion or focal, segmental, sclerotic lesions called **Kimmelstiel-Wilson nodules;** immunofluorescence localizes IgG, albumin, fibrinogen, and other plasma proteins, which represents non-immunological adsorption of these proteins to the GBM; electron microscopy shows thickening of the lamina densa of the GBM and dense deposits containing lipid debris corresponding to the Kimmelstiel-Wilson nodules.

c. **Clinical findings.** This is the leading cause of end-stage renal disease; earliest sign is microalbuminemia; overt proteinuria occurs 10–15 years after the onset of diabetes and causes nephritic syndrome; always progresses to end-stage renal disease.

5. **Renal amyloidosis.**

a. **General features.** Renal amyloidosis is caused by complications of **amyloidosis,** which is a group of diseases that have in common the deposition of **amyloid** protein in the intercellular space of various organs. Renal amyloidosis is associated with **AL amyloid protein** and **AA amyloid protein.** AL amyloid is derived from lambda immunoglobulin light chains and is associated with AL amyloidosis, multiple myeloma, light-chain deposition disease, and light-chain cast nephropathy. AA amyloid is derived from an inflammatory serum protein called SAA and is associated with rheumatoid arthritis, chronic tuberculosis, and familial Mediterranean fever.

b. **Pathologic findings** include amyloid appears as an amorphous, eosinophilic material that can be specifically stained with Congo red or thioflavine T; early deposition of amyloid occurs in the mesangium that eventually spreads to obliterate capillary lumens; increased size of glomeruli due to amyloid deposition; electron microscopy shows 10-nm non-branching amyloid fibrils within the mesangium that are oriented perpendicular to the GBM along with the loss of podocyte foot processes.

c. **Clinical findings** include proteinuria, nephrotic syndrome, and end-stage renal disease.

F. **MALIGNANT NEPHROSCLEROSIS**

a. **General features.** Malignant nephrosclerosis is caused by malignant hypertension (i.e., >125 mm Hg diastolic pressure, retinal blood vessel changes, papilledema, and renal functional impairment) whereby the endothelium is damaged, leading to thrombosis (a type of thrombotic microangiopathy).

b. **Pathologic findings.** Size of kidney varies from small to enlarged; cut surface of kidney has a red/yellow mottled appearance with small cortical infarcts; exhibits a microscopic background similar to benign nephrosclerosis; glomeruli show fibrinoid necrosis and consolidation; large arteries show edematous tunica intima expansion; afferent and efferent arterioles show fibrinoid necrosis; vascular thrombosis is present.

c. **Clinical findings** include headache, dizziness, visual disturbances, hematuria, proteinuria, occurs more frequently in men, aggressive antihypertensive medication controls this disease very well.

G. **PYELONEPHRITIS ("PYELO" = RENAL PELVIS).** Pyelonephritis is a type of infectious tubulointerstitial nephritis caused by bacterial infection with involvement of the renal parenchyma, calyces, and pelvis. The various types of pyelonephritis are indicated below:

1. **Acute pyelonephritis (APY)**

a. **General features.** APY is caused by bacterial infection either by the ascending route or hematogenous route. APY is a clinical syndrome. APY is characterized by an acute suppurative (purulent; pus-forming) inflammation of the kidney).

b. **Pathologic findings** include patchy suppurative inflammation of the renal interstitium and renal tubular necrosis (glomeruli are generally spared); suppuration causes discrete focal abscesses involving one or both kidneys or large, wedge-shaped areas in which the suppuration has coalesced; infiltration with predominantly neutrophils within the renal interstitium and renal tubules; renal papillary necrosis, in which the distal portion of the renal pyramids show gray-white to yellow necrosis that resembles infarction; pyonephrosis, in which the suppurative exudates fills the renal calyces, pelvis, and ureter; perinephric abscess, in which the suppurative inflammation breaks through the renal capsule into the perinephric tissue; pyelonephritic scar that is associated with fibrosis and deformation of the underlying renal calyx and pelvis.

c. **Clinical findings** include flank pain; costovertebral angle tenderness; fever; chills; nausea and vomiting; diarrhea; bacteriuria; pyuria; leukocyte casts (pus casts) within the urine that indicate renal involvement; urine and blood cultures are performed to determine infection; uncomplicated acute pyelonephritis follows a benign course and symptoms disappear within a few days after antibiotic treatment.

2. **Chronic pyelonephritis (CPY).**

a. **General features.** CPY is caused by recurrent or persistent bacterial infection secondary to either vesicoureteral reflux or urinary tract obstruction. CPY is a radiologic diagnosis. CPY is characterized by a chronic tubulointerstitial nephritis (inflammation) along with a blunting deformity and dilatation of renal calyces with overlying corticomedullary scarring of kidney parenchyma resulting in marked parenchymal loss. Of all the causes of tubulointerstitial nephritis, only CPY and analgesic nephropathy produce a deformity and dilatation of renal calyces with overlying corticomedullary scarring of kidney parenchyma.

b. **Pathologic findings include** kidneys scarring is irregular and asymmetric; deformed (blunted) and dilated renal calyces with coarse, discrete, overlying corticomedullary scarring; renal tubule atrophy, hypertrophy, and dilatation; dilated renal tubules contain colloidal casts that resemble thyroid follicles (called thyroidization); infiltration with neutrophils, lymphocytes, and plasma cells within the renal interstitium.

c. **Clinical findings** are usually nonspecific; some patients have recurrent acute symptomatic exacerbations of renal infection; some patients have no clear-cut symptoms despite persistent bacteriuria; some patients complain of vague flank pain, abdominal pain, or intermittent low-grade fever.

d. **Forms of CPY:** There are two main forms of CPY:

   i. **Chronic reflux-associated pyelonephritis (reflux nephropathy; CRPY).** CRPY is caused by recurrent or persistent bacterial infection secondary to vesicoureteral reflux and is the most common type of CPY. CRPY lacks an abrupt onset and is usually completely silent and diagnosed only during the investigation of acute UTIs, hypertension, or chronic renal failure especially in adult men who are seen for treatment of UTIs less often than women. Generally, renal involvement in CRPY occurs early in childhood as a result of congenital vesicoureteral reflux, which may be unilateral or bilateral. The scars associated with CRPY occur in the upper and lower poles of the kidney where the renal papillae are concave-shaped instead of the convex shape that occurs in the rest of the kidney.

   ii. **Chronic obstructive pyelonephritis (COPY).** COPY is caused by recurrent or persistent bacterial infection secondary to urinary tract obstruction (e.g., calculi; "kidney stones"). COPY may be insidious in onset and present with many of the clinical findings of acute pyelonephritis. The scars associated with COPY occur in all renal papillae.

H. **RENAL CELL CARCINOMA (RCC).** RCC is a malignant neoplasm involving the epithelium lining the renal tubules and ducts and is the most common cancer of the kidney. In 95% of the cases, RCC is sporadic and unilateral. In 5% of the cases, RCC is hereditary and arises in association with von Hippel-Lindau (VHL) disease, hereditary (autosomal dominant) clear cell carcinoma, or hereditary (autosomal dominant) papillary carcinoma and is multifocal and bilateral. **Clinical findings include** more frequent in men; risk factors include tobacco use and obesity; incidence peaks at about 60 years of age; hematuria is the most common presenting sign; the classic triad of hematuria, flank pain, and a palpable abdominal mass is observed in only 10% of patients; fever; weakness; malaise; weight loss; production of ectopic hormones (e.g., parathyroid-like hormone) leading to a number of paraneoplastic syndromes (e.g., hypercalcemia, polycythemia, hypertension, feminization or masculinization, or Cushing syndrome; one of the great mimics in medicine); tends to metastasize (to lungs and bones) before giving any clinical signs. The most common RCC is the **clear cell carcinoma** (70% frequency). The clear cell carcinoma tumor is solid, yellow-orange in color due to the presence of cytoplasmic lipid and glycogen, with cream-colored necrotic areas. A clear cell carcinoma shows spherical collections of neoplastic cells with a clear or granular cytoplasm that resemble proximal tubule cells. If the clear cell carcinoma is sporadic or hereditary, a deletion or an unbalanced chromosomal translocation (3; 6, 3; 8, 3; 11) is present resulting in a **deletion of chromosome 3** (3p 14-3p26 region). This region contains the VHL gene. The VHL gene is an anti-oncogene (tumor-suppressor gene) that encodes a protein that suppresses the cell cycle.

● **Figure 21-7 (A) Wilms tumor.** LM shows the following three components: a) metanephric blastema elements (blas) consisting of clumps of small, tightly packed embryonic cells; b) stromal elements (str); and c) epithelial elements generally in the form of abortive attempts at forming tubules (t) or glomeruli. **(B) Autosomal dominant polycystic kidney disease (ADPKD; also called adult polycystic kidney disease).** LM shows large, fluid cysts (cys) that are found throughout the substance of the kidney. In between the cysts, some functioning nephrons can be found. ADPKD is associated in about 10%–30% of the patients with a **Berry aneurysm** and subarachnoid hemorrhage. *RG*-renal glomerulus. **(C) Antiglomerular basement membrane glomerulonephritis (Goodpasture syndrome).** LM shows the accumulation of cells in the urinary space (Bowman's space) in the form of **"crescents"** (CR; *dotted lines*). The crescents are formed by an inflammatory exudate containing macrophages and fibrin filling the urinary space and the proliferation of simple squamous epithelium lining Bowman's capsule. These crescents eventually obliterate the urinary space and compress the renal glomerulus (RG). **(D) Diabetic glomerulosclerosis.** LM shows glomerular basement membrane thickening, a diffuse mesangial matrix expansion (*), and Kimmelstiel-Wilson nodules (*arrows*) that are hyaline masses situated at the periphery of the glomerulus. **(F) Acute polynephritis.** LM shows neutrophilic exudates within the collecting duct (*arrow*) and parenchyma. **(G) Chronic polynephritis.** LM shows that interstitial spaces are wide and contain lymphocytes, macrophages, plasma cells, and neutrophils (*). The renal tubules become atrophic and contain hyaline casts in their lumen (*arrow*). The entire kidney parenchyma may histologically resemble the thyroid gland (thyroidization). **(H) Renal cell carcinoma (clear cell carcinoma).** LM shows renal tubular epithelium consisting of clear, cuboidal cells arranged in tubules.

Case Study

A 30-year-old woman comes to your office complaining that "I feel like my body is swelling up. This has been going on for about 6 weeks now." She also tells you that "I'm feeling very tried and weak lately. I don't even feel like going out to the bars with my girlfriends." After some discussion, she informs you that she is an alcoholic who started abusing alcohol when she was 14 years old and "I'm not going to quit and go into any recovery program, so you can just forget about that. It's not going to happen." What is the most likely diagnosis?

Differentials

- Alcoholic cirrhosis, hypothyrodism, nephritic syndrome

Relevant Physical Exam Findings

- Tachypnea and tachycardia
- BP = 100/70 mm Hg
- Generalized 2+ pitting edema
- No enlargement of liver or spleen
- No ascites

Relevant Lab Findings

- Blood chemistry: Aspartate aminotransferase (AST) = 15U/L (Normal); Alanine amino-transferase (ALT) = 12 U/L (Normal); Albumin = 1.2 g/L (Low); Thyroid-stimulating hormone (TSH) = 3.5 μL/U/mL (Normal)
- Urinalysis: Protein = 5.1 g/24hr (High)
- Kidney Biopsy: silver staining shows spikes of basement membrane

Diagnosis

Membranous glomerulopathy (MG). MG is caused by the deposition of IgG and C3 immune complexes in a subepithelial (beneath the podocytes) location within the glomerulus whose etiology is unknown but may be secondary to systemic lupus erythematosus (SLE), hepatitis B, cancer, or penicillamine. Membranous glomerulopathy is the most common primary renal cause of nephritic syndrome in young adults. Pathological findings of MG include slightly increased size of glomeruli; no hypercellularity of glomeruli; silver staining shows spikes of basement membrane; glomerular sclerosis in advanced stages; immunofluorescence localizes IgG and C3 to subepithelial domes that lie between the spikes of basement membrane; electron microscopy shows spikes of basement membrane and dome-like subepithelial dense deposits ("spike and dome" appearance). Clinical findings of MG include clinical course is highly variable; 25% of patients shows spontaneous remission; 50% of patients have persistent proteinuria and only partial loss of kidney function; 25% of patients develop end-stage renal disease. Glomerulopathy is a general term applied to kidney disease in which glomerular pathology can be observed but no inflammation is present.

Glomerulopathy causes nephritic syndrome whose clinical findings include proteinuria >3.5–4.0 g of protein/day (hallmark finding), edema, hypoalbuminemia, and hyperlipidemia. Glomerulopathy disorders include MG, minimal change disease (lipoid nephrosis), focal segmental glomerulosclerosis, diabetic glomerulosclerosis, and renal amyloidosis. Cirrhosis is the end stage of chronic liver disease. Cirrhosis is defined as the destruction of normal hepatic architecture by fibrous septae that encompass regenerative nodules of hepatocyte parenchyma. Cirrhosis can progress to liver failure and present with jaundice (caused by hyperbilirubinemia) and edema (caused by hypalbuminemia). The spectrum of alcoholic liver disease involves three major morphologic and clinical conditions: fatty liver, alcoholic hepatitis, and alcoholic cirrhosis. Alcoholic cirrhosis is differentiated from other types of cirrhosis by the elevation of both AST and ALT, with AST twice that of ALT. The most common cause of cirrhosis is alcohol related. Severe hypothyroidism is called myxedema in adults or cretinism in children. Clinical findings of myxedema include cold intolerance; weight gain; mental and physical slowness; non-pitting edema; hair loss; and a dry, waxy swelling of the skin. The most common cause of myxedema is hyperthyroid therapy (surgery, radiation, or drugs). Glomerulonephritis is a general term applied to kidney diseases in which inflammation is prominent because of the deposition of immune complexes within the glomeruli, *in situ* formation of immune complexes, or antineutrophil cytoplasmic autoantibodies. The inflammation may cause proliferation of endothelial cells lining the glomerular capillaries, mesangial cells, or epithelial cells (both simple squamous epithelium lining Bowman's capsule and podocytes). In severe cases, glomerular necrosis occurs. Glomerulonephritis causes nephritic syndrome, whose clinical findings include hematuria (hallmark finding), proteinuria, edema, hypoalbuminemia, and hypertension. Glomerulonephritis disorders include IgA nephropathy (Berger's disease), acute poststreptococcal glomerulonephritis, Type I membranoproliferative glomerulonephritis, Type II membranoproliferative glomerulonephritis (dense deposit disease), lupus glomerulonephritis, antiglomerular basement membrane glomerulonephritis (Goodpasture syndrome), anti-neutrophil cytoplasmic autoantibody glomerulonephritis, and hereditary nephritis (Alport syndrome).

Hypophysis

The Adenohypophysis (Figure 22-1) has three subdivisions, called the **pars distalis,**
pars tuberalis, and **pars intermedia.**

A. **PARS DISTALIS** contains the following endocrine cells:

1. **Somatotrophs** secrete **growth hormone (GH)** under the control of hypothalamic
   factors **growth hormone-releasing factor (GHRF)** and **growth hormone-inhibiting**
   factor (somatostatin). GH binds to the GH receptor, which is a receptor tyrosine
   kinase. The functions of GH include the following:
   a. **In muscle,** GH decreases glucose uptake and increases protein synthesis.
   b. **In adipose tissue,** GH decreases glucose uptake and increases lipolysis.
   c. **In hepatocytes,** GH increases gluconeogenesis, increases glycogen degradation, and stimulates release of IGF-1 (somatomedin C).
   d. **IGF-1 (somatomedin C)** increases protein synthesis in chondrocytes at the epiphyseal growth plate and therefore causes **linear bone growth (pubertal growth spurt).**
   e. **Hyposecretion** of GH causes dwarfism.
   f. **Hypersecretion** of GH causes giantism or acromegaly.
2. **Mammotrophs** secrete **prolactin (PRL)** under the control of the hypothalamic
   factors **thyrotropin-releasing factor (TRF)** and **prolactin-inhibiting factor**
   (dopamine). PRL binds to the PRL receptor, which is a **receptor tyrosine kinase.**
   The functions of PRL include the following:
   a. Promotes milk secretion in lactating women.
   b. Promotes growth of mammary gland during pregnancy.
   c. Inhibits release of gonadotropin-releasing factor (GnRF) and thereby prevents
   ovulation (in women) or spermatogenesis (in men).
3. **Thyrotrophs** secrete **thyroid-stimulating hormone (TSH)** under the control of
   hypothalamic factor **thyrotropin-releasing factor (TRF).** TSH binds to the TSH
   receptor, which is a **G protein-linked receptor.** The function of TSH is to stimulate triiodothyronine (T_3) and thyroxine (T_4) secretion from thyroid follicular cells.
4. **Corticotrophs** secrete **adrenocorticotropin (ACTH)** under the control of hypothalamic factor **corticotropin-releasing factor (CRF).** ACTH binds to the ACTH
   receptor, which is a **G protein–linked receptor.** ACTH is derived from a large
   precursor protein called **pro-opiomelanocortin (POMC).** POMC is cleaved into
   ACTH and **β-lipotrophic hormone (β-LPH).** β-LPH is further cleaved into **γ-LPH**
   and **β-endorphin.** γ-LPH may give rise to **β-melanocyte-stimulating hormone**
   (β-MSH), which explains the hyperpigmentation observed in Addison disease.
   The functions of ACTH include the following:
   a. Stimulates the mitochondrial enzyme desmolase that converts cholesterol $\rightarrow$
   pregnenolone, a key step in the synthesis of all steroids.
   b. Stimulates the zona fasciculata and zona reticularis to secrete cortisol,
   androstenedione, and dehydroepiandrosterone (DHEA).

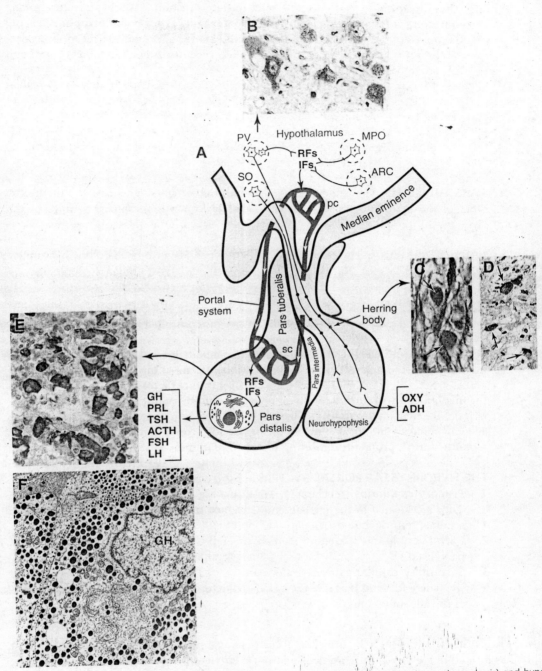

● **Figure 22-1 (A) Diagram of the hypophysis** (consisting of the adenohypophysis and neurohypophysis) and hypo-thalamus. Releasing factors (*RFs*) or inhibitory factors (*IFs*) from the arcuate nucleus (*ARC*), medial preoptic nucleus (*MPO*), and paraventricular nucleus (*PV*) of the hypothalamus enter the primary capillaries (*pc*) of the portal system. RFs and IFs travel to the secondary capillaries (*sc*), where they either stimulate or inhibit endocrine cells of the pars distalis. Oxytocin (*OXY*) and antidiuretic hormone (*ADH*) from the supraoptic nucleus (*SO*) and PV nucleus of the hypothalamus travel down axons to the neurohypophysis, where they are secreted at axon terminals into the blood. *ACTH* = adrenocorticotropin; *ADH* = antidiuretic hormone; *FSH* = follicle-stimulating hormone; *GH* = growth hormone; *LH* = luteinizing hormone; *OXY* = oxytocin; *PRL* = prolactin; *TSH* = thyroid-stimulating hormone. **(B)** LM of neuronal cell bodies immunocytochem-ically stained for ADH within the PV nucleus of the hypothalamus. **(C)** LM of Herring bodies (*arrows*) that characterize axons of the neurohypophysis (*H&E stain*). **(D)** LM of Herring bodies (*arrows*) immunocytochemically stained for ADH. **(E)** LM of somatotrophs of the adenohypophysis immunocytochemically stained for GH. **(F)** EM of a somatotroph of the ade-nohypophysis. Note the abundant secretory granules that contain GH.

5. **Gonadotrophs** secrete **follicle-stimulating hormone (FSH)** and **luteinizing hormone (LH)** under the control of hypothalamic factor **gonadotropin-releasing factor (GnRF).** FSH and LH bind to the FSH receptor and LH receptor, respectively, both of which are **G protein–linked receptors.** The functions of FSH and LH are indicated below.

   a. **FSH.** In women, FSH promotes the growth of secondary follicles → Graafian follicles. In men, FSH maintains spermatogenesis and stimulates synthesis of androgen-binding protein (ABP) in Sertoli cells.

   b. **LH.** In women, LH promotes ovulation (LH surge), formation of corpus luteum (luteinization), and progesterone secretion. In men, LH stimulates testosterone secretion from Leydig cells.

B. **PARS TUBERALIS.** The pars tuberalis surrounds the median eminence and infundibular stem of the neurohypophysis. The par tuberalis contains the portal venules of the hypophyseal portal system.

C. **PARS INTERMEDIA.** The pars intermedia (rudimentary in humans) contains numerous colloid-filled cysts **(Rathke's cysts).**

Ⅱ Hormonal Secretion from the adenohypophysis is controlled by hypothalamic neurons and the hypophyseal portal system.

A. **HYPOTHALAMIC NEURONS.** Neuronal cell bodies are located in the **arcuate nucleus, medial preoptic nucleus,** and **paraventricular nucleus** of the hypothalamus. The cell bodies synthesize **releasing factors (RFs)** and **inhibiting factors (IFs).** Axons project to the **median eminence,** where axon terminals secrete RFs and IFs into the primary capillaries of the hypophyseal portal system. RFs and IFs control hormone secretion from the adenohypophysis and include the following: **GHRF, growth hormone-inhibiting factor (somatostatin), prolactin-inhibiting factor (dopamine), TRF, CRF, and GnRF.**

B. **THE HYPOPHYSEAL PORTAL SYSTEM** has three components:
   1. **Primary capillaries** (fenestrated) are formed by the superior hypophyseal artery. They are located in the median eminence and are the site where RFs and IFs are secreted into the bloodstream.
   2. **Portal venules** are located in the pars tuberalis. They transport RFs and IFs to the pars distalis.
   3. **Secondary capillaries** (fenestrated) are located in the pars distalis. They are the site where RFs and IFs leave the bloodstream to stimulate or inhibit endocrine cells of the adenohypophysis.

Ⅲ The Neurohypophysis (Figure 22-1) receives axonal projections from neurons that have cell bodies located in the **supraoptic nucleus** and **paraventricular nucleus** of the hypothalamus. The cell bodies synthesize **oxytocin,** which causes **milk ejection** (by stimulating myoepithelial cells in the mammary gland to contract) and **uterine contraction during childbirth** (by stimulating smooth muscle cells of the myometrium). The cell bodies also synthesize **antidiuretic hormone (ADH),** which increases water reabsorption from tubular fluid to blood by the cortical and medullary collecting ducts of the kidneys. As axons project to the neurohypophysis, large aggregations of neurosecretory vesicles (called **Herring bodies)** containing either oxytocin or ADH (plus a carrier protein called **neurophysin)** can be observed. Axon terminals secrete oxytocin and ADH into a capillary network formed by the inferior hypophyseal artery. **Pituicytes** also are found within the neurohypophysis and may function as glial-type cells.

Chapter 23

Thyroid

I **Thyroid Follicles** are bounded by **follicular cells** and **parafollicular cells**. They are filled with a colloid that consists of **iodinated thyroglobulin**.

II **Follicular Cells** (Figure 23-1). These cells:

A. Contain **thyroid-stimulating hormone (TSH) receptors**, which are G protein-linked receptors ($\uparrow$cAMP)

B. Synthesize **thyroglobulin** and secrete thyroglobulin into the follicular lumen.

C. Take up iodide (I^-) from the blood using a **Na^+-I^- cotransporter** and transport it to the follicular lumen.

D. Oxidize iodide ($2I^- + H_2O_2 \rightarrow I_2$) using the enzyme **thyroid peroxidase** and **iodinate tyrosine residues in thyroglobulin,** thereby forming monoiodotyrosine (MIT) and diiodotyrosine (DIT), which are then coupled to form triiodothyronine (T_3) and thyroxine (T_4).

E. Are stimulated by **TSH** to begin endocytosis of iodinated thyroglobulin. TSH is secreted from the adenohypophysis and is under the control of **thyrotropin-releasing factor (TRF)** released from hypothalamic neurons.

F. Break down iodinated thyroglobulin into MIT, DIT, T_3, and T_4 through **lysosomal degradation.**

G. Deiodinate MIT and DIT using the enzyme **deiodinase** to recycle iodide (I^-); and secrete T_3 and T_4 into the bloodstream, which then circulate bound to **thyroid-binding globulin (TBG).**

H. T_3 (more potent) accounts for 10% of the thyroid output and has a half-life of 1 day. T_4 (less potent) accounts for 90% of the thyroid output and has a half-life of 8 days.

I. T_3 and T_4 function like **steroid hormones** in that they use a cytoplasmic receptor that belongs to the steroid-hormone receptor superfamily.

245

● **Figure 23-1 Diagram of triiodothyronine (T_3) and thyroxine (T_4) synthesis and secretion by follicular cells.** The secretion of calcitonin by parafollicular cells also is shown. Note the location of drug action. *DIT* = diiodotyrosine; *MIT* = monoiodotyrosine; *TBG* = thyroid-binding globulin; *TG* = thyroglobulin; *TSH* = thyroid-stimulating hormone; *TRF* = thyrotropin-releasing factor; *rER* = rough endoplasmic reticulum; *PTU* = propylthiouracil.

III Functions of T_3 and T_4 include the following:

A. Increase basal metabolic rate (BMR); i.e., rate of oxygen consumption and heat production.

B. Increase cardiac output, increase systolic blood pressure, and decrease diastolic blood pressure.

C. Increase gluconeogenesis, glycogen degradation, glucose oxidation, and lipolysis.

D. Increase eating and glucose absorption.

E. Stimulate cartilage growth.

F. Stimulate endochondral ossification and linear growth of bone.

G. Play a crucial role in central nervous system (CNS) development (a deficiency of T_3 and T_4 results in permanent brain damage).

IV Parafollicular Cells secrete **calcitonin,** which acts directly on osteoclasts to decrease bone resorption, thereby lowering blood $Ca2^+$ levels. Calcitonin binds to the calcitonin receptor, which is a G protein–linked receptor.

V Clinical Considerations

A. **GRAVES' DISEASE (GD)** is hyperthyroidism caused by a diffuse, hyperplastic (toxic) goiter. GD is relatively common in women. GD is an autoimmune disease that produces **TSH receptor-stimulating autoantibodies**. Clinical characteristics include: ophthalmopathy (lid stare, eye bulging), heat intolerance, nervousness, irritability, and weight loss in the presence of a good appetite.

B. **SECONDARY HYPERTHYROIDISM** is relatively uncommon and may be caused by a TSH adenoma in the adenohypophysis.

C. **HASHIMOTO THYROIDITIS (HT)** is the most common cause of goitrous hypothyroidism. HT is relatively common in middle-aged women. HT is an autoimmune disease that produces **thyroid peroxidase autoantibodies**. Clinical characteristics include: goiter and hypothyroidism. In some variants of Hashimoto thyroiditis, only hypothyroidism exists, no goiter.

D. **PRIMARY HYPOTHYROIDISM (PH)** is most commonly idiopathic, whereby **TSH receptor-blocking autoantibodies** are present. Clinical characteristics include: low blood pressure, low heart rate, low respiratory rate, reduced body temperature, and myxedema (peripheral nonpitting edema).

E. **SECONDARY HYPOTHYROIDISM** is relatively uncommon and is caused by a deficiency in the adenohypophysis (low TSH secretion) or hypothalamus (low TRF secretion).

F. ESTROGEN EFFECT. The use of oral contraceptive pills or the use of diethylstilbestrol for treatment of prostatic cancer increases synthesis of TBG.

G. DIFFUSE NONTOXIC (SIMPLE) GOITER is an enlargement of the entire thyroid gland in a diffuse manner without producing nodules. A simple goiter occurs most commonly in particular geographic areas (called **endemic goiter**), most often caused by deficiency of iodine in the diet. Wherever endemic goiter is prevalent, endemic **cretinism** occurs. A severe iodine deficiency during fetal development results in growth retardation and severe mental retardation.

H. DIAGNOSIS. Table 23-1 shows the laboratory findings used for diagnosis.

TABLE 23-1	LABORATORY FINDINGS USED FOR DIAGNOSIS OF THYROID DISORDERS					
Disorder	Mechanisms	Total T$_4$*	T$_3$RU (TBG)**	FTI†	TSH	I^{131}Uptake
Graves' disease	Production of TSH receptor–stimulating autoantibodies	High	High (Low)	High	Undetectable	High
Secondary hyperthyroidism	TSH adenoma	High	High (Low)	High	High	High
Factitious thyrotoxicosis	Excessive exogenous thyroid hormone intake	High	High (Low)	High	Low	Low
Thyroiditis	Inflammation of bacterial or viral origin	High	High (Low)	High	Low	Low
Hashimoto thyroiditis	Production of thyroid peroxidase autoantibodies	Low	Low (High)	Low	High	Low
Primary hypothyroidism	Production of TSH receptor-blocking antibodies	Low	Low (High)	Low	Very High	Low
Secondary hypothyroidism	Low TSH secretion by adenohypophysis or low TRF secretion by the hypothalamus	Low	Low (High)	Low	Low	Low
Increased TBG (increased estrogen)	Oral contraceptives, DES therapy for prostate cancer	High	Low (High)	Normal	Normal	Normal
Decreased TBG (increased androgens)	Steroid abuse	Low	High (Low)	Normal	Normal	Normal

DES = diethylstilbestrol; *T$_3$* = triiodothyronine; *T$_4$* = thyroxine; *TRF* = thyrotropin-releasing factor; *TSH* = thyroid-stimulating hormone; *TBG* = thyroid binding globulin.

*Total T$_4$ measures both bound and free T$_4$.

**The T$_3$ resin uptake (T$_3$RU) test is not a measure of serum T$_3$ levels; rather, it measures the percentage of free T$_4$. This test evaluates TBG levels via a competition assay between a resin and TBG for radioactive T$_3$. If TBG levels are low, then more radioactive T$_3$ will bind to the resin. TBG has an inverse relationship to T$_3$RU.

†Free thyroxine (T$_4$) Index (FTI) is a measure of free T$_4$. It is calculated by multiplying the total T$_4$ × T$_3$RU. FTI is rapidly becoming obsolete as major medical centers are using assays that directly measure free T$_4$.

I^{131} = radioactive iodine I^{131} uptake.

Pharmacology of the Thyroid

A. PROPYLTHIOURACIL (PTU) inhibits thyroid peroxidase and the peripheral conversion of $T_4 \rightarrow T_3$. It is used clinically to treat hyperthyroidism (e.g., Graves' disease) and thyrotoxicosis in pregnant women because it crosses the placenta to a lesser degree than methimazole.

B. METHIMAZOLE (TAPAZOLE) inhibits thyroid peroxidase. It is used clinically to treat hyperthyroidism (e.g., Graves' disease) but not thyrotoxicosis in pregnant women because it crosses the placenta to a greater degree than PTU.

C. LUGOL'S SOLUTION AND POTASSIUM IODIDE (THYRO-BLOCK, PIMA) inhibit the secretion of T_3 and T_4 and inhibit the iodination of thyroglobulin (Wolff-Chaikoff effect). They are used clinically to treat hyperthyroidism (e.g., Graves' disease).

D. THIOCYANATE AND PERCHLORATE competitively inhibit iodide (I^-) transport in thyroid follicular cells. They are used clinically to treat hyperthyroidism (e.g., Graves' disease).

E. IOPANOIC ACID (TELEPAQUE) AND SODIUM IPODATE (ORAGRAFIN) inhibit the peripheral conversion of $T_4 \rightarrow T_3$. They are used clinically to treat hyperthyroidism (e.g., Graves' disease).

F. LIOTHYRONINE SODIUM (CYTOMEL; TRIOSTAT) is T_3. It is used clinically to treat myxedema coma, which is a medical emergency caused by long-standing hypothyroidism.

G. LEVOTHYROXINE SODIUM (SYNTHROID; LEVOTHROID) is T_4. It is used clinically as hormone replacement therapy to treat hypothyroidism or to prevent cretinism in newborns.

Selected Photomicrographs

A. Normal thyroid, Hashimoto thyroiditis, and Graves' disease (Figure 23-2)

B. Papillary carcinoma and medullary carcinoma (Figure 23-3)

● **Figure 23-2 Normal and pathological thyroid. (A)** LM of a normal thyroid gland showing numerous thyroid follicles (*TF*) containing colloidal material. The follicles are lined by follicular cells arranged as a simple cuboidal epithelium. **(B)** LM of a normal thyroid gland showing a cluster of parafollicular cells that secrete calcitonin. **(C)** LM of Hashimoto thyroiditis (*HT*). HT is characterized by a high lymphocytic infiltration that may form lymphoid follicles with germinal centers (*L*). Normal thyroid follicles (*TF*) also are observed. **(D)** LM of Graves' disease (*GD*). Graves' disease is caused by a diffuse, hyperplastic goiter. The follicular cells are increased in number (hyperplasia) and arranged as a simple tall columnar epithelium. In addition, the follicular cells can form buds that encroach into the colloidal material (*arrows*).

● **Figure 23-3 Thyroid carcinomas. (A)** LM of papillary carcinoma (*PC*). Normal thyroid parenchyma can be observed (*Nor*). PC infiltrates normal thyroid parenchyma and forms elaborate branching papillae that are lined by single-to-multiple layers of follicular cells. The nuclei of follicular cells do not contain nucleoli ("Orphan Annie eyes"). Psammoma bodies sometimes surrounded by calcific lamellations are generally found within the core of the papillae. *Inset:* Gross photograph of a papillary carcinoma showing a yellow-white infiltrative mass (*arrow*) with some fibrous strands. **(B)** LM of medullary carcinoma (*MC*). MC is an endocrine neoplasm of the parafollicular cells that secretes calcitonin. The parafollicular cells are usually arranged in cell nests (*arrow*) surrounded by bands of stroma (*str*) containing amyloid. Inset: LM of medullary carcinoma cells immunocytochemically stained for calcitonin.

CASE STUDY

A 40-year-old woman comes to your office complaining that "About 4 weeks ago, I started feeling very nervous for no good reason. And, sometimes my heart starts to pump so fast it feels like it is going to jump out of my chest." She also tells you that "I have a real good appetite and have been eating a lot lately; but I still lost 15 pounds." After some discussion, she informs you that she can't stand this hot weather, has not had a period in 3 months, and frequently has diarrhea. What is the most likely diagnosis?

Differentials

- Hashimoto thyroiditis, menopause, pheochromocytoma.

Relevant Physical Exam Findings

- Tachycardia
- Moist warm skin
- Mild exophthalmos
- Goiter
- Resting tremor of the hands

Relevant Lab Findings

- Blood chemistry: Total T_4 = 17.2 µg.mL (High); Free thyroxine index (FTI) = 5.8 (High); TSH = undetectable
- Urinalysis: catecholamine = Normal
- Thyroid scan: high I^{131} uptake
- Thyroid biopsy: follicular cells are increased in number (hyperplasia) and arranged as simple tall columnar epithelium; follicular cells form buds that encroach into the colloid material

Diagnosis

Graves' Disease (GD). GD is hyperthyroidism caused by a diffuse, hyperplastic (toxic) goiter. GD is the most common form of hyperthyroidism. GD is an autoimmune disease that produces TSH receptor–stimulating autoantibodies. These autoantibodies mimic TSH and cause increased secretion of T_3 and T_4. The normal negative feedback loop does not inhibit the autoantibodies so that the thyroid gland is constantly stimulated. Clinical findings of hyperthyroidism include restlessness, irritability, and fatigue; resting tremor in the hands; heat intolerance; sweating with warm, moist skin; tachycardia with palpitations; fat and muscle loss despite increased caloric intake; thinning of hair; diarrhea; and amenorrhea. Hashimoto thyroiditis (HT) is the most common cause of goitrous hypothyroidism. In some variants of Hashimoto thyroiditis, only hypothyroidism and no goiter exists. HT is relatively common in middle-aged women. HT is an autoimmune disease that produces thyroid peroxidase autoantibodies and destroys the thyroid gland. HT progresses from a euthyroid state → transient hyperthyroidism → hypothyroidism. Clinical findings of hypothyroidism include myxedema; cold intolerance; weight gain; low pitch of voice; mental slowing; increased menstrual bleeding; constipation; edema of face, eyelids, and hands; and brittle and dry hair that falls out. Menopause is the stoppage of the menstrual cycle in women around 50 years of age. Clinical findings of menopause include hot flashes, sweating, depression, and insomnia. It should be considered that menopause and GD may run concurrently. Pheochromocytoma is a relatively rare (usually not malignant) catecholamine-producing tumor (both epinephrine and norepinephrine) of the adrenal medulla. A pheochromocytoma occurs mainly in adults and is generally found in the region of the adrenal gland but also is found in extra-adrenal sites. It occurs within families as part of the MEN Type II syndrome. Clinical findings of pheochromocytoma include persistent or paroxysmal hypertension, anxiety, tremor, profuse sweating, pallor, chest pain, abdominal pain, increased urine vanillylmandelic acid (VMA) and metanephrine levels, inability to suppress catecholamines with clonidine, and hyperglycemia.

Parathyroid

I **Chief Cells** secrete **parathyroid hormone (PTH).** PTH binds to the PTH receptor, which is a G protein-linked receptor ($\uparrow$ cAMP).

II **Oxyphil Cells** are distinctly eosinophilic because of the numerous mitochondria within the cytoplasm, but they have no known function.

III **Calcium Homeostasis** (Figure 24-1). The body regulates blood Ca^{2+} levels closely because hypocalcemia results in tetanic convulsions and death. The hormones most important for controlling blood Ca^{2+} levels are the following:

A. PTH

1. PTH increases kidney reabsorption of Ca^{2+} from the tubular fluid $\rightarrow$ plasma by the distal convoluted tubule (DCT) and collecting duct (CD), thereby elevating blood Ca^{2+} levels.
2. PTH acts directly on osteoblasts to secrete **macrophage colony-stimulating factor (M-CSF)** and to express a cell surface protein called **RANKL.** M-CSF stimulates monocytes to differentiate into macrophages and to express a cell surface receptor called **RANK.** RANKL (on the osteoblast) and RANK (on the macrophage) interact and cause the differentiation of macrophages into osteoclasts. Osteoclasts increase bone resorption, thereby elevating blood Ca^{2+} levels.
3. PTH increases the synthesis of 1α-hydroxylase in the kidney by the proximal convoluted tubule (PCT), thereby elevating blood 1,25-hydroxyvitamin D [1,25-$(OH)_2$ vitamin D] levels.

B. 1,25-$(OH)_2$ VITAMIN D

1. 1,25-$(OH)_2$ vitamin D mainly stimulates absorption of Ca^{2+} and PO_4^{2-} ions from the intestinal lumen into the blood, thereby elevating blood Ca^{2+} and PO_4^{2-} levels.
2. 1,25-$(OH)_2$ vitamin D also acts directly on osteoblasts to secrete IL-1, which stimulates osteoclasts to increase bone resorption, thereby elevating blood Ca^{2+} levels.

C. CALCITONIN is secreted by parafollicular cells found within the thyroid gland. Calcitonin acts directly on osteoclasts to decrease bone resorption, thereby lowering blood Ca^{2+} levels.

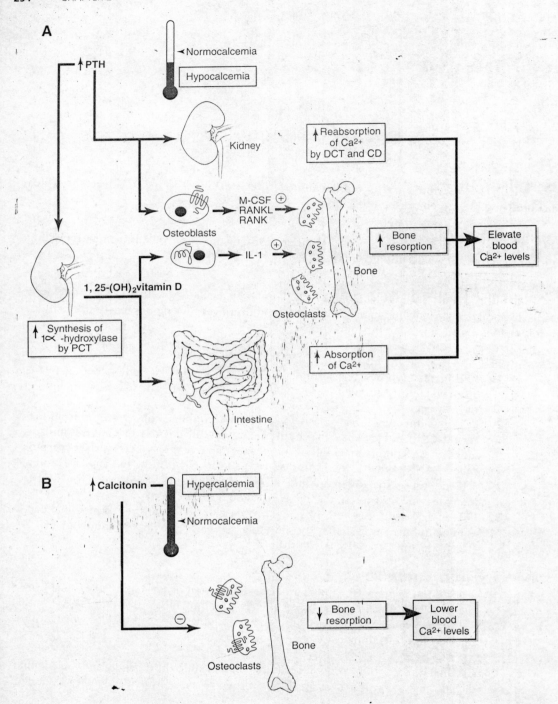

A

↑PTH

← Normocalcemia

Hypocalcemia

Kidney

↑ Reabsorption of Ca2+ by DCT and CD

M-CSF ⊕
RANKL
RANK

Osteoblasts

Bone resorption

Elevate blood Ca2+ levels

IL-1 ⊕

Bone

1, 25-(OH)₂vitamin D

Osteoclasts

↑ Synthesis of 1∝-hydroxylase by PCT

↑ Absorption of Ca2+

Intestine

B

↑Calcitonin — Hypercalcemia

← Normocalcemia

⊖

↓ Bone resorption

Lower blood Ca2+ levels

Bone

Osteoclasts

● **Figure 24-1 Calcium homeostasis. (A)** Blood calcium levels can be depicted on a thermometer such that when blood calcium levels are too low, PTH is released. PTH and 1,25-(OH)₂ vitamin D regulate blood calcium levels by acting on the kidney, bone, and intestine to elevate blood calcium levels. *M-CSF* = macrophage colony-stimulating factor; *RANKL* = RANK ligand; *RANK* = receptor for activation of nuclear factor kappa B. **(B)** Blood calcium levels can be depicted on a thermometer such that when blood calcium levels are too high, calcitonin is released. Calcitonin regulates blood calcium levels by acting on bone to lower blood calcium levels.

Clinical Considerations

A. PRIMARY HYPOPARATHYROIDISM (e.g., accidental surgical removal, DiGeorge syndrome, autoimmune destruction) is characterized by the absence of PTH, leading to **hypocalcemia.** Chronic renal failure and vitamin D deficiency also lead to hypocalcemia. Clinical findings include: carpopedal spasm, laryngospasm, **Chvostek sign** (tapping facial nerve elicits spasm of facial muscles), **Trousseau phenomenon** (inflated blood pressure cuff on arm elicits carpel tunnel spasm), calcification of basal ganglia, cataracts, and tetany. Seizures and cardiac arrest may occur in severe cases.

B. PSEUDOHYPOPARATHYROIDISM is a rare condition characterized by abnormal PTH receptors, leading to **hypocalcemia,** although there are high PTH levels.

C. PRIMARY HYPERPARATHYROIDISM (e.g., adenoma, hyperplasia, associated with multiple endocrine neoplasia [MEN] syndromes) is characterized by excessive secretion of PTH, leading to **hypercalcemia.** Clinical findings include osteitis fibrosa cystica (bone softening and painful fractures), urinary calculi, abdominal pain (caused by constipation, pancreatitis, or biliary stones), depression or lethargy, and cardiac arrhythmias. Think "painful bones, kidney stones, belly groans, mental moans."

D. MALIGNANT TUMORS (e.g., lung, breast, or ovarian carcinomas) may secrete a PTH-related protein, leading to **hypercalcemia.**

E. Diagnosis. Table 24-1 shows laboratory findings used for diagnosis.

TABLE 24-1	LABORATORY FINDINGS USED FOR DIAGNOSIS OF PARATHYROID DISORDERS		
Disorder	Calcium	Phosphorus	PTH
Hypocalcemia			
Primary hypoparathyroidism	Low	High	Low
Pseudohypoparathyroidism	Low	High	Normal → High
Secondary hypoparathyroidism (malabsorption)	Low	Low	High
Secondary hypoparathyroidism (renal failure)	Low	High	High
Hypoalbuminemia	Low (Normal ionized calcium)	Normal	Normal
Alkalosis	Normal (Decreased ionized calcium)	Normal	High
Hypercalcemia			
Primary hyperparathyroidism	High	Low	High
Malignant tumors	High	Low	Low

Pharmacology of Calcium Homeostasis

A. CALCIUM CARBONATE (TUMS), CALCIUM CHLORIDE, CALCIUM GLUCEPTATE, and **calcium gluconate** are calcium salt preparations. They are used to treat hypocalcemia.

B. **CALCIFEDIOL, CALCITRIOL, DIHYDROTACHYSTEROL,** and **ergocalciferol** are vitamin D preparations. They are used to treat hypocalcemia.

C. **ETIDRONATE (DIDRONEL) AND PAMIDRONATE (AREDIA)** are bisphosphonates that inhibit osteoclast activity. They are used to treat hypercalcemia.

D. **HUMAN CALCITONIN (CIBACALCIN) AND SALMON CALCITONIN (CALCIMAR)** are the 32-amino acid peptide secreted by the parafollicular cells of the thyroid gland that acts directly on osteoclasts to decrease bone resorption. They are used to treat hypercalcemia.

VI Selected Photomicrographs.
Isolated parathyroid glands, parathyroid embedded in the thyroid gland, LM of parathyroid, LM of chief cells immunocytochemically stained for PTH (Figure 24-2).

● **Figure 24-2 General features of the parathyroid gland. (A)** Four normal parathyroid glands dissected at autopsy of a 53-year-old man. **(B)** A normal parathyroid gland (*P*) embedded entirely within the thyroid gland (*THY*). **(C)** LM of a parathyroid gland. The chief cells (*arrows*) are arranged in sheets or cords. Chief cells contain lipid droplets, glycogen, and lysosomes. Chief cells synthesize and secrete the protein hormone PTH and therefore contain a distinct Golgi and rough endoplasmic reticulum (*rER*). Oxyphil cells (*Ox*) have a distinctly eosinophilic cytoplasm due to a large number of mitochondria. **(D)** LM of a parathyroid gland immunocytochemically stained for PTH. Note the staining of chief cells (*arrows*) arranged in sheets or cords.

Chapter 25

Adrenal

1 **Cortex.** Cortical cells of the adrenal gland synthesize and secrete steroid hormones. They have abundant smooth endoplasmic reticulum (sER), mitochondria with tubular cristae, and lipid droplets, which are characteristic of all steroid-secreting cells.

A. **ZONA GLOMERULOSA (ZG).** This region constitutes **15%** of the cortical volume. ZG cells are arranged in **glomerular-like clusters.** ZG cells synthesize and secrete **aldosterone.** The secretion of aldosterone is controlled by the **renin-angiotensin system.** Aldosterone has a **half-life of 20 minutes** as it is metabolized by the liver and excreted as a glucuronide. Urine levels of **aldosterone 3-glucuronide** are used for diagnostic purposes. The functions of aldosterone include the following:

   1. Increases Na^+ reabsorption from tubular fluid $\rightarrow$ plasma (water follows) by the cortical collecting ducts of the kidneys.
   2. Increases K^+ secretion from plasma $\rightarrow$ tubular fluid by the cortical collecting ducts of the kidneys.
   3. Increases H^+ secretion from plasma $\rightarrow$ tubular fluid by the cortical collecting ducts of the kidneys.
   4. Increases Na^+ absorption by enterocytes of the large intestine.
   5. Increases Na^+ reabsorption from excretory ducts of eccrine sweat glands.

B. **ZONA FASCICULATA (ZF).** This region constitutes **78%** of the cortical volume. ZF cells are arranged as two-cell wide **vertical cords.** ZF cells synthesize and secrete **cortisol.** The secretion of cortisol is controlled by **corticotropin-releasing factor (CRF)** and **adrenocorticotropin (ACTH)** from the hypothalamus and adenohypophysis, respectively. Abnormally high levels of ACTH (e.g., adenoma of adenohypophysis) cause hypertrophy of the ZF. Abnormally low levels of ACTH (e.g., hypophysectomy) cause atrophy of the ZF. Cortisol has a **half-life of 70 minutes** as it is metabolized by the liver and excreted in the urine as a glucuronide. Urine levels of **17-hydroxycorticoids** are used for diagnostic purposes. The functions of cortisol include the following:

   1. Inhibits glucose uptake and decreases insulin sensitivity in adipose tissue and muscle.
   2. Stimulates lipolysis in adipose tissue, which forms glycerol (used by the liver as substrate for gluconeogenesis) and fatty acids (which are metabolized by the liver for energy).
   3. Stimulates protein catabolism in muscle, which forms amino acids that are used by the liver as substrate for gluconeogenesis.
   4. Stimulates gluconeogenesis and glycogen synthesis in the liver. **Overall the most important metabolic effect of cortisol is the conversion of fat and muscle protein to glycogen.**

5. Inhibits bone formation, causing osteoporosis by reducing the synthesis of type I collagen and decreasing the absorption of Ca^{2+} by the intestinal tract by blocking the action of 1,25-(OH_2) vitamin D.
6. Produces anti-inflammatory response at high concentrations by inhibition of: **phospholipase A$_2$**, which releases arachidonic acid (a precursor for many immune mediators); **IL-2 production**, thereby preventing proliferation of T lymphocytes; and **histamine** and **serotonin release** from mast cells.
7. Stimulates surfactant production in the fetus.

C. **ZONA RETICULARIS (ZR).** This region constitutes 7% of the cortical volume. ZR cells are arranged as one-cell wide anastomosing rows and contain large amounts of **lipofuscin pigment.** ZR cells synthesize and secrete **dehydroepiandrosterone (DHEA)** and **androstenedione.** The secretion of DHEA and androstenedione is controlled by CRF and ACTH from the hypothalamus and adenohypophysis, respectively. Although DHEA and androstenedione are weak androgens, they are converted to testosterone by peripheral tissues. DHEA and androstenedione are metabolized by the liver to 17-ketosteroids. Urine levels of **17-ketosteroids** are used for diagnostic purposes. The functions of DHEA and androstenedione include the following:
1. In women, DHEA and androstenedione conversion to testosterone is a main source of testosterone. During puberty, DHEA and androstenedione also may serve as substrates for conversion to estrogen.
2. In men, DHEA and androstenedione conversion to testosterone is of little biologic significance because the testes produce most of the testosterone.

D. **SYNTHESIS OF ADRENOCORTICAL HORMONES** uses cholesterol as a precursor (Figure 25-1).

E. **CLINICAL CONSIDERATIONS**
1. **Primary hyperaldosteronism**
   a. **Cause.** Elevated levels of aldosterone (i.e., hyperaldosteronism) are commonly caused by an aldosterone-secreting adenoma (**Conn syndrome**) within the ZG.
   b. **Symptoms.** Primary hyperaldosteronism is characterized clinically by hypertension, hypernatremia as a result of increased Na^+ reabsorption, weight gain as a result of water retention, and hypokalemia as a result of increased K^+ secretion.
   c. **Treatment.** It is treated by **surgery or spironolactone,** which is an aldosterone receptor antagonist and therefore an effective antihypertensive and diuretic agent.
2. **Cushing syndrome**
   a. **Cause.** Cushing syndrome is most commonly caused by administration of **large doses of steroids** for treatment of primary disease. If not iatrogenic, elevated levels of cortisol (i.e., hypercortisolism) are caused by an **ACTH-secreting adenoma** within the adenohypophysis (75% of cases; strictly termed **Cushing disease**) or **adrenal cortical adenoma** (25% of cases).
   b. **Symptoms.** Cushing syndrome is characterized clinically by mild hypertension, impaired glucose tolerance, acne, hirsutism, oligomenorrhea, impotence and loss of libido (in men), osteoporosis with back pain and buffalo hump, central obesity, moon facies, and purple skin striae (bruise easily).
   c. **Treatment.** Surgery is an option. **Aminoglutethimide, metyrapone,** and **ketoconazole** are used in the treatment of Cushing syndrome.
3. **Congenital adrenal hyperplasia**
   a. **Cause.** Congenital adrenal hyperplasia is caused most commonly by mutations in genes for enzymes involved in adrenocortical steroid biosynthesis

● **Figure 25-1 Synthesis and metabolism of adrenocortical steroid hormones. Cholesterol** is the precursor of all steroid hormones. Most of the cholesterol is derived from **LDL** (low-density lipoprotein), which binds to the **LDL receptor** and enters the cell by **receptor-mediated endocytosis.** Cholesterol is then transported into the mitochondria by **StAR** (steroidogenic acute regulatory protein). Within the mitochondria, cholesterol is metabolized to pregnenolone by the enzyme desmolase. Pregnenolone is then transported to the cytoplasm. In general, enzymes for steroid biosynthesis are located either in the mitochondria or sER such that substrate intermediates are shuttled back and forth from mitochondria to the sER. Enzymes located in the mitochondria are indicated by the lighter shaded font. All other enzymes are located in the sER. The metabolic urine breakdown products (in *shaded boxes*) are used for diagnostic purposes. 21-Hydroxylase (*) and 11β-hydroxylase (**) are enzymes involved in congenital adrenal hyperplasia. *DHEA* = dehydroepiandrosterone.

(e.g., **21-hydroxylase deficiency, 11β-hydroxylase deficiency**). In 21-hydroxylase deficiency (90% of all cases), there is virtually no synthesis of aldosterone or cortisol, so that intermediates are funneled into androgen biosynthesis, thereby elevating androgen levels.

    b. **Symptoms.** The elevated levels of androgens lead to virilization of a female fetus, ranging from mild clitoral enlargement to complete labioscrotal fusion with a phalloid organ (female pseudointersexuality). In the male fetus, macrogenitosomia occurs. Because cortisol cannot be synthesized, negative feedback to the adenohypophysis does not occur, so ACTH continues to stimulate the adrenal cortex, resulting in adrenal hyperplasia.

    c. **Treatment.** Depending on the severity, treatment may include surgical reconstruction and steroid replacement.

  4. **Primary adrenal insufficiency (Addison disease)**

    a. **Cause.** Addison disease is commonly caused by autoimmune destruction of the adrenal cortex.

    b. **Symptoms.** It is characterized clinically by fatigue, anorexia, nausea, weight loss, hypotension, skin hyperpigmentation as a result of increased melanocyte-stimulating hormone (MSH) caused by an increase in ACTH secretion, hyponatremia, and hyperkalemia (may lead to fatal cardiac arrhythmias).

    c. **Treatment.** This condition is managed by steroid replacement therapy.

  5. **Secondary adrenal insufficiency**

    a. **Cause.** Secondary adrenal insufficiency is caused by a disorder of the hypothalamus or adenohypophysis that reduces the secretion of ACTH.

    b. **Symptoms.** It is clinically very similar to Addison disease except there is no hyperpigmentation of the skin.

F. **PHARMACOLOGY OF ADRENAL GLAND**

  1. **Aldosterone and fludrocortisone (Florinef)** are mineralocorticoids. They are used clinically in steroid replacement therapy (e.g., Addison disease).

  2. **Spironolactone** is an aldosterone receptor antagonist. It is used clinically to treat primary hyperaldosteronism (e.g., Conn syndrome).

  3. **Cortisol, cortisone,** and **corticosteroid** are glucocorticoids. They are used clinically in steroid replacement therapy (e.g., Addison disease).

  4. **Methylprednisolone (Medrol)** and **prednisone (Deltasone)** are glucocorticoids. They are used clinically as anti-inflammatory agents, immunosuppressive agents, and in chemotherapy (prednisone is part of the MOPP regimen).

  5. **Dexamethasone (Decadron)** is a glucocorticoid. It is used clinically as an anti-inflammatory agent, immunosuppressive agent, to suppress ACTH secretion, and in the diagnosis of Cushing disease (dexamethasone suppression test).

  6. **Aminoglutethimide (Cytadren)** inhibits desmolase thereby preventing synthesis of cortisol. It is used clinically to treat breast cancer and Cushing syndrome.

  7. **Metyrapone (Metopirone)** inhibits 11β-hydroxylase thereby preventing synthesis of cortisol. It is used clinically to treat Cushing syndrome.

  8. **Ketoconazole** inhibits the cytochrome P_{450} enzymes thereby preventing steroid biosynthesis in general. It is used clinically to treat Cushing syndrome.

  9. **Mitotane (Lysodren)** destroys the cells of the zona fasciculata and zona reticularis. It is used clinically to treat adrenocortical carcinoma.

G. **DIAGNOSIS.** Table 25-1 shows the laboratory findings used for diagnosis.

TABLE 25-1		LABORATORY FINDINGS USED FOR DIAGNOSIS OF ADRENAL DISORDERS				
		Plasma Levels				
Clinical Condition	Dex*	ALD	Cortisol	Androgens	ACTH	Other
Primary hyperaldosteronism (Conn syndrome)		High				
Cushing syndrome						
Normal patient	+		Normal		Normal	
ACTH adenoma	+		High		High	
Adrenal adenoma	−		High		Low	
Congenital adrenal hyperplasia						
21-Hydroxylase deficiency		Low	Low	High	High	Salt Loss with volume depletion
11β-Hydroxylase deficiency		Low	Low	High	High	Salt retention with hypertension
Addison disease (Primary adrenal insufficiency)		Low	Low	Low	High	
Secondary adrenal insufficiency		Normal	Low	Low	Low	

*Dex = **high-dose dexamethasone suppression test.** This test is based on the ability of dexamethasone (a synthetic glucocorti-coid) to inhibit ACTH and cortisol secretion. If the adenohypophysis-adrenal cortex axis is normal, dexamethasone will suppress ACTH and cortisol secretion and the test is considered positive (i.e., suppression occurred).
ALD = aldosterone; ACTH = adrenocorticotropin.

The Medulla contains **chromaffin cells,** which are **modified postganglionic sympathetic neurons.** Preganglionic sympathetic axons (via splanchnic nerves) synapse on chromaffin cells and on stimulation cause chromaffin cells to secrete catecholamines: epinephrine and norepinephrine. There are two types of chromaffin cells:

A. **EPINEPHRINE-CONTAINING CELLS** comprise a majority of the chromaffin cells in the medulla and contain small, homogeneous, light-staining granules. All of the circulating epinephrine in the blood is derived from the adrenal medulla. Epinephrine binds to α- and β-adrenergic receptors, which are G protein-linked receptors. Epinephrine has a **half-life of 1 to 3 minutes** as it is metabolized by the liver and excreted in the urine as **free epinephrine** or **metanephrine. Urinary levels of free epinephrine** are used for diagnostic purposes in problems of adrenal medulla function.

B. **NOREPINEPHRINE-CONTAINING CELLS** comprise a minority of the chromaffin cells in the medulla and contain large, electron-dense core granules. The majority of circulating norepinephrine in the blood is derived from the postganglionic sympathetic neurons and brain, with secretion from the adrenal medulla contributing only a minor portion. Norepinephrine binds to α- and β-adrenergic receptors, which are G protein-linked receptors. Norepinephrine has a **half-life of 1 to 3 minutes,** as it is metabolized by the liver and excreted in the urine as **free norepinephrine, normetanephrine, vanillylmandelic acid (VMA),** or **3-methoxy-4-hydroxyphenyglycol (MOPEG). Urinary levels of VMA and MOPEG** are used for diagnostic purposes in problems of the sympathetic nervous system.

C. **FUNCTIONS OF EPINEPHRINE AND NOREPINEPHRINE** basically include all the functions of the sympathetic nervous system as they elicit their effect via α- and β-adrenergic receptors. These functions include the following: contracts the dilator pupillae muscle causing dilation of the pupil (mydriasis), contracts the arrector pili muscle in skin, contracts vascular smooth muscle in skin and visceral vessels, relaxes vascular smooth muscle in skeletal muscle vessels, relaxes bronchial smooth muscle in the lung (bronchodilation), relaxes GI tract smooth muscle (decreases motility), contracts GI tract smooth muscle sphincters, relaxes smooth muscle in the urinary bladder, contracts smooth muscle in the urinary tract sphincter, contracts smooth muscle in the ductus deferens causing ejaculation, relaxes smooth muscle of the uterus, accelerates the SA node (increases heart rate), increases conduction velocity at the AV node, increases contractility of cardiac muscle, increases viscous secretion from salivary glands, increases eccrine sweat gland secretion (thermoregulation), increases apocrine sweat gland secretion, stimulates seminal vesicle and prostrate secretion during ejaculation, stimulates gluconeogenesis and glycogenolysis in hepatocytes, causes lipolysis in adipocytes, causes renin release from JG cells in the kidney (increases blood pressure), and inhibits insulin secretion from pancreatic beta cells.

D. BLOOD SUPPLY OF THE ADRENAL

1. The **superior and middle adrenal arteries** give rise to **capillaries** that supply the adrenal cortex and end in **medullary venous sinuses** within the adrenal medulla. This means that aldosterone, cortisol, androstenedione, and DHEA leave the adrenal cortex by first percolating through the adrenal medulla. This blood flow is significant because activation of **phenylethanolamine-N-methyltransferase (PNMT),** a key enzyme in the synthesis of epinephrine by chromaffin cells within the adrenal medulla, is dependent on high levels of cortisol.

2. The **inferior adrenal artery** gives rise to **medullary arterioles** that supply only the adrenal medulla (i.e., bypass the adrenal cortex) and end in **medullary venous sinuses.**

3. Medullary venous sinuses drain into the **central vein** by which aldosterone, cortisol, androstenedione, DHEA, epinephrine, and norepinephrine leave the adrenal gland.

E. SYNTHESIS OF CATECHOLAMINES uses tyrosine as a precursor (Figure 25-2).

F. CLINICAL CONSIDERATIONS

1. **Pheochromocytoma** is a relatively rare (usually not malignant) catecholamine-producing tumor (both epinephrine and norepinephrine) of the adrenal medulla.
   a. **Characteristics.** Pheochromocytoma occurs mainly in adults and is generally found in the region of the adrenal gland but also is found in extra-adrenal sites. It occurs within families as part of the multiple endocrine neoplasia (MEN) type II syndrome.
   b. **Symptoms.** It is associated with persistent or paroxysmal hypertension, anxiety, tremor, profuse sweating, pallor, chest pain, and abdominal pain.
   c. **Diagnosis.** Increased urine VMA and metanephrine levels, inability to suppress catecholamines with clonidine, and hyperglycemia are common laboratory findings.
   d. **Treatment.** Pheochromocytoma is treated by surgery or phenoxybenzamine (an α-adrenergic antagonist).

2. **Neuroblastoma** is a common extracranial neoplasm containing primitive neuroblasts of neural crest origin.
   a. **Characteristics.** Neuroblastomas occur mainly in children. They are found in extra-adrenal sites, usually along the sympathetic chain ganglia (60%) or within the adrenal medulla (40%). They metastasize widely.

● **Figure 25-2 Synthesis and metabolism of adrenomedullary catecholamines.** Synthesis begins with tyrosine as a precursor. The metabolic urine breakdown products (in *shaded boxes*) are used for diagnostic purposes. Urinary levels of vanillylmandelic acid (*VMA;* *) and 3-methoxy-4-hydroxyphenyglycol (*MOPEG;* **) are diagnostic of sympathetic nervous system function. Urinary levels of free epinephrine (†) are diagnostic of adrenal medulla function. The enzymes catecholamine O-methyltransferase (*COMT*) and monoamine oxidase (*MAO*) are key enzymes in the metabolism of catecholamines. When the adrenal medulla is stimulated, the secretion product is 90% epinephrine and 10% norepinephrine. All of the enzymes involved in catecholamine synthesis are found in the cytoplasm except dopamine β-hydroxylase, which is located within secretion granules. *PNMT* = phenylethanolamine-*N*-methyltransferase.

    b. Symptoms. It is associated with opsoclonus (rapid, irregular movements of the eye in horizontal and vertical directions; "dancing eyes").

    c. Diagnosis. A neuroblastoma contains small cells arranged in Homer-Wright pseudorosettes. Increased urine VMA and metanephrine levels are found.

    d. Treatment includes surgical excision, radiation, and chemotherapy.

� Selected Photomicrographs

A. Gross and histology of a normal adrenal gland (Figure 25-3)

B. Hyperadrenalism (Cushing syndrome), normal adrenal gland, hypoadrenalism (Addison disease) (Figure 25-4)

C. Pheochromocytoma and neuroblastoma (Figure 25-5)

● **Figure 25-3 General features of the adrenal gland. (A)** Gross photograph of a sliced normal adrenal gland. The zona glomerulosa and zona fasciculata appear as a light area (yellow color in fresh gross specimens) due to the large amount of lipid of these cells; whereas the zona reticularis appears as a dark area (dark brown color in fresh gross specimens) due to the eosinophilia and lipofuscin pigment of these cells. The medulla (*M*) appears as a gray area where dilated venules are observed (*arrows*). The boxed area is shown at higher magnification in **B. (B)** LM of a normal adrenal gland. A capsule is present on the exterior of the gland. The three zones of the adrenal cortex and the adrenal medulla are clearly apparent. *ZG* = zona glomerulosa; *ZF* = zona fasciculata; *ZR* = zona reticularis; *M* = medulla. **(C)** LM of the ZG. The ZG is a narrow, inconstant band (15% of the cortical volume) of cortex situated immediately below the capsule (*cap*). The cells of the ZG have distinct cell membranes and are arranged in glomerular-like clusters surrounded by small amounts of connective tissue. The ZG cells have a round nucleus and a faintly eosinophilic, vacuolated cytoplasm. **(D)** LM of the ZF. The ZF is a broad band of cortex (78% of the cortical volume). The ZF lies between the ZG and the ZR. The cells of the ZF have distinct cell membranes and are arranged as two-cell wide vertical cords that run perpendicular to the capsule and separated by parallel-running capillaries. The cells of the ZF have a round nucleus and a lipid-filled cytoplasm that give the ZF cells a vacuolated, clear appearance. The high lipid content of the ZF cells gives this zone a yellow color observed in fresh gross specimens. **(E)** LM of the ZR. The ZR is a band of cortex (7% of cortical volume). The ZR lies deep to the ZF and in the head and body of the adrenal gland abuts on the medulla. The cells of the ZR have a distinct cell membrane and are arranged as one-cell wide anastomosing rows of cells separated by capillaries. The cells of the ZR have a round nucleus and a lipid-sparse, distinctly eosinophilic cytoplasm. The deepest-located cells next to the medulla usually contain a yellow-brown lipofuscin pigment. The eosinophilia and lipofuscin pigment of the ZR cells give this zone a dark brown color in fresh gross specimens. **(F, G)** LM of the medulla. The medulla is located deep to the ZR in the head and body of the adrenal. The medulla is usually absent in the tail of the adrenal. The boundary between the cortex and medulla is quite distinct. At low magnification (*F*), venules (*) and nerve fibers (*arrows*) can be observed coursing through the medulla. At higher magnification **(G)**, chromaffin cells have an indistinct cell membrane and are arranged in tight clusters. The chromaffin cells have variable-shaped nuclei and generally a finely granular basophilic cytoplasm, although some cells appear vacuolated, which gives the medulla a mottled appearance.

● **Figure 25-4 Normal and pathological adrenal gland. (A)** Hyperplasia of the adrenal cortex (C) as might be found in congenital adrenal hyperplasia. *M* = adrenal medulla. **(B)** Normal adrenal gland showing the normal thickness of the adrenal cortex. **(C)** Hypoplasia of the adrenal cortex as might be found in Addison disease. All photomicrographs are taken at the same magnification so that the normal and pathologic changes may be compared.

● **Figure 25-5 Pathology of adrenal medulla. (A)** Gross photograph of a pheochromocytoma. Pheochromocytomas vary in size from 3 to 5 cm in diameter. They are gray-white to pink-tan in color. Exposure of the cut surface often results in darkening of the surface due to formation of yellow-brown adrenochrome pigment. **(B)** LM of a pheochromocytoma. A pheochromocytoma generally appears as a diffuse or nodular hyperplasia. The neoplastic cells are abundant cytoplasm with small centrally located nuclei. The neoplastic cells are separated into clusters by a slender stroma and numerous capillaries. **(C)** Gross photograph of a neuroblastoma. Neuroblastomas vary in size from 1 cm to filling the entire abdomen. They are generally soft and white to gray-pink in color. As the size increases, the tumors become hemorrhagic and undergo calcification and cyst formation. Note the nodular appearance of this tumor with the kidney apparent on the left border (*arrow*). **(D)** LM of a neuroblastoma, which is commonly composed of small, primitive-looking cells with dark nuclei and scant cytoplasm. The cells generally are arranged as solid sheets, and some cells arrange around a central fibrillar area, forming Homer-Wright pseudorosettes (*).

Case Study

A 30-year-old woman comes to your office complaining that "I'm getting fat, I have pimples like when I was a teenager, and I have a beard and mustache. What the hell is going on?" After some discussion, she informs you that she has not had a menstrual period in 4 months, she bruises easily, and she screams at her children over little things that never bothered her before. The woman is in an obvious high state of anxiety about her condition and begins to cry as she says, "Doc, I look like a circus freak! My husband won't even look at me. You've got to do something." What is the most likely diagnosis?

Differentials

- Adrenal adenoma or hyperplasia, alcoholism, small cell carcinoma of the lung

Relevant Physical Exam Findings

- Blood pressure = 175/115 mm Hg (High)
- Muscle weakness
- Central obesity; thin limbs
- Moon facies
- Purple striae

Relevant Lab Findings

- Blood chemistry: Fasting blood glucose = 145 mg/dL (High); Morning plasma cortisol = 55 μg/dL (High); Plasma ACTH = 15 pg/mL (High)
- Urinalysis: 24 hour free cortisol = 375 μg (High); Glucosuria = +1
- High dose dexamethasone suppression test: positive
- MRI of head: small pituitary adenoma
- Chest radiograph: negative

Diagnosis

Cushing Disease. Cushing disease refers to high levels of cortisol caused by an ACTH-secreting adenoma within the adenohypophysis. Cushing syndrome refers to the constellation of clinical findings that appear secondary to high levels of cortisol. Clinical findings of Cushing syndrome include mild hypertension, impaired glucose tolerance, acne, hirsutism, oligomenorrhea, men complain of impotence and loss of libido, osteoporosis with back pain and buffalo hump, central obesity, moon facies, and purple skin striae (bruise easily). Cushing syndrome is caused by administration of large doses of steroids for treatment of primary disease (i.e., iatrogenic; most common cause), an ACTH-secreting adenoma within the adenohypophysis, an adrenal adenoma, or adrenal hyperplasia. A definitive diagnosis of Cushing disease is indicated by a positive dexamethasone suppression test, high cortisol levels, high levels of ACTH, and MRI indication of a pituitary adenoma. An adrenal adenoma will also cause Cushing syndrome. A definitive diagnosis of an adrenal adenoma is indicated by a negative dexamethasone suppression test, high cortisol levels, low levels of ACTH, and CT scan indication of an adrenal adenoma. An adrenal adenoma usually occurs unilaterally, whereas adrenal hyperplasia occurs bilaterally. In adrenal hyperplasia, both adrenal glands are enlarged while maintaining their normal anatomical shapes. Note that in adrenal hyperplasia, except for the increased size, the adrenal glands appear normal, which may confound the diagnosis. In some cases of adrenal hyperplasia, the adrenal glands may demonstrate bilateral nodularity. Chronic alcoholics can develop signs of Cushing syndrome because of high levels of cortisol. However, this is associated with a negative dexamethasone suppression test. The ascites associated with chronic alcoholism is centrally located but is composed of fluid located in the peritoneal cavity; not fat. A small cell carcinoma of the lung can produce ACTH, which leads to high levels of cortisol and Cushing syndrome. However, the chest radiograph is negative in this case and there is no history of smoking.

Case Study

A 40-year-old woman comes to your office complaining that "I always feel nauseated and I get tired real fast, even when I'm at home just puttering around. This has been going on for about 3 months." She also tells you that "I've been vomiting quite a bit and I don't have an appetite. The only good thing about all this is that I've lost 15 pounds." After some discussion, she informs you that she has been married for 10 years and denies any extramarital affairs. However, before she got married she admits that "I was pretty wild and would pick up the cutest guy in the bar and take him home for the night. I took megadoses of antibiotics to prevent sexually transmitted diseases and I loved to use amyl and butyl nitrite to heighten my orgasm." The woman does not seem to be very concerned about her condition as she says, "Doc, just give me something for this nausea and vomiting and I'll be good to go. I want to lose another 15 pounds." What is the most likely diagnosis?

Differentials

- AIDS, hemochromatosis, pituitary hypofunction

Relevant Physical Exam Findings

- Blood pressure = 100/70 mm Hg reclined; 80/60 mm Hg standing (orthostatic hypotension)
- Increased pigmentation on her knuckles, knees, and elbows
- Areolae are bluish-black
- Axillary and public hair is sparse
- No lymphadenopathy

Relevant Lab Findings

- Blood chemistry: Hgb = 16 g/dL (High); Hct = 53% (High); Na^+ = 105 mEq/L (Low); K^+ = 6.5 mEq/L (High); HCO_3^- = 19 mEq/L (Low); BUN = 26 mg/dL (High); Fasting glucose = 45 mg/dL (Low); Serum ferritin = 200 ng/mL (Normal); Morning plasma cortisol = 3 mg/dL (Low); Morning plasma ACTH = 200 pg/mL (High)
- HIV test: Negative
- Purified protein derivative (PPD) test: Negative
- CT scan: small, non-calcified adrenal glands

Diagnosis

Addison Disease (AD; Primary adrenocortical insufficiency). AD is commonly caused by the autoimmune destruction of the adrenal cortex resulting in a deficiency of cortisol, aldosterone, and dehydroepiandrosterone. Skin hyperpigmentation is seen as a result of increased melanocyte-stimulating hormone (MSH), which is a byproduct of adrenocorticotropin hormone (ACTH) synthesis in the adenohypophysis. The deficiency of cortisol results in the following: contributes to orthostatic hypotension; mild pressor effect on the heart and vasculature; hypoglycemia because cortisol plays a role in gluconeogenesis; nausea; vomiting; anorexia; weight loss; and increase in ACTH levels because cortisol controls ACTH secretion by a negative feedback loop. The deficiency of aldosterone results in the following: hyponatremia; hypovolemia; decreased cardiac output; decreased renal blood flow; azotemia; hyperkalemia (which can lead to cardiac dysrhythmia). Aldosterone acts on the principal cells of the cortical collecting ducts in the kidney and causes increased Na^+ reabsorption (tubular fluid $\rightarrow$ plasma). Aldosterone also acts on the principal cells of the cortical collecting ducts in the kidney and causes increased K^+ secretion (plasma $\rightarrow$ tubular fluid). A definitive diagnosis of AD is indicated by low cortisol levels, low aldosterone levels, low dehydroepiandrosterone levels, and high ACTH levels. Some AIDS patients (20%) present with cortisol resistance and adrenal insufficiency. The HIV test rules out AIDS in this case. Some believe that megadoses of antibiotics, amyl and butyl nitrites, and multiple blood transfusions may destroy $CD4^+$ lymphocytes and lead to AIDS. Hemosiderin is a golden brown hemoglobin-derived pigment consisting of iron. Iron is absorbed mainly by surface absorptive cells within the duodenum, transported in the plasma by a protein called transferrin, and is normally stored in cells as ferritin, which is a protein–iron complex. During iron overload, intracellular ferritin undergoes lysosomal degradation, in which the ferritin protein is degraded and the iron aggregates within the cell as hemosiderin in a condition called hemosiderosis. The more extreme accumulation of iron is called hemochromatosis, which is associated with liver and pancreas damage. Hemochromatosis can be observed in patients with increased absorption of dietary iron, impaired utilization of iron, hemolytic anemias, and blood transfusions. Clinical findings of hemochromatosis include cirrhosis of the liver, diabetes, and increased skin pigmentation (bronze diabetes). Pituitary hypofunction (secondary adrenocortical insufficiency) presents with many of the same symptoms as AD because the adrenal cortex is under control of the adenohypophysis. A definitive diagnosis of pituitary hypofunction is indicated by low cortisol levels, normal aldosterone levels (because the zona glomerulosa of the adrenal cortex is controlled by the renin–angiotensin system), low dehydroepiandrosterone levels, and low ACTH levels. Since ACTH levels are low, MSH will not be increased so that no increased skin pigmentation would be observed.

Chapter 26

Female Reproductive System

Ovary (Figure 26-1). The ovaries are almond-shaped structures located posterior to the broad ligament. The ovaries are covered by a surface epithelium (simple cuboidal) called the **germinal epithelium** with a subjacent connective tissue layer called the **tunica albuginea.** The ovaries are divided into a **cortex** and **medulla.**

A. CORTEX. The cortex contains follicles in various stages of development including the **primordial follicle, primary follicle, secondary follicle,** and **Graafian follicle.** Follicles are composed of an oocyte, follicular cells, and thecal cells.

B. MEDULLA. The medulla lies deep to the cortex and contains: connective tissue, occasional smooth muscle cells, and numerous tortuous arteries (and veins) from which small branches radiate to the cortex.

C. CLINICAL CONSIDERATIONS

1. **Ovarian cysts.** Functional cysts in the ovary are so common as to be virtually physiologic and resolve spontaneously. A functional cyst is physiologically and hormonally an active cyst that has not yet involuted. They originate from either unruptured Graafian follicles or in Graafian follicles that have ruptured and immediately sealed. Ovarian cysts are nonneoplastic, fluid-filled cavities that may be solitary or multiple (up to 2 cm in diameter). There are three main types of cysts:
   a. **Follicular cysts** are generally large cysts (>2 cm) that may be diagnosed by palpation or ultrasound. Histologically, granulosa lutein cells can be identified if the pressure is not too great and theca lutein cells may be conspicuous.
   b. **Corpus luteum cysts** are lined by a conspicuous rim of granulosa lutein cells.
   c. **Theca lutein cysts** are caused by elevated levels of **β-human chorionic gonadotropin (β-hCG)** produced by the placenta during pregnancy. This causes a proliferation of theca lutein cells, which form small nodules in the ovary.

2. **Polycystic ovary syndrome** is characterized biochemically by increased levels of androgens and luteinizing hormone (LH), but decreased levels of follicle-stimulating hormone (FSH). This results in bilateral ovarian enlargement, cortical fibrosis, and multiple follicular cysts. Clinical findings include: chronic anovulation with menstrual irregularities such as oligomenorrhea or amenorrhea, oily skin and acne, hirsutism, and obesity.

3. **Ovarian tumors** originate from four cell types (germinal epithelium, oocyte, follicular cells, or stromal cells).
   a. **Germinal epithelium tumors** are the most common type. These tumors are cystic and may be filled with either a serous fluid or mucus. **Serous tumors** are generally malignant and bilateral with a poor prognosis.

Stage of Follicle	Oocyte	Follicular Cells	Thecal Cells
Primordial	**Primary oocyte** (46,4N) • Arrested in prophase of meiosis I	**Squamous cells** • 1 layer	**Fibroblasts**
Primary	**Primary oocyte** (46,4N) • Arrested in prophase of meiosis I	**Granulosa cells** • 11 → multiple layers	**Fibroblasts**
Secondary	**Primary oocyte** (46,4N) • Arrested in prophase of meiosis I • Zona pellucida present	**Granulosa cells** • Multiple layers • Secrete estrogens by aromatase conversion of androgens from theca interna • FSH receptors present • Antrum appears	**Theca interna** • Secrete androgens • LH receptors present **Theca externa** • Fibrous and vascular
FSH dependent Resumes meiosis I ↓ Graafian	**Secondary oocyte** (23,2N) • Arrested in metaphase of meiosis II • Zona pellucida present		

● **Figure 26-1 Development of the ovarian follicles.** The table shows the stages of follicle development along with the changes in the oocyte, follicular cells, and thecal cells. Diagram of the entire ovary shows the cycle of ovarian follicle maturation, luteinization, and residual scarring. *Curved arrows* point to LMs of primordial follicles, a primary follicle, a secondary follicle, and corpus luteum. *PO* = primary oocyte; *GC* = granulosa cells; *Th* = theca; *A* = antrum; *ZP* = zona pellucida; *GL* = granulosa lutein cells; *TL* = theca lutein cells.

   b. **Oocyte tumors (or germ cell tumors)**
   c. **Follicular cell tumors (or sex cord cell tumors)**
   d. **Stromal cell tumors**

Ⓓ **Corpus Luteum** is a temporary endocrine gland whose formation is **LH dependent**. After ovulation, the wall of the follicle collapses and becomes extensively infolded. Blood vessels and stromal cells invade the previously avascular granulosa cells. The granulosa and theca interna cells hypertrophy, develop sER, and accumulate lipid droplets (a process called luteinization), thereby becoming lutein cells.

A. **CELLULAR COMPOSITION.** There are two kinds of lutein cells:
   1. **Granulosa lutein cells** secrete **progesterone** and **estradiol** in response to FSH and LH stimulation. Granulosa lutein cells lack the steroidogenic enzymes required for the complete synthesis of estradiol. Theca lutein cells cooperate with the granulosa lutein cells by providing androstenedione, which is then converted into estradiol within the granulosa lutein cells. Progesterone maintains the endometrium of the uterus in the secretory (luteal) phase so that implantation and nutritional support of the blastocyst may occur. **Mifepristone (RU-486)** is a drug that binds to progesterone receptors and blocks progesterone action. RU-486 used in combination with **misoprostol (a PGE1$_1$ analogue)** is an effective and safe abortifacient.
   2. **Theca lutein cells** secrete **androstenedione** and **progesterone** in response to LH stimulation.

B. **EFFECT OF FERTILIZATION.** If fertilization occurs, the corpus luteum enlarges and becomes the predominant source of steroids needed to sustain pregnancy for approximately **8 weeks.** Thereafter, the placenta becomes the major source of the steroids required. If fertilization does not occur, the corpus luteum regresses and forms a **corpus albicans.**

Ⅲ **Uterine tubes (fallopian tubes; oviducts)** (Figure 26-2) are tubular structures that provide a channel for the transport of the preimplantation embryo to the uterus and the site of fertilization.

A. **REGIONS OF THE UTERINE TUBES**
   1. **Infundibulum** is the flared open end of the uterine tube next to the ovary. Fimbria are delicate, fingerlike projections that extend from the infundibulum toward the ovary.
   2. **Ampulla** is the longest segment of the uterine tube and has the largest diameter. This region is where **fertilization** occurs.
   3. **Isthmus** is the narrow segment of the uterine tube between the ampulla and uterus.
   4. **Intramural segment** is the portion of the uterine tube contained within the wall of the uterus.

B. **HISTOLOGIC LAYERS**
   1. **Mucosa.** The mucosa consists of an epithelium and lamina propria, but no muscularis mucosa. The **mucosal epithelium** consists of:
       a. **Secretory cells** (nonciliated; peg cells) that secrete a nutrient-rich medium for the nourishment of the sperm and preimplantation embryo.
       b. **Ciliated cells** whose cilia beat toward the uterus. The rate of ciliary beat is influenced by progesterone and estrogen and assists in transport of the preimplantation embryo to the uterus.

● **Figure 26-2 Normal and pathological uterine tube. (A)** LM (low magnification) of the ampulla of the uterine tube. Note the long slender mucosal folds that project into the lumen. The muscularis layer (M) is also shown. The boxed area is shown at higher magnification in B. **(B)** LM of the mucosal folds shows the epithelial lining and connective tissue of the lamina propria. The boxed area is shown at higher magnification in C. **(C)** LM of the mucosal folds shows the epithelial lining (*EPI*) consisting of secretory nonciliated cells (peg cells; *arrow*) and ciliated cells along with the lamina propria (*LP*). **(D)** Gross photograph of acute and chronic salpingitis. The uterine tube is markedly distended, the fimbriated end is closed, and there is hemorrhage on the serosal surface. **(E)** Gross photograph of an ectopic tubal pregnancy.

2. **Muscularis layer** consists of smooth muscle oriented in an inner circular layer and an outer longitudinal layer. Peristaltic contractions may help to move the preimplantation embryo toward the uterus.
3. **Serosa** consists of simple squamous epithelium (visceral peritoneum).

C. CLINICAL CONSIDERATIONS

1. **Acute and chronic salpingitis** is a bacterial infection (most commonly *Neisseria gonorrhea* or *Chlamydia trachomatis*) of the uterine tube with acute inflammation

(neutrophil infiltration) or chronic inflammation, which may lead to scarring of the uterine tube predisposing to **ectopic tubal pregnancy.**

2. **Ectopic tubal pregnancy** most often occurs in the **ampulla** of the uterine tube. Risk factors include salpingitis, pelvic inflammatory disease, pelvic surgery, or exposure to DES (diethylstilbestrol). Clinical signs include: sudden onset of abdominal pain which may be confused with appendicitis in a young woman, last menses 60 days ago, positive hCG test, and culdocentesis showing intraperitoneal blood. Ectopic tubal pregnancy is a medical emergency and should always be considered when a cycling female (no matter how young) presents with abdominal pain.

IV. Uterus

A. REGIONS OF THE UTERUS

1. The **body** is the expanded part of the uterus below the entrance of the uterine tubes.
2. The **fundus** is the rounded superior part of the uterus above the entrance of the uterine tubes.
3. The **cervix** is the most inferior part of the uterus that projects into the vagina.

B. HISTOLOGIC LAYERS. The uterine wall consists of:

1. **Endometrium** consists of simple columnar epithelium, which invaginates into the endometrial stroma to form **endometrial glands.** The endometrium can be divided into two layers:
   a. **Basal layer** regenerates the functional layer each month during the menstrual cycle. The basal layer is NEVER sloughed off.
   b. **Functional layer** undergoes alterations during the menstrual cycle. The functional layer is sloughed off each month during menses.
2. **Myometrium** consists of smooth muscle cells that are connected by gap junctions and contract on stimulation by **oxytocin** and **prostaglandins (PGE_2 and $PGF_{2\alpha}$)** at parturition. During pregnancy, the myometrial smooth muscle cells hypertrophy and increase in number. The myometrium contains the **stratum vasculare,** which is highly vascular and is the source of the endometrial blood supply.
3. **Perimetrium** consists of connective tissue covered by peritoneal mesothelium.

V. The Menstrual Cycle (Figure 26-3) is a series of phases that repeats ideally every 28 days.

A. THE MENSTRUAL PHASE (DAYS 1–4) is characterized by the **necrosis and shedding** of the functional layer of the endometrium. Spiral arterioles constrict episodically for a few days and finally constrict permanently, resulting in ischemia that leads to necrosis of endometrial glands and stroma. The spiral arterioles subsequently dilate and rupture, resulting in hemorrhage that sheds the necrotic endometrial glands and stroma.

B. THE PROLIFERATIVE (FOLLICULAR) PHASE (DAYS 4–15) is characterized by the **regeneration** of the functional layer of the endometrium from the devastating effects of the menstrual phase. This phase is controlled by **estrogen** secreted by the granulosa cells of the secondary and Graafian follicle. Epithelial cells and fibroblasts of the basal layer of the endometrium regenerate to form **straight endometrial glands** and stroma, respectively.

C. THE OVULATORY PHASE (DAYS 14–16) is characterized by **ovulation** of the secondary oocyte arrested in metaphase of meiosis II that coincides with **peak levels of LH (LH surge).**

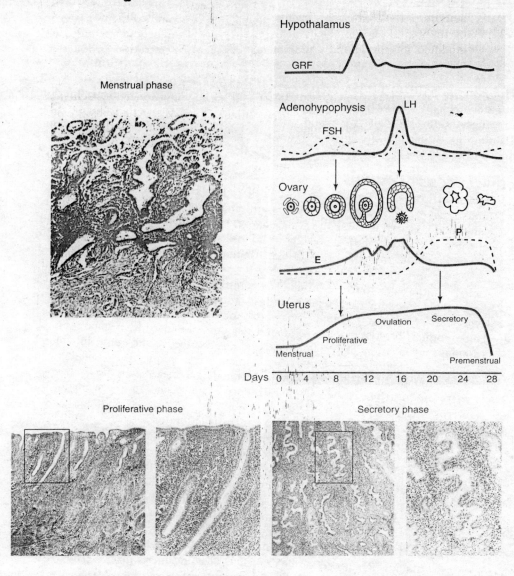

● **Figure 26-3 Hormonal control of the menstrual cycle.** The hypothalamus secretes gonadotropin-releasing factor (*GRF*). In response to GRF, the adenohypophysis secretes follicle-stimulating hormone (*FSH*) and luteinizing hormone (*LH*). In response to FSH, the development of a secondary follicle to a Graafian follicle is stimulated in the ovary. The granulosa cells within the secondary follicle and Graafian follicle secrete estrogen (*E*). In response to estrogen, the endometrium of the uterus enters the proliferative phase. In response to LH (LH surge), ovulation occurs. After ovulation, the granulosa lutein cells of the corpus luteum secrete progesterone (*P*). In response to progesterone, the endometrium of the uterus enters the secretory phase. LM of the proliferative phase of the endometrium showing straight endometrial glands. The boxed area is shown at higher magnification. LM of the secretory phase of the endometrium showing convoluted endometrial glands with secretion product within the lumen. The boxed area is shown at higher magnification. LM of the menstrual phase of the endometrium showing endometrial glands undergoing necrosis and shedding. Conditions that impair the secretion of GnRH from the hypothalamus will prevent the secretion of FSH that is necessary for follicle development and will result in infertility. **Female infertility** is usually treated with **clomiphene (Clomid, Serophene).** Clomiphene is an estrogen receptor antagonist in the hypothalamus and adenohypophysis which blocks feed back inhibition by endogenous estrogens and thereby increases FSH and LH secretion so that ovulation occurs. In **polycystic ovary syndrome,** increased LH secretion from the adenohypophysis stimulates excessive production of androgens by the theca interna cell of secondary and Graafian follicles, resulting in numerous atretic or cystic follicles.

D. **THE SECRETORY (LUTEAL) PHASE (DAYS 15–25)** is characterized by the **secretory activity** of the endometrial glands. This phase is controlled by **progesterone** secreted by the granulosa lutein cells of the corpus luteum. The endometrial glands become modified to **convoluted endometrial glands with secretion product** within their lumen.

E. **THE PREMENSTRUAL PHASE (DAYS 25–28)** is characterized by **ischemia** as a result of reduced blood flow to the endometrium. This phase is controlled by the **reduction in progesterone and estrogen** as the corpus luteum involutes. As the endometrial glands begin to shrink, the spiral arterioles are compressed, thereby reducing blood flow and causing ischemic damage.

F. **CLINICAL CONSIDERATIONS**

1. **Endometriosis** is the appearance of foci of endometrial tissue in abnormal locations outside the uterus (e.g., ovary, uterine ligaments, pelvic peritoneum). The ectopic endometrial tissue shows cyclic changes synchronous with the endometrium of the uterus. Endometriosis results in infertility, dysmenorrhea, and pelvic pain (most pronounced at the time of menstruation). The serosal surfaces of pelvic organs are sprinkled with red, bluish, or yellow punctate lesions. Bluish lesions are called **"gunpowder mark" lesions.** The ectopic endometrial tissue consists of a hemorrhagic endometrial stroma and glands. Blood-filled cysts (**"chocolate cysts"**) up to 3–5 cm in diameter may be found on the ovaries.

2. **Leiomyoma (fibroids)** is a very common benign tumor derived from smooth muscle within the myometrium of the uterus. They may be classified as subserosal, intramural, or submucosal. Subserosal and submucosal tumors may be pedunculated and therefore protrude from the uterine surface or protrude into the uterine cavity, respectively.

3. **Primary amenorrhea** is the complete absence of menstruation in a woman from puberty.

4. **Secondary amenorrhea** is the absence of menstruation for at least 3 months in a woman who previously had normal menstruation.

   a. **Causes.** The most common cause of secondary amenorrhea is pregnancy, which can be determined by assaying urine **β-hCG.** Other pathologic causes of secondary amenorrhea include hypothalamic or pituitary malfunction (e.g., **anorexia nervosa**), ovarian disorders (e.g., **ovariectomy**), and end-organ disease (e.g., **Asherman syndrome**, in which the basal layer of the endometrium has been removed by repeated curettages).

   b. **Diagnosis.** These causes are evaluated clinically by assaying serum FSH and LH levels along with a progesterone challenge. Bleeding after a **progesterone withdrawal test** indicates that the endometrium was primed by estrogen, thereby indicating that the hypothalamic–pituitary axis and the ovaries are functioning normally. The results of such clinical evaluations are indicated in Table 26-1.

TABLE 26-1	RESULTS OF CLINICAL EVALUATIONS FOR SECONDARY AMENORRHEA		
Test*	Serum FSH	Serum LH	Bleeding After Progesterone Withdrawal
Anorexia nervosa	Low	Low	No
Ovariectomy	High	High	No
Asherman syndrome	Normal	Normal	No

*10 mg of medroxyprogesterone is given daily for 5 days. Withdrawal bleeding suggests that sufficient estrogen production is present for uterine proliferation.
FSH = follicle stimulating hormone; LH = luteinizing hormone.

5. **Menorrhagia** is excessive bleeding at menstruation in either the amount of blood or number of days. It is usually associated with a leiomyoma (fibroids).

6. **Dysmenorrhea** is excessive pain during menstruation. It is commonly associated with endometriosis and an increased level of PGF in the menstrual fluid.

7. **Metrorrhagia** is bleeding that occurs at irregular intervals. It is commonly associated with cervical carcinoma or cervical polyps.

8. **Prepubertal bleeding** is bleeding that occurs before menarche. It is commonly associated with vaginitis, infection, sexual abuse, or embryonal rhabdomyosarcoma.

9. **Postmenopausal bleeding** occurs approximately 1 year after the cessation of the menstrual cycle. It is commonly associated with malignant tumors of the uterus.

VI **Cervix.** The cervix is the lower part of the uterus that measures about 2.5 to 3.0 cm in length. The cervix is divided into a **supravaginal portion** (lying above the vaginal vault) and a **vaginal portion (portio vaginalis)** that protrudes into the vagina. The junction between the cervix and uterus is at the **internal os.** Histologically, the cervical wall consists of:

A. **A SIMPLE COLUMNAR EPITHELIUM,** which invaginates into the cervical stroma to form **mucus-secreting cervical glands.** This epithelium and cervical glands do not slough off during the menstrual cycle and are relatively unaffected by the menstrual cycle except that the cervical mucus produced during the proliferative phase is **watery** and the cervical mucus produced during the secretory phase is **viscous.**

B. The wall of the cervix is predominatly **connective tissue** with very little smooth muscle (very different compared with the uterine wall, which is predominately smooth muscle). During pregnancy, the cervix undergoes little or no expansion. However, during childbirth, the connective tissue becomes pliable (called **"cervical softening"**) owing to the action of **relaxin.**

VII **Ectocervix** (Figure 26-4). The outer epithelial surface of the vaginal portion of the cervix (portio vaginalis) is called the **ectocervix.** The epithelial surface lining the lumen of the **endocervical canal** is called the **endocervix.**

A. During prepuberty, the **ectocervix** is covered by a **nonkeratinized, stratified squamous epithelium** that is continuous with the vaginal epithelium.

B. The **endocervical canal** connects the uterine cavity with the vaginal cavity and extends from the internal os to the **external os.** The endocervical canal is lined by **simple columnar epithelium,** which invaginates into the cervical stroma to form **mucus-secreting cervical glands.**

C. At puberty, the simple columnar epithelium of the endocervical canal extends onto the ectocervix. However, exposure of the simple columnar epithelium to the acidic (pH 3) environment of the vagina induces a transformation from columnar to squamous epithelium (i.e., **squamous metaplasia**) and the formation of a **transformation zone.**

D. The transformation zone is the site of **Nabothian cysts,** which develop as stratified squamous epithelium grows over the mucus-secreting simple columnar epithelium and entraps large amounts of mucus.

● Figure 26-4 Diagram of the cervical–vaginal junction. During prepuberty, the ectocervix is covered by nonkeratinized stratified squamous epithelium that is continuous with vaginal epithelium (*dark shaded area*). At puberty, the simple columnar epithelium and cervical glands extend onto the ectocervix. In the adult, exposure of the simple columnar epithelium to the acidic (pH 3) environment of the vagina induces a squamous metaplasia, forming the transformation zone (*clear area*). Nabothian cysts (*NB*) may form in the transformation zone. LM of the ectocervix shows a nonkeratinized, stratified squamous epithelium. Note the luminal cells have a clear cytoplasm indicative of large amounts of glycogen storage. LM of the endocervix shows a simple columnar epithelium (*SC*) and prominent mucus-secreting cervical glands (*GL*). LM of the transformation zone in the adult shows nonkeratinized, stratified squamous epithelium and Nabothian cysts. *TZ* = transformation zone.

    E. The transformation zone is the most common site of **squamous cell carcinoma of the cervix,** which is usually preceded by epithelial changes called **cervical intraepithelial neoplasia (CIN)** diagnosed by a Pap smear. **Human papillomavirus (HPV)** has also been linked as an important factor in cervical oncogenesis and is often tested for.

VIII **Vagina** (Figure 26-5). The vagina is a fibromuscular tube that is kept moist by mucus produced by cervical glands that drains down through the cervical canal and additional mucus produced by the **greater vestibular glands (of Bartholin)** and **lesser vestibular glands.** Histologically, the vaginal wall consists of a mucosa (epithelium and lamina propria), muscularis layer, and adventitia.

● **Figure 26-5 Vaginal changes and infections. (A)** In the absence of estrogen, a decreased thickness of the vaginal epithelium is observed. **(B)** In the presence of estrogen, an increased thickness of the vaginal epithelium is observed. A vaginal smear contains three basic cell types from various levels of the vaginal epithelium: superficial squamous cells (*SSC*), intermediate squamous cells (*ISC*), and parabasal cells (*PBC*). **(C)** *Trichomonas vaginalis*. The presence of the flagellated protozoan is shown in a vaginal smear. **(D)** *Candida albicans*. The presence of the yeast is shown in a vaginal smear. **(E)** *Gardnerella vaginalis*. A "clue cell," which is a squamous cell with a clumped nucleus and folded cytoplasm covered with bacteria, is shown.

TABLE 26-2	MATURATION INDEX* IN VARIOUS CLINICAL SITUATIONS		
	SSC	ISC	PBC
Normal nonpregnant adult woman	70	30	0
Estrogen tumor or therapy Polycystic ovarian syndrome	100	0	0
Pregnant woman Prepubescent girl	0	100	0
Menopausal woman	0	0	100

*Maturation index is based on the morphology of 100 observed cells.
ISC = intermediate squamous cells; *PBC* = parabasal cells; *SSC*= superficial squamous cells.

A. **EPITHELIUM.** The vagina is lined by **nonkeratinized, stratified squamous epithelium.**

1. The most superficial layer of cells is continuously exfoliated during the menstrual cycle, but exfoliation increases during the late secretory phase and menstrual phase.

2. Under the influence of estrogen, the epithelial cells accumulate large amounts of glycogen and undergo cell proliferation in the basal and parabasal layers.

3. The exfoliated cells contain **glycogen**, which is metabolized by commensal lactobacilli to lactic acid, which forms an **acidic (pH = 3) environment.** The acidic environment deters the invasion of bacterial pathogens and fungi (e.g., *Candida albicans*, which causes vaginal thrush).

4. A vaginal smear (stained with Schorr's trichrome and Harris hematoxylin) may be used clinically to evaluate the hormonal status of a woman (Table 26-2). A vaginal smear contains three basic cell types.

   a. **Superficial squamous cells** (40–65 μm diameter) are flat with an irregular border and a light-orange cytoplasm. These cells form under the influence of estrogen.

   b. **Intermediate squamous cells** (20–40 μm diameter) are flat with an irregular border and a blue cytoplasm. These cells form under the influence of progesterone.

   c. **Parabasal cells** (12–15 μm diameter) are oval with a large nucleus with prominent chromatin and a blue cytoplasm. Parabasal cells in a vaginal smear imply the absence of estrogen or progesterone influence.

B. The **lamina propria** is comprised of connective tissue and contains a rich network of blood vessels that is thought to help moisten the vagina.

C. The **muscularis layer** consists of ill-defined bundles of **smooth muscle** and a rich network of **elastic fibers** that are responsible for the great distensibility of the vagina during childbirth.

D. The **adventitia** consists of connective tissue.

IX **Histopathology of the Vagina.** Vaginitis is a chronic infection most often caused by *Trichomonas vaginalis* (15% of cases), *Candida albicans* (25%), or *Gardnerella vaginalis* (30%). The vaginal epithelium is resistant to bacterial, fungal, and protozoan invasion so that the pathogens remain within the lumen of the vagina.

A. *TRICHOMONAS VAGINALIS* is a **flagellated protozoan** that is sexually transmitted. It produces a vaginitis characterized by an inflammatory vaginal smear with numerous neutrophils, fiery-red appearance of the vaginal and cervical mucosa ("strawberry mucosa"), and a **thin, gray-white, frothy, purulent, malodorous discharge (pH >4.5).** Postcoital bleeding is a common complaint. The organism is best seen in fresh preparations diluted with warm saline in which the tumbling motility of the organism can be observed.

B. **CANDIDA ALBICANS** is a **yeast** that produces pseudohyphae and true hyphae in tissues. It produces superficial white patches or large fluffy membranes that easily detach, leaving a red, irritated underlying surface and a **thick, white, "cottage cheese" discharge (pH <4.5).** The organism can be observed on potassium hydroxide (KOH) preparations of the discharge.

C. **GARDNERELLA VAGINALIS** (a **Gram-negative bacillus**) is a bacterial infection generally called **bacterial vaginosis** in which higher than normal levels of the bacteria are present. It is not sexually transmitted. It produces a vaginitis characterized by no inflammatory vaginal smear, no changes in the mucosa, and a **thin, homogenous, somewhat adherent, fishy-odor discharge (pH >4.5).** The discharge gives a positive amine test ("whiff test"; fishy amine smell) when mixed with KOH. A vaginal smear will show increased number of bacteria and "clue cells," which are squamous cells with a clumped nucleus and a folded cytoplasm covered with bacteria.

X Breast. The breast lies in the superficial fascia of the anterior chest wall overlying the **pectoralis major** and **serratus anterior muscles** and extends into the **superior lateral quadrant** of the axilla as the **axillary tail** in which a high percentage of tumors occur. The breast is covered by **skin** (epidermis and dermis), which is modified at the nipple and areola and contains **suspensory (Cooper) ligaments, adipose tissue** (which contributes to size and contour), and **mammary gland tissue.**

A. **NIPPLE AND AREOLA**
   1. The nipple is a round, raised area of modified skin in the center of the **areola.** The skin has a lightly **keratinized stratified squamous epithelium** and a dermis of **connective tissue with elastic fibers and smooth muscle fibers** arranged circularly around the base of the nipple and longitudinally that parallel the lactiferous ducts. Contraction of the smooth muscles because of cold, tactile, or emotional stimulation results in **erection of the nipple.** The base of the epithelium is invaded by deep dermal papillae containing numerous capillaries that bring blood close to the surface and impart a **pinkish color** to the nipple in children and blonde individuals. At puberty, the epithelium becomes pigmented (melanin) and changes the color to **light → dark brown.**
   2. The skin around the nipple is called the **areola,** which is modified skin that contains large sebaceous glands that form small nodular elevations in the areola called **Montgomery tubercles.** The color of the areola is initially pinkish (like the nipple), but during pregnancy the color changes to light → dark brown as a result of increased pigmentation (melanin). After delivery, the areola may lighten in color but rarely returns to its original shade. The **sensory innervation** of the nipple and areola are important because stimulation of the nipple and areola by the suckling infant triggers a sequence of neurohormonal events that result in **ejection of milk (oxytocin)** and **production of milk (prolactin).**
   3. **Clinical considerations.** Nipple secretion typically contains exfoliated duct cells, α-lactalbumin, immunoglobulins, lactose, cholesterol, steroids, and fatty acids, along with ethanol, caffeine, nicotine, barbiturates, pesticides, and technetium.
      a. A nipple discharge that is green, milky, yellow, or brown, not spontaneous, bilateral, and affects multiple ducts is usually a **benign situation.**

   b. A milky discharge (galactorrhea) along with a headache and peripheral vision loss may indicate a **pituitary adenoma (prolactinoma)**.

   c. A nipple discharge that is bloody or clear (serous), spontaneous, unilateral, and affects a single duct usually indicates a **malignant situation**.

B. MAMMARY GLAND (Figure 26-6). In general, the mammary gland is a compound, tubuloalveolar gland, which develops as downgrowths of the epidermis along the **milk line**, which runs from the axilla to the groin on each side. The mammary gland consists of **alveoli**, which are ultimately drained by **15–20 lactiferous ducts** that open onto the tip of the **nipple arranged in a ring.** Just deep to the surface of the nipple, each lactiferous duct expands into a **lactiferous sinus**, which serves as a reservoir for milk during lactation. The histology of the mammary gland changes as the female progresses through prepuberty, puberty, pregnancy, and lactation.

● **Figure 26-6 Mammary gland. (A) Prepuberty.** Breast tissue from a 4-month-old female infant. Note the simple system of ducts or epithelial downgrowths. **(B) At puberty.** Breast tissue from an 11-year-old girl. Note the branching system of ducts (D) and the solid masses of epithelial cells (M). **(C) During pregnancy.** Breast tissue taken from a pregnant woman. Note the lobule (*dotted line; L*) consisting of alveoli distended with colostrum. An interlobular duct (*inter*) is shown. **(D) During lactation.** Breast tissue taken from a lactating woman. Note that the alveoli (A) and ducts (D) are filled with milk. **(E)** Diagram of an alveolar epithelial cell from an alveolus of a breast during lactation. Note that the alveolar epithelial cell secretes both a lipid product and protein product as components of the milk.

1. **Prepuberty.** At birth and prepuberty, the nipple and a simple system of ducts (or epithelial downgrowths) embedded in connective tissue are present. The full development of epithelial downgrowths begins at puberty.

2. **At puberty.** The development of breasts at puberty is one of the secondary sex characteristics of women. Under the influence of **estrogen** from the ovary, the breast accumulates **adipose tissue,** which is largely responsible for variations in breast size. In addition, epithelial downgrowths begin in earnest and branch into the connective tissue to form a system of ducts. There are no alveoli present, only **solid masses of epithelial cells.**

3. **During pregnancy.** Under the influence of estrogen and progesterone, the duct system grows prolifically in length and branching. Eventually, the characteristic structure of the mammary gland takes shape: **15–20 lobules** drained by **intralobular ducts** that empty into **interlobular ducts** and eventually into the **lactiferous ducts.** In addition, the solid masses of epithelial cells grow and form **alveoli,** which are surrounded by **myoepithelial cells.** Ducts and alveoli distend as alveoli secrete **colostrum.** This proliferation of glandular tissue takes place at the expense of the adipose tissue, which concurrently decreases as glandular tissue increases.

4. **During lactation.** The epithelial cells of the alveoli become active in **milk production.** Numerous fat droplets and secretory vacuoles containing dense aggregates of milk proteins can be observed ultrastructurally at the apical end of the alveolar epithelial cells. Human breast milk is produced 1–3 days after childbirth. Breast milk contains a substantial amount of lipid, protein, lactose, vitamins, and secretory IgA (which affords temporary enteric passive immunity). Although milk is produced continuously by the alveoli (milk production), it is delivered only in response to suckling **(milk letdown).** Suckling stimulates afferent neurons, which relay the information to the hypothalamus such that the following actions occur: 1) **oxytocin** is released from the posterior hypophysis, which causes the contraction of myoepithelial cells and milk letdown; and 2) **prolactin-inhibiting hormone (PIH; dopamine)** is inhibited, which causes the release of **prolactin** from the adenohypophysis and further milk production.

XI   Selected Photomicrographs

A. Cervical biopsy of cervical intraepithelial neoplasia (CIN I, CIN II, CIN III), Pap smears of cervical intraepithelial neoplasia (CIN I, CIN II, CIN III), human papilloma virus (HPV), and squamous cell carcinoma (Figure 26-7)

B. Fibroadenoma of the breast, infiltrating duct carcinoma of the breast (Figure 26-8)

● **Figure 26-7 Cervical biopsy and pathology of the cervix. (A)** Cervical biopsy panel ranging from normal to CIN III. A normal cervical biopsy shows a typical appearance of stratified squamous epithelium. CIN I shows superficial keratinization and koilocytotic atypia as evidenced by prominent perinuclear halos (*small arrows*). CIN III shows atypical oblong nuclei, vertical orientation of epithelial cells, and mitotic figures near the surface (*arrows*). **(B)** Pap smear panel ranging from normal to CIN III. A normal Pap smear shows typical superficial squamous epithelial cells with relatively small nucleus and with a large cytoplasmic area. Progression from CIN I to CIN III is generally reflected in a reduction in the amount of cytoplasm and an increase in the nucleus-to-cytoplasm ratio. CIN I shows nuclear enlargement, hyperchromatism, and binucleation disproportionate to cytoplasmic maturity. CIN III shows nuclei that vary in size and shape. The chromatin material is coarse and granular. **(C)** Human papilloma virus (HPV) localized in cervical biopsy by in situ hybridization for DNA sequences specific for HPV. **(D)** Squamous cell carcinoma of the cervix. CIN I → CIN III usually precedes the appearance of squamous cell carcinoma. Stratified squamous epithelium (*asterisk*) in the transformation zone has invaded the underlying stroma, forming nests of malignant cells (*arrows*). High magnification of the nests (boxed area) is shown. *CIN* = cervical intraepithelial neoplasia.

● **Figure 26-8 Breast pathology. (A–C) Fibroadenoma of the breast. (A)** A mediolateral oblique mammogram. A benign mass is shown. A benign mass has the following characteristics: **shape** is round or oval, **margins** are well-circumscribed, density is low-medium contrast, it becomes smaller over time, and **calcifications** are large, smooth, and uniform. **(B, C)** LM of a fibroadenoma, which is a benign proliferation of the connective tissue stroma (*str*). As a consequence, the glands (*gl*) are compressed into cords of epithelium with slitlike spaces. A fibroadenoma presents clinically as a sharply circumscribed, spherical nodule that is freely movable. **(D–F) Infiltrating duct carcinoma. (D)** A cranio-caudal mammogram. A malignant mass is shown. A malignant mass has the following characteristics: **shape** is irregular with many lobulations, **margins** are irregular or spiculated, density is medium-high, breast architecture may be distorted, it becomes larger over time, and **calcifications** (not shown) are small, irregular, variable , and found within ducts (ductal casts). *Arrows* indicate a clear zone around the tumor with spicules. **(E, F)** LM of infiltrating duct carcinoma of the breast. The tumor cells are arranged in cell nests (*), cell cords (*arrows*), anastomosing masses, or a mixture of all of these. The cells are surrounded by fairly thick bands of connective tissue stroma (*arrowheads*). This is the most common type of breast cancer, accounting for 65%–80% of all breast cancers. Some features that are common to all infiltrative breast carcinomas include: fixed in position, retraction and dimpling of the skin, thickening of the skin (peau d'orange), and retraction of the nipple. The presence of estrogen receptors or progesterone receptors within the carcinoma cells indicates a good prognosis for treatment. Tamoxifen is an estrogen receptor blocker and is the drug of choice for treatment. The presence of the c-erb B2 oncoprotein (similar to the epidermal growth factor receptor) on the surface of the carcinoma cells indicates a poor prognosis for treatment. *BRCA*-1 (breast cancer susceptibility gene) is an antioncogene (tumor suppressor gene) located on chromosome 17 (17q21) that encodes for BRCA protein (a zinc finger gene-regulatory protein) containing phosphotyrosine, which will suppress the cell cycle. A mutation of the *BRCA*-1 gene is present in 5%–10% of women with breast cancer and confers a very high lifetime risk of breast and ovarian cancer.

Case Study

A 55-year-old woman comes to your office complaining that "I'm having real bad pains in my stomach. I feel bloated and uncomfortable even though I've lost a few pounds recently." She also tells you that "I've got to pee a lot more often lately." After some discussion, she informs you that she has never been pregnant and her menstrual periods have always been regular. Her mother and sister both died of breast cancer. The woman does not seem to be very concerned about her condition as she says, "Doc, I've had regular breast exams ever since my mom died and they have always been negative, thank God. You know, my mother and sister got a bad break with breast cancer and I'm very lonely without them. I really feel lucky that I only have a little stomach ache to deal with." What is the most likely diagnosis?

Differentials

- Cancer metastasis to the ovary, endometrial carcinoma

Relevant Physical Exam Findings

- Mass in the pelvis
- Ascites in the abdomen
- No vaginal discharge

Relevant Lab Findings

- Blood chemistry: serum CA-125 high
- CT scan: 7-cm right ovarian mass; 5-cm left ovarian mass
- Biopsy: extensive network of papillae projecting from the wall of the mass along with invasion of the stroma and capsule; many laminated calcified concretions (psammoma bodies) are observed

Diagnosis

Ovarian serous cystadenocarcinoma (OS). OS is the most common ovarian neoplasm ($\approx$50% of ovarian cancers) and are commonly bilateral. OS is a multiloculated tumor with soft, delicate papillae lining the entire surface. Solid areas with necrosis and hemorrhage are commonly present. The majority of ovarian tumors do not secrete hormone but are associated with serum CA-125 antigen. Risk factors for ovarian cancer are nulliparity and a family history of cancer associated with the BRCA1 mutation. Clinical findings for ovarian tumors include abdominal distention, lower abdominal pain, pelvic pressure, compression of regional organs, ascites, increased urinary frequency, and weight loss. The most common cancer metastasis to the ovary occurs from tumors of the uterus, uterine tubes, contralateral ovary, breast, and GI tract. The Krukenberg tumor describes stomach cancer that metastasizes to the ovaries. Endometrial carcinoma is the most common gynecologic malignancy in the United States and has been linked to prolonged estrogen stimulation of the endometrium (e.g., estrogen replacement therapy during menopause). Endometrial carcinoma often presents with vaginal bleeding. Risk factors for endometrial carcinoma are nulliparity, obesity, diabetes, late menopause, early menarche, and unopposed estrogen stimulation.

Chapter 27

Male Reproductive System

Testes. The testes (plural) are paired, ovoid organs located in the scrotum. Each mature adult testis (singular) is 4–5 cm in length; 2.5 cm in width; 3 cm in thickness; and weighs about 11–17 g. The right testis is commonly slightly larger and heavier than the left. The testes are surrounded incompletely (medially, laterally, and anteriorly—but not posteriorly) by a sac of peritoneum called the **tunica vaginalis.** Beneath the tunica vaginalis, the testes are surrounded by a thick connective tissue capsule called the **tunica albuginea** because of its whitish color. Beneath the tunica albuginea, the testes are surrounded by a highly vascular layer of connective tissue called the **tunica vasculosa.** The tunica albuginea projects connective tissue **septae** inward toward the mediastinum that divides the testis into about **250 lobules,** each of which contains **1–4 highly coiled seminiferous tubules.** These septae converge toward the midline on the posterior surface where they meet to form a ridgelike thickening called the **mediastinum.** The septae are continuous with the **interstitial connective tissue** that contains the Leydig (interstitial) cells that secrete testosterone. The testes contain the **seminiferous tubules, straight tubules, rete testes,** and the **Leydig (interstitial) cells.**

A. **SEMINIFEROUS TUBULES** (Figures 27-1 and 27-2, Table 27-1). In a sexually mature male, a seminiferous tubule is about 30–80 cm in length and 150 μm in diameter, and has a lumen. (In a sexually immature boy, the seminiferous "tubules" have no lumen and are therefore more appropriately referred to as **seminiferous cords.**) The combined total length of all the seminiferous tubules in each testis is about 300–900 m. The seminiferous tubules are lined by a complex stratified epithelium **(germinal epithelium)** consisting of two basic cell types: **Sertoli cells** and **spermatogenic cells.**

1. **Sertoli cells.** Sertoli cells are columnar cells with unusually ruffled apical and lateral surfaces owing to the fact that these surfaces surround the developing spermatogenic cells. Sertoli cells extend the full thickness of the germinal epithelium. The functions of sertoli cells include:

   a. Provide mechanical and nutritional support for developing spermatogenic cells.
   b. Phagocytose excess cytoplasm discarded by spermatids.
   c. Form the **blood-testes barrier** through **tight junctions** on their lateral surfaces.
   d. Secrete **inhibin** that inhibits release of follicle-stimulating hormone (FSH) from adenohypophysis.
   e. Secrete **MIF (müllerian inhibitory factor)** during fetal development that inhibits development of the paramesonephric duct in a genotypic XY fetus.
   f. Synthesize **androgen-binding protein (ABP)** that binds testosterone so that high levels of testosterone are present in the seminiferous tubules, which is necessary for spermatogenesis to occur.
   g. Possess **FSH receptors** (G protein–linked receptor) so that FSH from the adenohypophysis stimulates spermatogenesis and synthesis of ABP.

2. **Spermatogenic cells.** Spermatogenic cells are the "male germ cells" that are undergoing the transformation from type A spermatogonia → sperm. This transformation

● **Figure 27-1 General features of the testes. (A)** Diagram of the testis and duct system. **(B)** LM of a seminiferous tubule within the testis. The seminiferous tubule contains spermatogonia (1), primary spermatocytes (2), secondary spermatocytes (3), early spermatids (4), late spermatids (5), and Sertoli cells (6). In addition, the three stages of spermatogenesis (spermatocytogenesis, meiosis, and spermiogenesis) are indicated by the brackets (correlated with Table 27-1). The level of the blood-testes barrier is indicated by the dotted line. **(C)** Diagram of the Sertoli cell. Note the close relationship of the Sertoli cell and spermatogenic cells (*arrows*) whereby the spermatogenic cells indent the surface of the Sertoli cell so that the cell border of the Sertoli is quite irregular. **(D–G)** Diagram of the four phases of spermiogenesis. **(D) Golgi phase.** 1 = Golgi; 2 = Golgi vesicles; 3 = acrosomal granule with the acrosomal vesicle; 4 = nucleus; 5 = centrioles and developing axoneme (cilium). **(E) Cap phase.** 1 = Golgi; 2 = acrosomal cap; 3 = centrioles and developing axoneme (cilium). **(F) Acrosome phase.** 1 = acrosome; 2 = nucleus; 3 = manchette; 4 = Golgi. **(G) Maturation phase.** 1 = nucleus; 2 = mitochondrial sheath; 3 = annulus (a dense ring that separates the middle piece from the principal piece); 4 = principal piece; 5 = excess cytoplasm.

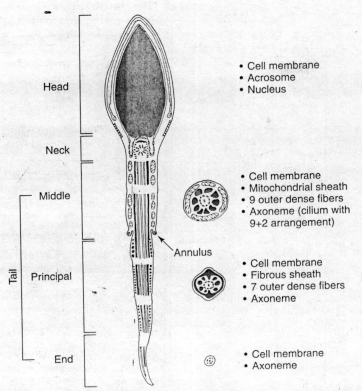

- Head
  - Cell membrane
  - Acrosome
  - Nucleus
- Neck
- Middle
  - Cell membrane
  - Mitochondrial sheath
  - 9 outer dense fibers
  - Axoneme (cilium with 9+2 arrangement)

Annulus

- Principal
  - Cell membrane
  - Fibrous sheath
  - 7 outer dense fibers
  - Axoneme
- Tail
- End
  - Cell membrane
  - Axoneme

● **Figure 27-2 Ultrastructural morphology of a mature spermatozoon.** The spermatozoon consists of a **head region, neck region,** and **tail region** (which is further divided into the **middle piece, principal piece,** and **end piece**). Cross sections of the middle piece, principal piece, and end piece are shown. Note the list of components from outside to inside. The annulus is a dense ring that separates the middle piece from the principal piece. Newly ejaculated sperm are incapable of fertilization until they undergo capacitation. Capacitation is a reversible process whereby freshly ejaculated sperm develop the capacity to fertilize a secondary oocyte. Capacitation normally occurs in the female reproductive tract and takes 7 hours. It involves the following: unmasking of glycosyltransferases on the sperm cell membrane and removal of surface-coating proteins derived from seminal fluid.

is called **spermatogenesis.** As the spermatogenic cells undergo spermatogenesis, they migrate from the basal layer to the luminal layer of the germinal epithelium and consist of the following cell types: **type A spermatogonia (dark type A and pale type A), type B spermatogonia, primary spermatocytes, secondary spermatocytes, spermatids (early and late stages), and spermatozoa (sperm).** Spermatogenesis is divided into three stages: **spermatocytogenesis, meiosis, and spermiogenesis.**

a. **Spermatocytogenesis.** Dark type A spermatogonia undergo *mitosis* to provide a continuous supply of stem cells throughout the reproductive life of the male. Then, pale type A spermatogonia undergo mitosis and differentiate to form **type B spermatogonia.** Type B spermatogonia may also undergo mitosis to produce more type B spermatogonia. Type B spermatocytes then enter meiosis.

b. **Meiosis.** Meiosis is a cell division process that occurs only in the production of the male and female gametes (do not confuse meiosis with mitosis). **MEIOSIS OCCURS ONLY IN THE OVARY AND TESTES.** Meiosis consists of two cell divisions **(meiosis I and meiosis II)** and results in the formation of four

SUMMARY OF SPERMATOGENESIS

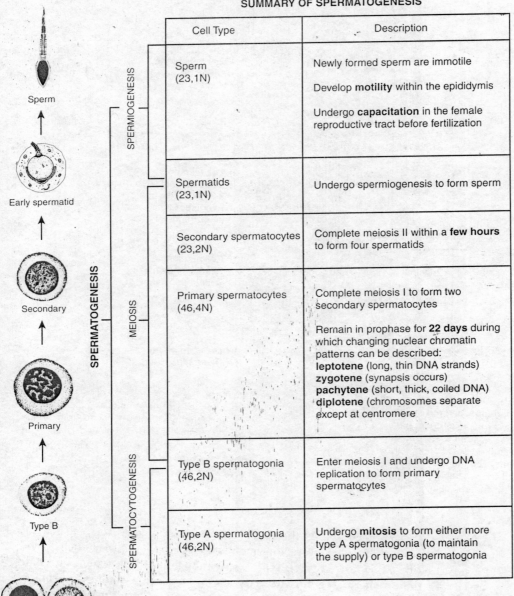

Cell Type	Description
Sperm (23,1N)	Newly formed sperm are immotile Develop **motility** within the epididymis Undergo **capacitation** in the female reproductive tract before fertilization
Spermatids (23,1N)	Undergo spermiogenesis to form sperm
Secondary spermatocytes (23,2N)	Complete meiosis II within a **few hours** to form four spermatids
Primary spermatocytes (46,4N)	Complete meiosis I to form two secondary spermatocytes Remain in prophase for **22 days** during which changing nuclear chromatin patterns can be described: **leptotene** (long, thin DNA strands) **zygotene** (synapsis occurs) **pachytene** (short, thick, coiled DNA) **diplotene** (chromosomes separate except at centromere
Type B spermatogonia (46,2N)	Enter meiosis I and undergo DNA replication to form primary spermatocytes
Type A spermatogonia (46,2N)	Undergo **mitosis** to form either more type A spermatogonia (to maintain the supply) or type B spermatogonia

Left-side diagram labels (bottom to top):

Dark   Pale
Type A

Type B

Primary

Secondary

Early spermatid

Sperm

Vertical labels: SPERMATOGENESIS, SPERMIOGENESIS, MEIOSIS, SPERMATOCYTOGENESIS gametes containing 23 chromosomes and 1N amount of DNA. Meiosis does three important things: **(i)** reduces the number of chromosomes within the gametes to ensure that the human species number of chromosomes (46) can be maintained from generation to generation, **(ii)** redistributes maternal and paternal chromosomes to ensure genetic variability, and **(iii)** promotes the exchange of small amounts of maternal and paternal DNA via **crossover** during meiosis I.

c. **Spermiogenesis.** Spermiogenesis is a **postmeiotic** series of morphologic changes by which spermatids (round-shaped cells) are transformed into sperm ("sleek swimmers"). The transformation is divided into four phases.

   (1) Golgi phase. Numerous **pro-acrosomal granules** appear in the Golgi vesicles and coalesce to form a single **acrosomal granule** within the **acrosomal vesicle.** The centrioles migrate to the posterior pole of the spermatid and initiate assembly of the 9+2 microtubule arrangement of the axoneme (i.e., cilium) of the sperm tail.

   (2) Cap phase. The acrosomal vesicle flattens and spreads over the anterior two thirds of the nucleus and is now called the **acrosomal cap.**

   (3) Acrosome phase. The large acrosomal granule diffuses throughout the acrosomal vesicle thereby forming the **acrosome.** The nuclear chromatin begins to condense as the nucleus begins to elongate. Cytoplasmic microtubules organize into a cylindrical sheet called the **manchette,** which assists in the elongation of the spermatid and extends from the posterior rim of the acrosome toward the developing tail. Centrioles migrate to the posterior pole of the spermatid and initiate the formation of the **outer dense fibers** around the axoneme. Cytoplasmic mitochondria migrate to form a **helical sheath** around the outer dense fibers. The spermatid rotates so that the acrosomal cap orients toward the basal lamina of the seminiferous tubule and the tail orients toward the lumen.

   (4) Maturation phase. The nucleus acquires its final elongated and condensed state. Excess spermatid cytoplasm is discarded and phagocytosed by Sertoli cells. The manchette disassembles. Intercellular bridges are lost.

B. **STRAIGHT TUBULES.** Toward the terminal portion of each seminiferous tubule, the spermatogenic cells disappear such that the germinal epithelium lining the seminiferous tubule consists solely of Sertoli cells. At the end of each seminiferous tubule, there is an abrupt narrowing or transition to the **straight tubules** (also called **tubuli recti**), which are lined by **simple cuboidal epithelium.**

C. **RETE TESTES.** The straight tubules empty into an anastomosing labyrinth of channels located at the mediastinum called the rete testes. The rete testes are lined by **simple cuboidal epithelium.**

D. **LEYDIG CELLS** (Figure 27-3). The Leydig cells (or interstitial cells) of the testes are located in the loose connective tissue between the seminiferous tubules. Leydig cells are large, irregularly shaped, polygonal, acidophilic cells. Leydig cells have an elaborate sER, lipid droplets, mitochondria with tubular cristae, and highly refractive, rod-shaped crystals called crystals of Reinke. Leydig cells are steroid-secreting cells (i.e., testosterone) and therefore have all the cell organelles that are typically found in steroid-secreting cells. The functions of the Leydig cells include:

1. Possess **LH receptors** (G protein–linked receptor) so that luteinizing hormone (LH) from the adenohypophysis stimulates testosterone secretion.

Figure 27-3 **(A)** LM of Leydig cells (*Ley*) found in the connective tissue between the seminiferous tubules (*SEM*) near capillaries (*cap*). **(B)** EM of Leydig cells. Smooth endoplasmic reticulum (*SER*), mitochondria with tubular cristae (*M*), and lipid droplets (*arrows*) are typically found in a steroid-secreting cell. *CR* = crystals of Reinke. **(C)** Flow chart of androgen biosynthesis. *StAR* = steroidogenic acute regulatory protein. Deficiencies of enzymes with an * are clinically important. **(D)** Diagram of hormonal control of the male reproductive system. Gonadotropin releasing factor (*GRF*) from the hypothalamus stimulates the adenohypophysis. In response to GRF, the adenohypophysis (*AD*) secretes follicle-stimulating hormone (*FSH*) and luteinizing hormone (LH). FSH binds to FSH receptors (□) on the Sertoli cells, which stimulates the synthesis of androgen-binding protein (*ABP*). The Sertoli cells secrete inhibin (*INH*) that inhibits FSH secretion (a feedback loop). LH binds to LH receptors (△) on the Leydig cells, which stimulates the secretion of testosterone (*T*). T circulates in the blood bound to sex steroid–binding globulin (*SSBG*). T binds to ABP within Sertoli cells to maintain high levels of T necessary for spermatogenesis.

2. Secrete **testosterone.** Testosterone gives rise to two other potent androgens via the following pathways:

$$\text{Testosterone} \xrightarrow{\text{5}\alpha\text{-reductase}} \textbf{dihydrotestosterone (DHT)}$$

$$\text{Testosterone} \xrightarrow{\text{3}\alpha\text{-reductase}} \textbf{5}\alpha\textbf{-androstanediol}$$

3. Aromatization of testosterone and androstenedione within the liver and adipose tissue by P_{450} **aromatase** produces significant amounts of estradiol and estrone in males.
4. During fetal life, testosterone is essential in the development of the epididymis, ductus deferens, seminal vesicle, and ejaculatory duct. DHT is essential in the development of the penis and scrotum (external genitalia) and prostate gland.
5. During puberty and adult life, androgens are essential for: spermatogenesis, function of prostate, seminal vesicle, and bulbourethral glands, appearance of secondary sex characteristics, closure of the epiphyseal growth plate, increase in muscle mass, lipid metabolism (testosterone increases low-density lipoprotein [LDL] and decreases high-density lipoprotein [HDL]), and stimulation of cartilage growth.
6. One to two percent of circulating testosterone is in the free form; the remainder is bound to a liver-derived **sex steroid–binding globulin** or **albumin.**
7. Testosterone is degraded in the liver by conversion to various metabolites with the addition of glucuronide (e.g., 3α-androstanediol glucuronide) and excreted in the urine.

E. CLINICAL CONSIDERATIONS OF THE TESTES

1. **5α-Reductase 2 deficiency** is caused by a mutation in the 5α-reductase 2 gene that renders the 5α-reductase 2 enzyme inactive. Normally, 5α-reductase 2 catalyzes the conversion of **testosterone (T)** → **DHT.** 5α-Reductase 2 deficiency produces the following clinical findings: underdevelopment of the penis and scrotum (microphallus, hypospadias, and bifid scrotum) and prostate gland. The epididymis, ductus deferens, seminal vesicle, and ejaculatory duct are normal. These clinical findings have led to the inference that DHT is essential in the development of the penis and scrotum (external genitalia) and prostate gland in genotypic XY fetus. At puberty, these individuals demonstrate a striking virilization. An increased T:DHT ratio is diagnostic (normal = 5; 5α-reductase 2 deficiency = 20–60).
2. **17β-Hydroxysteroid dehydrogenase 3 (HSD) deficiency** is caused by a mutation in the **17β-HSD 3 gene** that renders 17β-HSD 3 enzyme inactive. Normally, 17β-HSD 3 catalyzes the conversion of **androstenedione** → **testosterone.** This is the most common defect in androgen biosynthesis. 17β-HSD deficiency produces the following clinical findings: underdevelopment of the penis and scrotum (microphallus, hypospadias, and bifid scrotum) and prostate gland. The epididymis, ductus deferens, seminal vesicle, and ejaculatory duct are normal. The clinical findings in 17β-HSD deficiency and 5α-reductase 2 deficiency are very similar.
3. **Complete androgen insensitivity (CAIS; testicular feminization syndrome)** is caused by a mutation in the **androgen receptor (AR) gene** that renders AR inactive. Normally, AR is a **nuclear transcription factor** that is activated by androgens to bind DNA promoter regions that regulate transcription of other genes. CAIS produces the following clinical findings: 46,XY genotype, testes, and normal-appearing female external genitalia; the uterus and uterine tubes are

absent. These individuals present as normal-appearing females and their psychosocial orientation is female despite their genotype.

4. **Seminoma** (Figure 27-4A) is the most common type of germ cell neoplasm in men 20–40 years of age. About 90% of all testicular cancers arise from germ cells. Almost all germ cell neoplasms involve the isochromosome of the short arm of chromosome 12 [i(12p)], which is virtually diagnostic. Seminoma causes either a painless testicular mass (usually on the right side) or a diffuse nodularity throughout the testis. Seminoma is associated with **elevated human chorionic gonadotropin (hCG) levels.**

5. **Testicular teratocarcinoma** (Figure 27-4B) is a germ cell neoplasm. In its early histologic stages, a testicular teratocarcinoma resembles a blastocyst (!!!) with three primary germ layers and may be loosely referred to as "male pregnancy." Later, the tumor comprises well-differentiated cells and structures from each of the three primary germ layers: e.g., colon glandular tissue (endoderm), cartilage (mesoderm), and squamous epithelium (ectoderm). Testicular teratocarcinoma is associated with **elevated hCG and α-fetoprotein (AFP) levels.**

Ⅱ Duct System

A. **EFFERENT DUCTULES.** About 15 efferent ductules leave the testis by penetrating the tunica albuginea and connect the rete testis to the proximal portion of the epididymis. The efferent ductules are lined by a **simple columnar epithelium** that contains both **tall columnar cells** and **short columnar cells,** which give the luminal surface a sawtoothed appearance. The tall columnar cells are **ciliated** and have a role in the movement of sperm through the ductule. The short columnar cells are not ciliated but have numerous **microvilli, apical invaginations,** and **numerous pinocytotic vesicles** (indicating intense endocytotic activity). Eighty percent of the testicular fluid secreted in the seminiferous tubules is reabsorbed in the efferent ductules. The efferent ductules also have a thin **circular layer of smooth muscle** that aids in the movement of sperm.

B. **EPIDIDYMIS.** The epididymis is a very long (6 m) and highly coiled duct that is described as having a **head region, body region,** and **tail region. Sperm maturation (i.e., motility) and storage** occur in the epididymis. Histologically, the epididymis has an epithelial lining and muscular coat.
   1. **Epithelium.** The epididymis is lined by a **pseudostratified columnar epithelium** consisting of tall columnar **principal cells** and **basal cells.** The epididymis has a **smooth luminal surface** (in contrast to the saw-toothed pattern of the efferent ductules).
      a. **The principal cells** are characterized by **stereocilia,** apical invaginations, numerous pinocytotic vesicles, coated vesicle, lysosomes, well-developed rER, and Golgi. The principal cells have the following functions: resorption of testicular fluid begun in the efferent ductules, phagocytosis of degenerating sperm or spermatid residual bodies not phagocytosed by the Sertoli cells, and secretion of glycoproteins, which bind to the surface of the cell membrane of the sperm, sialic acid, and glycerophosphocholine (which inhibits capacitation thus preventing sperm from fertilizing a secondary oocyte until the sperm enter the female reproductive tract).
      b. **The basal cells** act as a stem cell population to resupply the principal cells.
   2. **Muscular coat.** In the head and body region of the epididymis, the muscular coat consists of a **circular layer of smooth muscle** that aids in the movement of sperm. In the tail region of the epididymis, the muscular coat consists of an **inner**

● **Figure 27-4 Testicular neoplasms. (A) LM of seminoma.** About 95% of testicular neoplasms arise from germ cells. Almost all germ cell neoplasms involve the isochromosome of the short arm of chromosome 12 [i(12p)], which is virtually diagnostic. Seminoma is the most common type of germ cell neoplasm. Low-power LM of a seminoma showing normal testicular tissue at the periphery (*Nor*) with typical seminiferous tubules and seminoma (*Sem*). High-magnification LM of a seminoma that consists of clusters of moderately sized round cells with large centrally located nuclei with prominent nucleoli (*outlined areas*). Mitotic figures can be observed (*arrow*). The cell clusters are separated by fibrous cords (*double arrows*). The fibrous cords are heavily infiltrated with lymphocytes (*arrowhead*), which may play a role in the immune rejection of seminomas and contribute to the favorable prognosis of these neoplasms. **(B) LM of testicular teratocarcinoma (TC).** TC is another type of germ cell neoplasm that is composed of a collection of well-differentiated cells or structures from each of the three primary germ layers. TC is composed of a fibrous stroma with many cystlike structures (*). In addition, well-differentiated glandular structures resembling colon glandular epithelium (endoderm; *box 1*), cartilage (mesoderm; *box 2*), and squamous epithelium (ectoderm; *box 3*) are shown.

longitudinal layer, middle circular layer, and **outer longitudinal layer of smooth muscle.** These three layers contract as a result of neural stimulation during sexual excitation and force sperm from the tail of the epididymis to the ductus deferens. This is the initial muscular component that contributes to the force of ejaculation.

C. DUCTUS DEFERENS. The ductus deferens begins at the inferior pole of the testis, ascends to enter the spermatic cord, transits the inguinal canal, and enters the abdominal cavity by passing through the deep inguinal ring. The distal end of the ductus deferens enlarges to form the **ampulla,** where it is joined by a short duct from the seminal vesicle and then continues as the ejaculatory duct. The epithelium is similar to the epididymis, i.e., **pseudostratified columnar epithelium with principal cells and basal cells.** The smooth muscular coat is similar to the tail region of the epididymis, i.e., **inner longitudinal layer, middle circular layer,** and **outer longitudinal layer of smooth muscle,** and contributes to the force of ejaculation.

D. EJACULATORY DUCT. The ejaculatory duct passes through the prostate gland and opens into the prostatic urethra at the **seminal colliculus** of the urethral crest. The epithelium is similar to the epididymis and ductus deferens. However, the ejaculatory duct has no smooth muscular coat. The force for ejaculation is derived primarily by the smooth muscular coat of the tail region of the epididymis and ductus deferens.

E. URETHRA
  1. Female urethra. The female urethra is about 3–5 cm long and begins at the **internal urethral orifice** of the bladder where the detrusor muscle extends longitudinally into the urethra but does not form a significant internal urethral sphincter. The female urethra courses through the **urogenital diaphragm** where it becomes related to the **deep transverse perineal muscle** and **sphincter urethrae muscle** (also called external urethral sphincter) both of which are skeletal muscle innervated by the **pudendal nerve.** The posterior surface of the female urethra fuses with the anterior wall of the vagina such that the **external urethral sphincter** does not completely surround the female urethra. This may explain the high incidences of stress incontinence in women, especially after childbirth. The female urethra terminates as the **navicular fossa** at the **external urethral orifice,** which opens into the **vestibule of the vagina** between the labia minora just below the clitoris. The female urethra develops endodermal outgrowths into the surrounding mesoderm to form the **urethral glands** and **paraurethral glands of Skene** (which are homologous to the prostate gland in the male). The paraurethral glands of Skene open on each side of the external urethral orifice. The vestibule of the vagina develops endodermal outgrowths into the surrounding mesoderm to form the **lesser vestibular glands** and the **greater vestibular glands of Bartholin** (which are homologous to the bulbourethral glands of Cowper in the male). The greater vestibular glands of Bartholin open on each side of the vaginal orifice. The female urethra is lined proximally by **transitional epithelium.** The remainder of the urethra is lined by **non-keratinized stratified squamous epithelium.** At the external urethral orifice the stratified epithelium becomes slightly keratinized. The wall of the urethra consists of an **inner layer of smooth muscle** and an **outer layer of skeletal muscle.** The inner layer of smooth muscle is continuous with the detrusor muscle of the bladder and is present throughout the course of the urethra. The outer layer of skeletal muscle is formed from skeletal muscle fibers derived from the external urethral sphincter.

Although the outer layer of skeletal muscle is obviously most prominent near the urogenital diaphragm, the outer layer of skeletal muscle is present throughout the course of the urethra.

2. **Male urethra.** The male urethra is about 18–20 cm long and begins at the **internal urethral orifice** of the bladder where the detrusor muscle extends longitudinally into the prostatic urethra and forms a complete collar around the neck of the bladder called the **internal urethral sphincter.** The male urethra is divided into five parts:

a. **Prostatic urethra.** The prostatic urethra courses through and is surrounded by the **prostate gland.** The posterior wall has an elevation called the **urethral crest.** The **prostatic sinus** is a groove on either side of the urethral crest that receives most of the prostatic ducts from the prostate gland. At a specific site along the urethral crest there is an ovoid enlargement called the **seminal colliculus** (also called the **verumontanum**) where the ejaculatory ducts open and the **prostatic utricle** (a vestigial remnant of the paramesonephric duct in males that is involved in the embryological development of the vagina and uterus) is found. The prostatic urethra is lined by a **transitional epithelium.** The wall of the prostatic urethra consists of an inner layer of smooth muscle (continuous with the detrusor muscle), an outer layer of skeletal muscle (derived from the external urethral sphincter), and the prostate gland.

b. **Membranous urethra.** The membranous urethra courses through the **urogenital diaphragm** where it becomes related to the **deep transverse perineal muscle** and **sphincter urethrae muscle** (also called **external urethral sphincter**) both of which are skeletal muscle innervated by the **pudendal nerve.** The external urethral sphincter completely surrounds the male urethra. The prostatic urethra plus the membranous urethra are called the **posterior urethra** by radiologists. The membranous urethra is lined by a **stratified columnar epithelium.** The wall of the membranous urethra consists of an inner layer of smooth muscle (continuous with the detrusor muscle) and an outer layer of skeletal muscle (derived from the external urethral sphincter).

c. **Bulbous urethra.** The bulbous urethra courses through the **bulb of the penis** and develops endodermal outgrowths into the surrounding mesoderm to form the **bulbourethral glands of Cowper.** The bulbous urethra contains the openings of the bulbourethral glands of Cowper. The bulbous urethra is lined by a **stratified columnar epithelium.** The wall of the bulbous urethra is a highly vascularized, loose connective tissue with elastic fibers that is a part of the corpus spongiosum.

d. **Proximal part of the penile (spongy or cavernous) urethra.** The proximal part of the penile urethra courses through and is surrounded by the **corpus spongiosum.** The proximal part of the penile urethra develops endodermal outgrowths into the surrounding mesoderm to form the **urethral glands of Littre.** The proximal part of the penile urethra is lined by a **stratified columnar epithelium.** The wall of the proximal part of the penile urethra is a highly vascularized, loose connective tissue with elastic fibers that is a part of the corpus spongiosum.

e. **Distal part of the penile urethra.** The distal part of the penile urethra courses through the **glans penis** and terminates as the **navicular fossa** at the **external urethral orifice** which opens onto the surface of the glans penis. The bulbous urethra plus the proximal and distal parts of the penile urethra are called the **anterior urethra** by radiologists. The distal part of the penile urethra is lined by a **stratified squamous epithelium.** The wall of the distal part of the penile urethra is a highly vascularized, loose connective tissue with elastic fibers that is a part of the corpus spongiosum.

III Accessory Glands

A. SEMINAL VESICLE. The seminal vesicles are highly coiled tubular diverticula that originate as evaginations of the ductus deferens distal to the ampulla. The mucosa (epithelium and lamina propria) is thrown into highly convoluted folds forming labyrinth-like cul-de-sacs, all of which open into a central lumen. The **lamina propria** consists of connective tissue. The **muscular coat** consists of an inner circular layer and an outer longitudinal layer. Contraction of the smooth muscle during ejaculation discharges the secretory product (seminal fluid) into the ejaculatory duct. The **adventitia** consists of connective tissue. The seminal vesicles are lined by a **pseudostratified columnar epithelium** consisting of **columnar cells** and **basal cells.**

1. **Columnar cells** have numerous microvilli, rER, Golgi, lipid droplets, secretory granules, and lipochrome pigment. These are characteristics of cells active in secretion. The secretion product is a whitish-yellow viscous material that contains fructose (the principal metabolic substrate for sperm) and other sugars, choline, proteins, amino acids, ascorbic acid, citric acid, and prostaglandins. Seminal vesicle secretion (i.e., seminal fluid) accounts for 70% of the volume of the ejaculated semen. The characteristic pale yellow color of semen is caused by the lipochrome pigment secreted by the columnar cells. In forensic medicine, the presence of fructose (which is not produced elsewhere in the body) and choline crystals is used to determine the presence of semen.

2. **Basal cells.** The basal cells are stem cells.

B. BULBOURETHRAL (BU) GLANDS OF COWPER. The BU glands are located in the deep perineal space embedded in the skeletal muscles of the urogenital diaphragm (i.e., deep transverse perineal muscle and sphincter urethrae muscle) and adjacent to the membranous urethrae. The ducts of the BU glands open into the penile urethra. The BU glands are compound tubuloalveolar glands (resembling mucus-secreting glands) surrounded by a connective tissue capsule that extends septae that divide the BU gland into many lobules. The compound tubuloalveolar glands are lined by a simple cuboidal epithelium. The epithelium produces a clear, mucouslike, slippery fluid, which contains galactose, galactosamine, galacturonic acid, sialic acid, and methylpentose. This fluid makes up a major portion of the preseminal fluid (or pre-ejaculate fluid) and probably serves to lubricate the penile urethra.

C. PROSTATE GLAND (Figure 27-5).

1. **General features.** The prostate gland is located between the base of the urinary bladder and the urogenital diaphragm. The anterior surface of the prostate is related to the retropubic space. The posterior surface of the prostate is related to the seminal vesicles and rectum. The prostate gland can be easily palpated by a digital examination via the rectum. The prostate gland consists of five lobes: **right and left lateral lobes, right and left posterior lobes,** and a **middle lobe.** The prostate gland is a collection of 30–50 compound tubuloalveolar glands that are arranged in three zones: the **peripheral zone** (contains the largest glands and highest number of glands), **central zone,** and **transitional (periurethral) zone.** The compound tubuloalveolar glands are lined by a simple columnar epithelium (however, it may vary from pseudostratified to cuboidal epithelium). The prostatic epithelium contains **basal cells, secretory**

cells, and **endocrine cells.** The **basal cells** are the stem cells or proliferative compartment of the prostatic epithelium normally dividing and maturing into secretory cells. The **secretory cells** contain rER, Golgi, small clear secretory vacuoles, and lysosomes. The epithelium produces the prostatic fluid, which contains citric acid, prostatic acid phosphatase (PAP), prostaglandins, fibrinogen, and prostatic-specific antigen (PSA). Serum levels of **PSA** and **PAP** are used as a diagnostic tool for prostatic carcinoma. PSA is a serine protease that liquifies semen after ejaculation. The **endocrine cells** are randomly scattered and contain serotonin, somatostatin, calcitonin, and bombesin. The lumen of the glands contains **corpora amylacea (or prostatic concretions),** which are calcified or precipitated prostatic fluid, the significance of which is not understood. The number of prostatic concretions increases with age. The prostate gland is surrounded by a **capsule** consisting of connective tissue and smooth muscle. The capsule is highly vascularized (important in carcinoma metastasis). The capsule (both connective tissue and smooth muscle) extends into the prostate gland forming the **stroma.**

2. **Clinical considerations of the prostate gland**
   a. **Benign prostatic hyperplasia (BPH)** (Figure 27-6). **BPH** is characterized by hypertrophy of the **transitional (periurethral) zone,** which generally involves the lateral and middle lobes. BPH compresses the prostatic urethra and obstructs urine flow. The hypertrophy may be related to increased sensitivity of prostate to **DHT.** BPH is NOT premalignant. Clinical signs include: increased frequency of urination, nocturia, difficulty starting and stopping urination, and a sense of incomplete emptying of the bladder. Treatment may include: 5α-reductase inhibitors (e.g., **finasteride [Proscar]**) to block conversion of T → DHT, or α-adrenergic antagonists (e.g., **terazosin, prazosin, doxazosin**) to inhibit prostate gland secretion.
   b. **Prostatic carcinoma (PC)** (Figure 27-7). **PC** is most commonly found in the **peripheral zone,** which generally involves the posterior lobes (which can be palpated on a digital rectal examination). Because PC begins in the peripheral zone, by the time urethral blockage occurs (i.e., patient complains of difficulty in urination), the carcinoma is in an advanced stage. **Prostatic intraepithelial neoplasia (PIN)** is frequently associated with PC. Serum **PSA levels** are diagnostic. Metastasis to bone (e.g., lumbar vertebrae, pelvis) is frequent. Treatment may include: **leuprolide (Lupron),** which is a gonadotropin-releasing factor (GRF) agonist that inhibits the release of FSH and LH when administered in a continuous fashion, thereby inhibiting secretion of testosterone, **cyproterone (Androcur)** or **Flutamide (Eulexin),** which are androgen receptor antagonists, radiation, or prostatectomy.

IV **Penis.** The penis consists of three columns of erectile tissue bounded together by the **tunica albuginea:** one **corpus spongiosum** and two **corpora cavernosa.** The penis is supported by the **suspensory ligament,** which arises from the linea alba and inserts into the deep fascia (of Buck). The arterial supply is from the internal pudendal artery via the **deep artery of the penis** (involved in the erection of the penis) and **dorsal artery of the penis.** The venous drainage is to the **deep dorsal vein of the penis** → prostatic venous plexus → internal iliac vein → inferior vena cava (IVC); venous drainage is also to the **superficial dorsal vein of the penis** → external pudendal vein → great saphenous vein → femoral vein → external iliac vein → IVC. The penis is innervated by the pudendal nerve via the **dorsal nerve of the penis.**

A. **CORPUS SPONGIOSUM.** The corpus spongiosum begins as the bulb of the penis and ends as the glans penis. It is ventrally situated in the penis and transmits the urethra.

During erection, the corpus spongiosum does not get as turgid as the corpora cavernosa.

B. **CORPORA CAVERNOSA.** The corpora cavernosa begin as the **crura of the penis** and end proximal to the glans. They are dorsally situated in the penis.

C. **ERECTILE TISSUE OF THE PENIS.** The erectile tissue of the penis found within the corpus spongiosum and corpora cavernosa consists of vascular channels that are lined by endothelium. The walls of these channels consist of connective tissue and smooth muscle. Within the walls, blood vessels and small nerves can be found. Erection of the penis is dictated by blood flow into the erectile tissue under parasympathetic neural control.

● **Figure 27-5 Normal prostate gland. (A)** Diagram of the prostate gland indicating the relationship of the peripheral zone, central zone, and periurethral zone to the prostatic urethra. **(B)** LM of prostate gland. Note the network tubuloalveolar glands (*gl*) surrounded by a connective tissue stroma (*str*). **(C)** LM of prostatic epithelium. Note the basal cells (*arrowheads*) with round nuclei adjacent to the basal lamina. Note the secretory cells (*arrows*) with more elongated nuclei joined by terminal bars near the lumen. **(D)** LM of the lumen of a tubuloalveolar gland within the prostate. Note the corpora amylacea or prostatic concretions (*pc*) within the lumen, which is a distinguishing histologic characteristic.

● **Figure 27-6 LM of benign prostatic hyperplasia (BPH).** BPH is the most common disorder of the prostate gland and generally occurs in elderly men. The glands in the periurethral zone and central zone (close to the urethra) are characteristically enlarged so that compression of the urethra occurs with resulting **difficulty in urination. (A)** Low magnification shows a proliferation of both glands within a fairly well-defined nodule (*dotted lines*) and the connective tissue stroma. The epithelium of the glands characteristically forms papillary buds or infoldings (*arrows*), which are much more prominent than in the normal prostate. Other glands are cystically dilated (*). **(B)** High magnification of the boxed area in A shows hyperplastic glands and stroma infiltrated by lymphocytes (*dotted area*). **(C)** High magnification of hyperplastic glands lined by a conspicuous epithelium of tall columnar cells that appear multilayered in some locations (*arrows*). Within the lumen, corpus amylacea and papillary buds or infoldings can be seen.

● Figure 27-7 LM of prostatic carcinoma (PC). PC generally starts in the glands of the peripheral zone near the capsule. Hence, by the time blockage of the urethra occurs, PC is already in an advanced state. The most reliable sign of malignancy is the invasion of the capsule that contains lymphatics, blood vessels, and nerves. The finding of osteoblastic metastasis in bone, particularly lumbar vertebral bodies, is diagnostic of PC. **(A)** Low magnification of PC showing the main glands of the prostate near the capsule. Numerous small malignant alveoli can be observed lying side-by-side to each other (*arrows*). **(B, C)** High magnification of the boxed area in A shows malignant alveoli lined by simple cuboidal epithelium (*arrows*). The alveoli may be filled with cell nests. In a poorly differentiated PC alveoli are not apparent; instead cords of neoplastic cells will invade the stroma.

Case Study

A 28-year-old married man comes to your office complaining that "I have a lump on my right testicle. It doesn't hurt, but I'm sure worried about it." He also tells you that "It can't be a venereal disease, because I swear to you that I have never cheated on my wife." After some discussion, he informs you that he can not recall any incident where he received trauma to the groin area (e.g., a straddle injury during bicycle riding or a kick to the groin). The man has an obvious grave look of foreboding on his face and says, "Doc, my wife and I want to have children but this lump is getting bigger. Am I going to lose my testicle and be sterile?" Which of the following is the most likely diagnosis?

Differentials

- Epididymitis, hydrocele, mumps, orchitis, spermatocele, testicular torsion

Relevant Physical Exam Findings

- Nodular enlargement of the right testicle
- Normal left testicle

Relevant Lab Findings

- Blood chemistry: ß-human chorionic gonadotropin (ß-hCG) levels = High; α-fetoprotein (AFP) levels = Normal
- CT scans: no metastatic lesions in the abdomen or pelvis
- Ultrasound reveals a solid mass (not fluid-filled)
- Nodular biopsy: sheet of moderately sized cells with copious cytoplasm and large centrally placed nuclei with prominent nucleoli.

Diagnosis

Seminoma. Seminoma is the most common type of germ cell neoplasm in men 20–40 years of age. About 90% of all testicular cancers arise from germ cells. Almost all germ cell neoplasms involve the isochromosome of the short arm of chromosome 12 [i(12p)], which is virtually diagnostic. Clinical findings of seminoma include either a painless testicular mass (usually on the right side) or a diffuse nodularity throughout the testis. Seminoma is associated with elevated ß-hCG levels. Epididymitis is usually caused by *Chlamydia trachomatis* or *Neisseria gonorrhoeae*. Clinical findings of epididymitis include epididymal pain, swelling, and fever. Hydrocele of the testes occurs when a small patency of the processus vaginalis remains so that peritoneal fluid can flow into the processus vaginalis, which results in a fluid-filled cyst near the testes. Mumps viral infection in postpubertal males may result in mumps orchitis where both testis become swollen and tender (rarely causes sterility). Clinical findings of mumps viral infection include malaise, fever, and shaking chills. A spermatocele is a cystic, fluid-filled mass containing sperm. Testicular torsion is the rotation of the testes about the spermatic cord usually toward the penis (i.e., medial rotation). The incidence is increased when the testes are positioned horizontally and the tunica vaginalis is attached high on the spermatic cord ("bell clapper deformity"). Because the pampiniform venous plexus collapses more easily than the testicular artery, the testis becomes distended with blood and very painful. This is a medical emergency since compression of the testicular vessels results in ischemic necrosis within 6 hours.

Skin

① General Features. Skin is the largest organ of the body. Skin consists of three layers: the outer **epidermis**, the middle **dermis**, and the deep **hypodermis** (or **subcutaneous layer**) that corresponds to the superficial fascia in gross anatomy. Skin is classified as **thick skin** (>5 mm; covering the palms of the hand and soles of the feet) and **thin skin** (1–2 mm; covering the rest of the body). In addition, skin has a number of epidermal derivatives (or skin appendages), namely, **hair, nails, eccrine sweat glands, apocrine sweat glands, and sebaceous glands.** Skin has the following functions: regulation of body temperature, a water barrier, nonspecific barrier to microorganisms, excretion of salt, synthesis of vitamin D, and a sensory organ.

⑪ Epidermis. This layer is classified as **stratified squamous keratinized epithelium.** A number of different cell types can be found in this epithelium as indicated below.

A. KERATINOCYTES are so named because their major product is **keratin (an intermediate filament).** Keratinocytes are arranged in five strata: **basale, spinosum, granulosum, lucidum, and corneum** (Figure 28-1).

B. NONKERATINOCYTES

1. **Melanocytes** are **clear cells** that have long, branching cytoplasmic processes and are found in the **stratum basale.**
   a. They are derived from **neural crest cells** and their differentiation is dependent on the **c-kit receptor** (a tyrosine kinase receptor).
   b. They synthesize **melanin** pigment in organelles called **melanosomes.** Melanosomes contain **tyrosinase**, which catalyzes the conversion of tyrosine → dopa → melanin. When melanin synthesis is completed, the melanosome loses its tyrosinase activity and the melanosome is now called a **melanin granule.** Melanin granules are transferred to neighboring keratinocytes within the stratum basale and spinosum via cytoplasmic processes.
2. **Merkel cells** are **mechanoreceptor cells** found in the **stratum basale.**
   a. They are derived from **neural crest cells.**
   b. They contain many **dense-core granules**, presumably containing neurotransmitters.
   c. They are in contact with sensory nerve fibers that project from the dermis into the epidermis and terminate in a platelike ending called the **nerve plate.**

Strata	Characteristics
Stratum corneum (C)	Keratinocytes are devoid of nuclei and organelles, have a thickened cell membrane because of deposition of an **involucrin, small proline-rich proteins, loricrin, and keratin/filaggrin complexes,** and have a cytoplasm filled with keratin/filaggrin complexes
Stratum lucidum (L)	This stratum is a highly refractive transitional zone that is apparent only in thick skin of palms and soles
Stratum granulosum (G)	Keratinocytes contain **keratohyaline granules,** numerous **lamellar bodies,** which secrete **glycolipid acyl glucosylceramide** to form an impermeable water barrier, keratin (tonofibrils associated with the keratohyaline granules), and **filaggrin** (a protein that cross-links keratin)
Stratum spinosum (S)	Keratinocytes are attached to each other by numerous **desmosomes,** contain keratin (called **tonofibrils,** which attach to the dense plaque of desmosomes), contain a few **lamellar bodies,** and are **postmitotic**
Stratum basale (B)	Keratinocytes are attached to basement membrane via **hemidesmosomes,** contain **keratin,** and are **mitotically active**

● **Figure 28-1 General features of the skin. (A)** Table of characteristics of keratinocytes within various strata of the epidermis. LM of thick skin indicating the various strata of the epidermis (*Epi*) and dermis (*Derm*). B = stratum basale; S = stratum spinosum; G = stratum granulosum; L = stratum lucidum; C = stratum corneum. **(B)** Diagram of a melanocyte (*Mel*), Langerhans cell (*Lang*), and keratinocyte (*Ker*). **(C)** LM of a Pacinian corpuscle (*PC*) within the dermis. Note the small nerve bundles nearby (*N*). **(D)** LM of a Meissner corpuscle (*MC*) within the dermis. **(E)** Diagram of skin appendages showing an eccrine sweat gland (*Ec*), apocrine sweat gland (*Ap*), sebaceous gland (*S*), and hair (*H*) with its associated arrector pili muscle (*M*).

3. **Langerhans cells** are **antigen-presenting cells** that have long, branching cytoplasmic processes and are found mainly in the **stratum spinosum.**
   a. They originate in the bone marrow (mesoderm) and participate in **type IV delayed-type reactions** (see Chapter 14, VII, D).
   b. They phagocytose antigens, leave the epidermis to enter the lymphatic system, enter a regional lymph node where they become **dendritic cells** that express MHC class I, MHC class II, and B7 molecules, and activate T cells.
   c. They contain **Birbeck granules.**

III **Dermis.** The dermis consists of connective tissue composed of fibroblasts, type I collagen, and elastic fibers. The epidermal–dermal junction is stabilized by **hemidesmosomes** between the keratinocytes of the stratum basale and the **basement membrane.**

IV # Glands

A. **ECCRINE SWEAT GLANDS** are widely distributed throughout the skin and are active throughout life.
   1. The **secretory portion** contains **clear cells** that secrete a product composed of H_2O, Na^+, Cl^-, K^+, urea, and NH_4^+. **Dark cells** secrete a glycoprotein by **merocrine** secretion.
   2. The **excretory portion (duct)** consists of **cuboidal cells** that reabsorb H_2O, Na^+, and Cl^- under the influence of **aldosterone** and open onto the skin surface as **sweat pores.**
   3. **They regulate body temperature** via postganglionic sympathetic neurons that use acetylcholine (cholinergic). Note: As a rule, postganglionic sympathetic neurons use norepinephrine as their neurotransmitter. However, there is an exception to the rule in the regulation of body temperature.
   4. **They regulate emotional sweating** via postganglionic sympathetic neurons that use norepinephrine (adrenergic).

B. **APOCRINE SWEAT GLANDS** are found in the axilla, mons pubis, and anal regions and are active at puberty.
   1. The **secretory portion** contains cells that secrete a viscous product via **merocrine** secretion.
   2. The **excretory portion (duct)** opens into the pilosebaceous canal of a hair shaft.
   3. Apocrine sweat glands are under the influence of **androgens** and **estrogens.**
   4. Modified apocrine sweat glands are found in the eyelids **(glands of Moll)** and external auditory meatus **(ceruminous glands,** which produce cerumen, i.e., ear wax).
   5. **They produce a malodorous body scent** (pheromones; for sexual attraction) via postganglionic sympathetic neurons that use norepinephrine (adrenergic).

C. **SEBACEOUS GLANDS** are widely distributed throughout the skin (except palms of the hands and soles of the feet) and are very active during puberty.
   1. The **secretory portion** contains cells with numerous lipid droplets that secrete **sebum** (composed of triglycerides, wax esters, squalene, and cholesterol) via **holocrine** secretion.
   2. The **excretory portion (duct)** opens into the pilosebaceous canal of a hair shaft.
   3. Sebaceous glands are under the influence of **androgens** (increase activity) and **estrogens** (decrease activity).

4. Hair-independent sebaceous glands are found on the lips, areolae of the nipple, labia minora, prepuce of the penis, and eyelids (tarsal glands of meibomian).
5. They lubricate the skin and play a role in **acne.**

Ⓥ Nerves

A. **MOTOR NERVES.** Postganglionic sympathetic neurons activate glands, contract arrector pili muscle, and control blood flow.

B. **SENSORY NERVES AND RECEPTORS**
1. **Free nerve endings.** Unmyelinated axons enter the epidermis and terminate in the stratum granulosum. They function in **pain and temperature sensation.**
2. **Merkel endings (mechanoreceptor).** Myelinated axons terminate in a platelike ending called the **nerve plate** that contacts Merkel cells in the stratum basale. They function in **tactile sensation (high resolution).**
3. **Meissner's corpuscles (mechanoreceptor).** A myelinated axon loses its myelin sheath, enters a connective tissue capsule within the dermal papillae, and pursues a zigzag course among disk-shaped epithelial cells. They function in **tactile two-point discrimination.**
4. **Pacinian corpuscles (mechanoreceptor).** A myelinated axon loses its myelin sheath in the dermis and enters a connective tissue capsule within the dermis and hypodermis. The unmyelinated axon is surrounded by 20–60 concentric layers of cells and gelatinous material ("onion appearance"). They function in **touch, vibration, and pressure sensation.**

Ⓥ Clinical Considerations (Figure 28-2)

A. **MALIGNANT MELANOMA** is a skin lesion with irregular borders and striking variations in pigmentation. Melanomas involve the transformation of melanocytes with long, branching cytoplasmic processes to oval cells that breach the basement membrane and grow in nests within the dermis. **Dysplastic nevi** are precursors of malignant melanoma.

B. **VITILIGO** is a disorder characterized by the **loss of melanocytes** because of autoimmune mechanisms, resulting in patches of hypopigmented skin most noticeable in darkly pigmented individuals. This disorder contrasts with **albinism** in which melanocytes are present but lack the enzyme tyrosinase so no melanin pigment is produced.

C. **BULLOUS PEMPHIGOID** is a disease that affects the epidermal–dermal adhesion and results clinically in **subepidermal blisters.** Mutations in the genes for keratin, laminin, integrin, bullous pemphigoid antigen (type XVII collagen), and type VII collagen have been implicated. Linear deposition of IgG along the basement has been observed.

D. **PSORIASIS** is a chronic disease that presents as recurrent eruptions of **red or silvery plaques.** Psoriasis is characterized by epidermal hyperplasia (acanthosis) as a result of abnormal cell proliferation, retention of nuclei in keratinized surface cells (parakeratosis), and elongation of dermal papillae.

● **Figure 28-2 Skin pathology. (A, B) Malignant melanoma. (A)** Photograph of a malignant melanoma showing the clinical warning signs: asymmetry, border irregularity, color variation, and diameter >6 mm. **(B)** LM of malignant melanoma shows the invasion of melanocytes into the dermis, forming cell nests (*arrow*). **(C)** LM of bullous pemphigoid shows the separation of the epidermis (*Epi*) from the dermis (*Der*), forming a subepidermal blister (*). Bullous pemphigoid presents clinically as prominent skin blisters usually found on the inner thigh, flexor surface of the arm, and oral mucosa. **(D)** LM of psoriasis showing the characteristic elongation of the dermal papillae (*arrows*). Psoriasis presents clinically as red or silvery plaques usually found on the elbows, knees, buttocks, or scalp.

Case Study

A 40-year-old man with freckles, a light complexion, and naturally blond hair comes to your office complaining that "I have a pink bump on my nose. I can tell that people are starting to stare at it because it looks funny." He also tells you that "the bump bleeds sometimes, but it heals pretty quickly." After some discussion, he informs you that he has been a professional golfer since he was 20 years old and he first noticed something on his nose about 1 year ago but it was "just a shiny, pearl-like bump and didn't look too bad so I ignored it." Although the man expressed concern only over his cosmetic appearance, his real worry becomes apparent when he says to you, "Doc, a few of my golfing buddies got skin cancer and they died pretty quick. Do you think I'm next?" What is the most likely diagnosis?

Differentials

- Actinic keratosis, malignant melanoma, squamous cell carcinoma

Relevant Physical Exam Findings

- A firm, non-tender nodule on the nose
- No other skin lesions found

Relevant Lab Findings

- Skin biopsy: multiple nests of deeply basophilic epithelial cells that protrude into the dermis and are attached to the epidermis; the periphery of the nests is composed of an organized layer of polarized, columnar keratinocytes with the long axis of each cell perpendicular to the surrounding basement membrane (i.e., palisading).

Diagnosis

Basal cell carcinoma (BCC). BCC is a locally invasive tumor that derives its names from the histologic similarity of the tumor cells to basal layer keratinocytes. BCC is the most common malignant skin neoplasm in persons with pale skin over 40 years of age with excessive exposure to sunlight. Although BCC is aggressive, it rarely metastasizes. Actinic keratosis (AK) presents as a rough, scaly, keratotic patch (wart-like appearance) on the face, neck, upper trunk, or extremities. AK is a premalignant lesion that may eventually develop into squamous cell carcinoma. A melanoma presents as a flat, dark brown or black lesion with irregular borders and alternating hypopigmentation. The most important clinical characteristic of a melanoma is a new or pre-existing lesion that enlarges or changes pigmentation. Melanomas involve the transformation of melanocytes with long, branching cytoplasmic processes to oval cells that breach the basement membrane and grow in nests in the dermis. Melanomas that demonstrate an aggressive vertical growth pattern will readily metastasize. Squamous cell carcinoma (SCC) presents as an ulcerating, scaling nodule on the back of hands, face, lips, and ears. SCC is the second most common malignant skin neoplasm and may be caused by sun exposure, ionizing radiation, chemical carcinogens, or human papilloma virus. SCC may begin as actinic keratosis. SCC rarely metastasizes. SCC is composed of cells that resemble the stratum spinosum and extend into the dermis with whorls of keratin present.

Eye

I **General Features** (Figure 29-1). The eye consists of three concentric tunics that make up the wall of the eye. The **corneoscleral tunic** (outermost fibrous tunic) consists of the white, opaque **sclera** and transparent **cornea**. The **uveal tunic** (middle vascular tunic) consists of the **choroid** and **stroma of the ciliary body and iris**. The **retinal tunic** (innermost tunic) consists of the **pigment epithelium and neural retina (posteriorly)** and **epithelium of the ciliary body and iris (anteriorly)**. The **lens** is suspended by **zonular fibers** (forming the suspensory ligament) from the ciliary body behind the iris. The **posterior chamber** and **anterior chamber** of the eye are filled with **aqueous humor,** which is a clear fluid secreted by the ciliary body epithelium. The **vitreous cavity** is filled with the **vitreous body,** which is a transparent gelatinous substance.

II **Cornea** is a transparent structure composed of five layers (Table 29-1). The central portion of the cornea receives nutrients from the **aqueous humor** within the anterior chamber of the eye, whereas the peripheral portion receives nutrients from **blood vessels of the limbus.** The cornea is an avascular structure, but is highly innervated by branches of cranial nerve V_1 (ophthalmic division of the trigeminal nerve).

III **Sclera** is a thick, opaque layer of collagen and elastic fibers produced by fibroblasts. The tendons of the extraocular muscles attach to the sclera.

IV **Limbus** (corneoscleral junction) is the junction of the transparent cornea and the opaque sclera. The limbus contains a **trabecular network** and the **canal of Schlemm,** which are involved in the flow of aqueous humor. The flow of aqueous humor follows this route: **posterior chamber $\rightarrow$ anterior chamber $\rightarrow$ trabecular network $\rightarrow$ canal of Schlemm $\rightarrow$ aqueous veins $\rightarrow$ episcleral veins.** The drainage rate of aqueous humor is balanced by the secretion rate of aqueous humor from the ciliary epithelium, thus maintaining a constant **intraocular pressure of 23 mm Hg.** An obstruction of aqueous humor flow will increase intraocular pressure, causing a condition called **glaucoma,** which may lead to blindness if untreated. There are two types of glaucoma:

A. **OPEN-ANGLE GLAUCOMA** (most common) occurs when the trabecular network is open but the canal of Schlemm is obstructed.

B. **CLOSED-ANGLE GLAUCOMA** occurs when the trabecular network is closed, usually because of an inflammatory process of the uvea (uveitis; e.g., infection by cytomegalovirus).

● **Figure 29-1 Diagram of the eye tunics. (A)** Corneoscleral tunic. **(B)** Uveal tunic. **(C)** Retinal tunic. **(D)** This diagram shows all three tunics combined into the adult structure of the eye. **(E)** Adult eye with its various components. *a* = anterior chamber; *p* = posterior chamber; *curved arrow* = flow of aqueous humor.

TABLE 29-1	LAYERS OF THE CORNEA
Layers	Characteristics
Corneal epithelium	Anterior aspect of cornea (exposed to air) Nonkeratinized stratified squamous epithelium Many free nerve endings (CN V_1) High capacity for repair (regeneration) Continuous with the conjunctiva at the limbus
Bowman layer	A distinctive portion of the corneal stroma Contains type I collagen Not a true basement membrane
Stroma	Connective tissue Contains type I and V collagen Thickest layer of the cornea
Descemet membrane	A basement membrane
Corneal endothelium	Posterior aspect of cornea (exposed to aqueous humor) Simple squamous epithelium Participates in active transport of nutrients into the stroma

CN = cranial nerve.

V **Iris.** The posterior surface is lined by two layers of simple columnar epithelium. The anterior surface of the iris lacks an epithelial covering and consists of the stroma. The stroma contains the dilator pupillae muscle and sphincter pupillae muscle.

A. **DILATOR PUPILLAE MUSCLE** is radially arranged around the entire circumference of the iris and is innervated by the sympathetic nervous system. Preganglionic sympathetic neurons project to the sympathetic trunk and ascend to the superior cervical ganglion. The superior cervical ganglion projects postganglionic sympathetic neurons through the perivascular plexus of the carotid system, entering the orbit through the superior orbital fissure. The postganglionic sympathetic neurons release **norepinephrine,** which stimulates contraction (i.e., **pupil dilation or mydriasis**) via **α-adrenergic receptors.** Any pathology that compromises this sympathetic pathway will result in **Horner syndrome,** which causes **miosis** (constriction of pupil as a result of paralysis of dilator pupillae muscle), **ptosis** (drooping of eyelid as a result of paralysis of superior tarsal muscle), and **hemianhydrosis** (loss of sweating on one side).

B. **SPHINCTER PUPILLAE MUSCLE** is circularly arranged around the entire circumference of the iris and is innervated by the parasympathetic nervous system. Preganglionic parasympathetic neurons from the **Edinger-Westphal nucleus of cranial nerve III** project to the **ciliary ganglion.** The ciliary ganglion projects postganglionic parasympathetic neurons to the sphincter pupillae muscle. The postganglionic parasympathetic neurons release **acetylcholine (ACh),** which stimulates contraction (i.e., **pupil constriction or miosis**) via **muscarinic acetylcholine receptors (mAChR).** Lesions involving **cranial nerve III** (oculomotor nerve) will result in a **fixed and dilated pupil.**

VI **Ciliary Body.** The ciliary body is lined by two layers of simple columnar epithelium called the **ciliary epithelium.** The ciliary epithelium **secretes aqueous humor** and **produces the zonular fibers** that attached to the lens. The stroma contains the **ciliary muscle.** The ciliary muscle is circularly arranged around the entire circumference of the ciliary body and is innervated by the parasympathetic nervous system. Preganglionic parasympathetic neurons from the **Edinger-Westphal nucleus of cranial nerve III** project to the **ciliary ganglion.** The ciliary ganglion projects postganglionic parasympathetic neurons to the ciliary muscle. The postganglionic parasympathetic neurons release **ACh,** which stimulates contraction (i.e., **accommodation**) via **mAChR.**

A. **ACCOMMODATION** is the process by which the lens becomes **rounder to focus a nearby object** or **flatter to focus a distant object.**

B. **FOR CLOSE VISION (E.G., READING),** the ciliary muscle contracts, which **reduces tension on the zonular fibers** attached to the lens and thereby allows the lens to take a **rounded shape.**

C. **FOR DISTANT VISION,** the ciliary muscle relaxes, which **increases tension on the zonular fibers** attached to the lens and thereby allows the lens to take a **flattened shape.**

VII **Lens.** The lens is a biconvex, transparent, and avascular structure that receives its nutrients from the aqueous humor. It consists of the following components:

A. **LENS CAPSULE** is a thick basement membrane that completely surrounds the lens.

B. **LENS EPITHELIUM** is a simple cuboidal epithelium located beneath the lens capsule only on the anterior surface (i.e., no epithelium is found on the posterior surface). The lens epithelium is mitotically active and migrates to the equatorial region of the lens, where the cells elongate and rotate so that they are parallel to the lens surface.

C. **LENS FIBERS** are prismatic remnants of the elongated lens epithelium that lose their nuclei and organelles. They are filled with cytoskeletal proteins called **filensin** and **α,β,γ-crystallin,** which maintain the conformation and transparency of the lens. The older lens fibers are displaced to the center of the lens whereas the newer lens fibers are found at the periphery.

D. **CATARACTS** are an opacity of the lens caused by a change in the solubility of lens proteins, filensin and α,β,γ-crystallin. This causes light scattering and impairs accurate vision. Cataracts are observed in elderly persons and are associated with diabetes. Glucose is the major metabolite of the lens. When glucose levels are high (diabetes), the byproduct sorbitol is formed in high concentration, which reduces the solubility of α,β,γ-crystallin, leading to lens opacity (cataracts).

VIII **Retina.** The posterior two thirds of the retina is a light-sensitive area **(pars optica)** and the anterior one third is a light-insensitive area **(par ciliaris and iridis)**; these two areas are separated by the **ora serrata.** The 10 layers that constitute the retina are described and illustrated in Figure 29-2. The retina has a number of specialized areas, which include the following:

A. **OPTIC DISK.** The optic disk is the site where axons of the ganglion cells converge to form the optic nerve (cranial nerve II) by penetrating the sclera, forming the **lamina cribrosa.** The optic disk lacks rods and cones and is therefore a **blind spot.** The central artery and vein of the retina pass through the optic disk.

B. **FOVEA.** The fovea is a shallow depression of the retina located 3 mm lateral (temporal side) to the optic disk along the visual axis. The **fovea centralis** is located at the center

Layers		Characteristics
10	Inner limiting membrane	Termination of Müller cells and their basement membrane
9	Optic nerve fibers	Unmyelinated axons of ganglion cells
8	Ganglion cells	Nuclei of ganglion cells
		Site of action potential generation
7	Inner plexiform layer	Synapses between bipolar and amacrine cells with ganglion cells
6	Inner nuclear layer	Nuclei of horizontal, bipolar, amacrine, and Müller cells
5	Outer plexiform layer	Synapses between bipolar and horizontal cells with rods and cones
		Retinal blood vessels may extend to this layer
4	Outer nuclear layer	Nuclei of rods and cones
3	Outer limiting membrane	Zonula adherens between rods/cones and Müller cells
2	Photoreceptor layer	Outer segment with membrane disks containing **Na+ ion channels,** connecting cilium, and inner segment of rods and cones
		Location of intraretinal space; detached retina occurs between 1 and 2
1	Pigment epithelium	Has tight junctions at apical border to form blood–retinal barrier, basal infoldings, and contains melanin
		Converts 11-trans retinal $\rightarrow$ 11-cis retinal
		Phagocytoses shed tips of rod outer segments
		Transports nutrients from choroid capillaries up to layer 4

Figure 29-2 Diagram of the retina. Tight junctions between the pigment epithelial cells establish a **blood-retinal barrier.** Therefore, blood supply to most of the retina (up to layer 5 [outer plexiform layer]) is from retinal blood vessels via the central artery of the retina (a branch of the ophthalmic artery). Retinal blood vessels are visible by ophthalmoscopic examination in which visible changes may be observed in hypertension or diabetic retinopathy. The central artery of the retina leaves the optic disk and travels between layer 10 (inner limiting membrane) and the vitreous body. Other layers of the retina (layers 1–4) are supplied by choroid capillaries. Müller cells act as supporting glial-type cells. Note the direction of the incident light and that it must pass through many layers of the retina before reaching the rods and cones. The asterisk indicates the site of retinal detachment; the double asterisk indicates the presence of Na+ ion channels; the triple asterisk indicates the site of action potential generation.

of the fovea and is the area of highest visual acuity and color vision. The fovea centralis contains **only cones (no rods or capillaries)** that are arranged **at an angle** so that light directly impinges on the cones without passing through other layers of the retina and are linked to a single ganglion, both of which contribute to visual acuity. The **macula lutea** is a yellowish area (as a result of xanthophyll pigment accumulation in ganglion cells) surrounding the fovea centralis.

IX Clinical Considerations

A. RETINITIS PIGMENTOSA (RP) is a genetic disease characterized by degeneration of rods, night blindness (nyctalopia), and "gun barrel" vision. RP may be caused by abetalipoproteinemia (Bassen-Kornzweig syndrome) and may be arrested by massive doses of vitamin A. In RP, blood supply to the retina is reduced and a pigment is observed on the surface of the retina (hence the name). The family of RP genes is located on chromosomes X, 3, and 6. Interestingly, the gene for rhodopsin also maps to chromosome 3.

B. DIABETIC RETINOPATHY. In patients with diabetes, retinal blood vessels frequently become leaky and exude fluid into the retina (particularly in the fovea), leading to loss of visual acuity. It is the leading cause of blindness in the developed world and may be reduced by strict regulation of blood glucose levels.

C. PAPILLEDEMA (CHOKED DISK) is a noninflammatory edema of the optic disk (papilla) as a result of increased intracranial pressure usually caused by brain tumors, subdural hematoma, or hydrocephalus. It usually does not alter visual acuity, but may cause bilateral **enlarged blind spots.**

D. NIGHT BLINDNESS (NYCTALOPIA) is a condition in which vision in poor illumination is defective because of vitamin A (retinol) deficiency. An aldehyde of vitamin A (retinol) called **retinal** is the chromophore component of rhodopsin.

E. RETINOBLASTOMA (Rb) is a tumor of the retina that occurs in childhood and develops from precursor cells in the immature retina. The *Rb* gene is located on chromosome 13 and encodes for Rb protein, which binds to a gene regulatory protein and causes suppression of the cell cycle (i.e., the *Rb* gene is a tumor-suppressor gene [also called an anti-oncogene]). A mutation in the *Rb* gene encodes an abnormal Rb protein such that there is no suppression of the cell cycle. This leads to the formation of retinoblastoma. Hereditary retinoblastoma causes multiple tumors in both eyes. Nonhereditary retinoblastoma causes one tumor in one eye.

X Selected Photomicrographs

A. CORNEA, RETINA, IRIS, AND CILIARY BODY (Figure 29-3)

B. ROD PHOTORECEPTOR CELL (Figure 29-4)

● **Figure 29-3 General features of the eye. (A) LM of cornea.** The five layers of the cornea are indicated. *epi* = corneal epithelium; *bl* = Bowman layer; *str* = stroma; *dm* = Descemet membrane; *endo* = corneal endothelium. **(B) LM of retina.** The 10 layers of the retina are indicated. The asterisk indicates the site of retinal detachment; the double asterisk indicates the presence of Na^+ ion channels; the triple asterisk indicates the site of action potential generation. **(C) LM of iris.** The posterior surface of the iris is lined by two layers of simple columnar epithelium, which are derived embryologically from the outer pigment layer (*out*) and inner (*in*) neural layer of the optic cup. Both of these layers are so highly pigmented that the two cell layers cannot be distinguished (see *dotted line* for boundary). The iris contains the dilator pupillae muscle and sphincter pupillae muscle, which are formed from the epithelium of the outer pigment layer (*out*) by the transformation of the epithelial cells into contractile cells. The stroma (*str*) of the iris contains connective tissue, blood vessels, nerves, and melanocytes. **(D) LM of ciliary body.** The ciliary body is lined by two layers of simple columnar epithelium, which are derived embryologically from the outer pigment layer (*out*) and the inner neural layer (*in*) of the optic cup. The outer pigment layer is pigmented, but the inner neural layer is nonpigmented. The ciliary body is thrown into folds called ciliary processes (*cp*). Both layers of epithelium are involved in the production of aqueous humor and zonular fibers of the lens. The stroma (*str*) of the ciliary body contains connective tissue and the ciliary muscle.

● **Figure 29-4 The photoreceptor cell. (A) Diagram of a rod photoreceptor cell.** Note the various regions of the rod: outer segment, which contains Na⁺ ion channels and membrane disks; connecting cilium, which contains the cilium, basal body, and centriole; inner segment, which contains mitochondria, rER, sER, and Golgi; cell body, which contains the nucleus; and synaptic body, which contains synaptic vesicles. **(B)** EM of the outer segment and connecting cilium regions. Note the cilium, basal body, and centriole. **(C)** Diagram of the boxed area in A and B depicting the process of visual transduction. In the dark, rod photoreceptor cells have open Na⁺ ion channels, which maintain the rod in a constant state of **depolarization. Rhodopsin** (photopigment) consists of a chromophore called **11-cis-retinal** bound to a glycoprotein called **scotopsin.** After light stimulation, 11-cis-retinal is isomerized to **11-trans-retinal,** which is released from scotopsin in a process called **bleaching.** Bleaching activates a G protein called **transducin** that activates **cGMP phosphodiesterase** (converts cGMP → GMP), thereby lowering cGMP levels. Low cGMP levels close Na⁺ ion channels, thereby eliciting a **hyperpolarization.** 11-Trans-retinal is converted back to 11-cis-retinal by the pigment epithelium and transported back to the rod photoreceptor cell by **interstitial retinoid-binding protein (IRBP),** where it combines with scotopsin to regenerate rhodopsin. Note that visual transduction is quite different from the way action potentials in muscle and nerve are generated. In muscle and nerve, stimuli open Na⁺ ion channels, thereby eliciting a depolarization. In rod photoreceptor cells, stimuli close Na⁺ ion channels, thereby eliciting hyperpolarization.

Ear

I **General Features.** The ear is the organ of hearing and balance. The ear consists of the external ear, middle ear, and inner ear.

II **External Ear** consists of the following:

A. **EXTERNAL AUDITORY MEATUS** is an air-filled tubular space. The lateral portion is supported by cartilage and lined by skin that contains hair follicles, sebaceous glands, and ceruminous glands (produce ear wax). The medial portion is supported by the temporal bone and is lined by thinner skin. The external auditory meatus develops from **pharyngeal groove 1**, which becomes filled with ectodermal cells, forming a temporary **meatal plug** that disappears before birth. The external auditory meatus is innervated by **cranial nerve (CN) V$_3$** and **CN IX**.

B. **AURICLE** (known as "the ear" by laypeople) is supported by elastic cartilage and covered by skin. The auricle develops from **six auricular hillocks** that surround pharyngeal groove 1. The auricle is innervated by **CN V$_3$, CN VII, CN IX, and CN X,** and **cervical nerves C2 and C3.**

III **Middle Ear** consists of the following:

A. **OSSICLES**
1. **Malleus** develops from cartilage of **pharyngeal arch 1** (Meckel's cartilage). The malleus is attached to the **tympanic membrane** and is moved by the **tensor tympani muscle,** which is innervated by CN V$_3$.
2. **Incus** develops from the cartilage of **pharyngeal arch 1** (Meckel's cartilage). The incus articulates with the malleus and stapes.
3. **Stapes** develops from the cartilage of **pharyngeal arch 2** (Reichert's cartilage). The stapes is attached to the **oval window** of the vestibule and is moved by the **stapedius** muscle, which is innervated by CN VII.

B. **AUDITORY TUBE AND MIDDLE EAR CAVITY** develop from **pharyngeal pouch 1.**

C. **TYMPANIC MEMBRANE (EARDRUM)** develops from **pharyngeal membrane 1.** The tympanic membrane separates the middle ear from the external auditory meatus of the external ear, has a conical depression at its center because of the attachment of the malleus, and is innervated (sensory) by CN V$_3$ and CN IX. The tympanic membrane consists of three layers:

1. Keratinized stratified squamous epithelium covers the external surface.
2. Connective tissue, which is vascularized and innervated, constitutes the middle layer.
3. Simple squamous epithelium covers the internal surface.

IV Internal Ear. The internal ear consists of the semicircular ducts, utricle, saccule, and cochlear duct, all of which are referred to as the **membranous labyrinth** containing **endolymph.** The membranous labyrinth is initially surrounded by mesoderm that later becomes cartilaginous and ossifies to become the **bony labyrinth** of the temporal bone. The mesoderm closest to the membranous labyrinth degenerates, thus forming the **perilymphatic space** containing **perilymph.** Thereby, the membranous labyrinth is suspended within the bony labyrinth by perilymph. Perilymph, which is similar in composition to **cerebrospinal fluid (CSF),** communicates with the subarachnoid space via the **perilymphatic duct.**

A. **SEMICIRCULAR DUCTS (KINETIC LABYRINTH)** (Figure 30-1). **Type I** and **type II hair cells** that cover the **cristae ampullaris** (a prominent ridge within the ampulla) have numerous stereocilia and a single **kinocilium** on their apical border. These cells synapse with bipolar neurons of the vestibular ganglion of CN VIII. The kinetic labyrinth also contains **supporting cells.** Hair cells and supporting cells are covered by a gelatinous mass called the **cupula.** The semicircular ducts respond to **angular acceleration** and **deceleration of the head.**

B. **UTRICLE AND SACCULE (STATIC LABYRINTH)** (Figure 30-1). **Type I** and **type II hair cells** within **maculae** (a specialized receptor area within the wall) have stereocilia and a single **kinocilium** on their apical border. These cells synapse with bipolar neurons of the vestibular ganglion of CN VIII. The static labyrinth also contains **supporting cells.** Hair cells and supporting cells are covered by a gelatinous mass called the **otolithic membrane,** which contains $CaCO_3$ crystals **(otoliths).** The utricle and saccule respond to the position of the head with respect to **linear acceleration** and the **pull of gravity.**

C. **COCHLEAR DUCT** (Figure 30-2). This triangular duct comprises a **vestibular membrane** (roof), **basilar membrane** (floor), and **stria vascularis** (lateral wall). The stria vascularis participates in the formation of endolymph. The cochlear duct contains the **organ of Corti.** The organ of Corti contains a single row of **inner hair cells** and three rows of **outer hair cells** that have stereocilia (but no kinocilium) on their apical border and synapse with bipolar neurons of the cochlear (spiral) ganglion of CN VIII (90% of these bipolar neurons synapse with inner hair cells). It also contains **pillar** and **phalangeal supporting cells.** The outer hair cells are in contact with a gelatinous mass called the **tectorial membrane** (contains **α- and β-tectorin protein**). The organ of Corti responds to **sound.**

V Clinical Considerations

A. **RUBELLA VIRUS.** The organ of Corti may be damaged by exposure to rubella virus during week 7 and week 8 of embryologic development.

B. **MENIERE DISEASE** is caused by an increase in endolymph. Clinical findings include: vertigo (the illusion of rotational movement), nausea, positional nystagmus (involuntary rhythmic oscillations of the eye), vomiting, and tinnitus (ringing of the ears).

C. **WAARDENBURG SYNDROME** is an autosomal dominant congenital deafness associated with pigment abnormalities resulting from abnormal neural crest cell migration.

● **Figure 30-1 (A) Diagram of the membranous labyrinth.** Note the location of specialized sensory areas (*black color*) for angular acceleration (cristae ampullaris), linear acceleration (maculae), and hearing (organ of Corti). **(B) Cristae ampullaris** of the semicircular ducts (kinetic labyrinth). The deflection of the cupula by endolymph movement during angular acceleration stimulates the hair cells. When stereocilia move toward the kinocilium, hair cells are depolarized and afferent nerve fibers are stimulated. When stereocilia move away from the kinocilium, hair cells are hyperpolarized and afferent nerve fibers are not stimulated. **(C) Macula** of the utricle and saccule (static labyrinth). The displacement of otoliths by endolymph movement during linear acceleration stimulates hair cells.

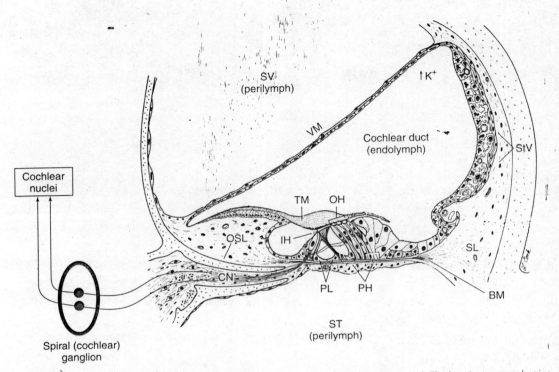

● **Figure 30-2 Organ of Corti of the cochlear duct.** The organ of Corti responds to sound. The hearing process begins when airborne sound waves cause vibration of the tympanic membrane, which moves the stapes against the oval window. This produces waves of perilymph within the scala vestibuli and scala tympani. The waves of perilymph cause an upward displacement of the basilar membrane such that the stereocilia of the hair cells hit the tectorial membrane. As a result, K^+ ion channels open, hair cells are depolarized, and afferent nerve fibers are stimulated. Note that the endolymph has a high K^+ concentration, which is maintained by the stria vascularis (*StV*). Note the vestibular membrane (*VM*), stria vascularis (*StV*), basilar membrane (*BM*), cochlear nerve fibers (*CN*), scala vestibuli (*SV*) containing perilymph, scala tympani (*ST*) containing perilymph, cochlear duct containing endolymph, three rows of outer hair cells (*OH*), one row of inner hair cells (*IH*), tectorial membrane (*TM*), spiral ligament (*SL*), outer phalangeal cells (*PH*), pillar cells (*PL*), and osseous spiral lamina (*OSL*). The basilar membrane extends between the osseous spiral lamina and the spiral ligament.

Credits

Figure 1-1: A, B From Dudek RW: *High-Yield Cell and Molecular Biology*. Philadelphia: Lippincott Williams & Wilkins, 1999; fig. 9-1. **C** From Miller OL, Beatty BR: *Science*, the cover, 164:955, 1969.

Figure 1-2: From Dudek R: *High-Yield Cell and Molecular Biology*. Baltimore: Lippincott Williams & Wilkins, 1999:1-1. Original source: Reproduced with permission from Marks D: *BRS Biochemistry*. 3rd ed. Baltimore: Williams & Wilkins, 1998.

Figure 1-3: From Dudek RW: *High-Yield Cell and Molecular Biology*. Baltimore: Lippincott Williams & Wilkins, 1999:2-2.

Figure 1-4: Modified from Dudek RW: *High-Yield Cell and Molecular Biology*. Baltimore: Lippincott Williams & Wilkins, 1999, fig. 15-1.

Figure 1-5: From Dudek RW: *High-Yield Cell and Molecular Biology*. Baltimore: Lippincott Williams & Wilkins, 1999:14-1.

Figure 1-6: From Dudek RW: *High-Yield Cell and Molecular Biology*. Baltimore: Lippincott Williams & Wilkins, 1999:14-2.

Figure 1-7: From Dudek RW: *High-Yield Cell and Molecular Biology*. Baltimore: Lippincott Williams & Wilkins, 1999:14-3.

Figure 1-8: From Dudek RW: *High-Yield Cell and Molecular Biology*. Baltimore: Lippincott Williams & Wilkins, 1999:7-1. Original source; Redrawn from Alberts et al. *Essential Cell Biology*, Garland, NY, 1998, p. 264.

Figure 1-9: From Dudek RW: *High-Yield Cell and Molecular Biology*. 2nd ed. Baltimore: Lippincott Williams & Wilkins, 2006, fig. 4-2.

Figure 1-10: A From Dudek RW: *High-Yield Histology*. 3rd ed., Baltimore: Lippincott Williams & Wilkins, 2004:1-7A. Original source: Cormack D: *Essential Histology*. 2nd ed. Philadelphia: Lippincott Williams & Wilkins, 2001, p. 26, fig. 2-2. **B** From Cormack D: *Essential Histology*. 2nd ed. Philadelphia: Lippincott Williams & Wilkins, 2001:2-3. **C** Cormack D: *Essential Histology*. 2nd ed. Philadelphia: Lippincott Williams & Wilkins, 2001:2-4. **D** From Dudek RW: *High-Yield Histology*. 3rd ed. Baltimore: Lippincott Williams & Wilkins, 2004:1-7C. Original source. Reprinted with permission from Stafstrom J, Stahelin L: *J Cell Biol* 98:699, 1984. **E** From Dudek RW: *High-Yield Histology*. 3rd ed. Baltimore: Lippincott Williams & Wilkins, 2004:1-7B. Original source. Reprinted with permission from Feldherr C, Kallenbach E, Schultz N: *J Cell Biol* 99:2216, 1984. **F** Courtesy of Dr. RW Dudek. **G** Courtesy of Dr. RW Dudek. **H** From Ross MH, Kaye GI, Pawlina W: *Histology: A Text and Atlas*. 4th ed. Baltimore: Lippincott Williams & Wilkins, 2003:2.70c. Courtesy of Dr. Scott H. Kaufmann, Mayo Clinic. **Table 1-2**. Modified from Alberts B, et al: *Molecular Biology of the Cell*, 3rd ed. New York: Garland, 1994:18-1.

Figure 2-2: Dudek RW: *High-Yield Cell and Molecular Biology*. 2nd ed. Baltimore: Lippincott Williams & Wilkins, 2001:4-3. Original source; Redrawn from Alberts B, et al: *Essential Cell Biology*: NY, Garland, 1998:230.

322

Figure 3-1: From Dudek RW: *High-Yield Cell and Molecular Biology*. 2nd ed. Baltimore: Lippincott Williams & Wilkins, 2001:1-1.

Figure 3-2: From Dudek RW: *High-Yield Cell and Molecular Biology*. 2nd ed. Baltimore: Lippincott Williams & Wilkins, 2001:1-2.

Figure 3-3: From Dudek RW: *High-Yield Cell and Molecular Biology*. 2nd ed. Baltimore: Lippincott Williams & Wilkins, 2001:1-3.

Figure 3-4: From Dudek RW: *High-Yield Cell and Molecular Biology*. 2nd ed. Baltimore: Lippincott Williams & Wilkins, 2001:1-4.

Figure 4-2: A, B, F, G Reprinted with permission from Cormack DH: *Essential Histology*. 2nd ed. Philadelphia: Lippincott Williams & Wilkins, 2001, p. 101, fig. 4-6; p. 101, fig. 4-5; and p. 83, fig. 3-22. **C** From Ross MH, Pawlina W, Kaye GI: *Histology: A Text and Atlas*. 4th ed. Philadelphia: Lippincott Williams & Wilkins, 2003, p. 103, fig. 4-14A. **D** Reprinted with permission from Arias IM et al: *The Liver: Biology and Pathobiology*. 4th ed. Philadelphia: Lippincott Williams & Wilkins, 2001, p. 30, fig. 3-1C. **E** Reprinted with permission from Dellmann HD, Eurell J: *Textbook of Veterinary Histology*. 5th ed. Philadelphia: Lippincott Williams & Wilkins, 1998, p. 3, fig. 1-4.

Figure 5-1: A-1, B-1, and E From Ross MH, Pawlina W, Kaye GI: *Histology: A Text and Atlas*. 4th ed. Philadelphia: Lippincott Williams & Wilkins, 2003, p. 131, fig. 5-5; p. 138, fig. 5-12; and p. 145, fig. 5-18. **A-2, B-2** Reprinted with permission from Dudek RW: *High-Yield Embryology*. 2nd ed. Philadelphia: Lippincott Williams & Wilkins, 2000, p. 94, fig. 16-1 and p. 104, fig. 17-5. **C** Reprinted with permission from Gartner L, Hiatt J: *Color Atlas of Histology*. 3rd ed. Philadelphia: Lippincott Williams & Wilkins, 2000, p. 60, fig. 1. **D** Reprinted with permission from Dellmann HD, Eurell J: *Textbook of Veterinary Histology*. 5th ed. Philadelphia: Lippincott Williams & Wilkins, 1998, p. 36, fig. 3-8. **F** Courtesy of Dr. RW Dudek.

Figure 7-1: A Reprinted with permission from Rohen JW, Yokochi C, Lutjen-Drecoll E: *Color Atlas of Anatomy*. 4th ed. Baltimore: Williams & Wilkins 1998, p. 9 (no figure number). **B, C** Courtesy of Dr. RW Dudek. **D** Reprinted with permission from Cormack DH: *Essential Histology*. 2nd ed. Philadelphia: Lippincott Williams & Wilkins, 2001, Plate 8-6 (no page number). **E** Reprinted with permission from Cormack DH: *Clinically Integrated Histology*. Philadelphia: Lippincott-Raven, 1998, p. 89, fig. 4-16.

Figure 7-2: A–E Courtesy of Dr. RW Dudek.

Figure 7-3: A, B Reprinted with permission from Cormack DH: *Clinically Integrated Histology*. Philadelphia: Lippincott-Raven, 1998, p. 73, fig. 4-5D and p.73, fig. 4-5C. **D** Reprinted with permission from Damjanov I: *Histopathology: A Color Atlas and Textbook*. Baltimore: Williams & Wilkins, 1996, p. 432, fig. 17-9.

Figure 7-4: A, D Reprinted with permission from Damjanov I: *High-Yield Pathology*. Philadelphia: Lippincott Williams & Wilkins, 2000, p. 126, fig. 17-3 and p. 127, fig. 17-4. **B, E** Reprinted with permission from Damjanov I: *Histopathology: A Color Atlas and Textbook*. Baltimore: Williams & Wilkins, 1996, p. 441, fig. 17-20A and p. 443, fig. 17-21A. **C** Reprinted with permission from Cormack DH: *Clinically Integrated Histology*. Philadelphia: Lippincott-Raven, 1998, p. 74, fig. 4-6.

Figure 8-1: A Reprinted with permission from Ross MH, Romrell LJ, Kaye GI: *Histology: A Text and Atlas*. 2nd ed. Philadelphia: Lippincott Williams & Wilkins, 1992, p. 249, fig. 10-2.

Figure 8-4: A, F: Reprinted with permission from Cormack DH: *Essential Histology*. 2nd ed. Philadelphia: Lippincott Williams & Wilkins, 2001, p. 240, fig. 10-2 and p. 251, fig. 10-15. **B, C** Reprinted with permission from Dellmann HD, Eurell J: *Textbook of Veterinary Histology*. 5th ed. Philadelphia: Lippincott Williams & Wilkins, 1998, p. 86, fig. 5-9.

Figure 8-5: A Reprinted with permission from Cormack DH: *Essential Histology*. 2nd ed. Philadelphia: Lippincott Williams & Wilkins, 2001, p. 242, fig. 10-5. **B, C** Dudek RW: *High-Yield Histology*. 2nd ed. Philadelphia: Lippincott Williams & Wilkins, 2000, p. 49, figs. 6-4A and 6-4B. **D** Reprinted with permission from Gartner L, Hiatt J: *Color Atlas of Histology*. 3rd ed. Philadelphia: Lippincott Williams & Wilkins, 2000, p. 117, fig. 1.

Figure 8-6: A, B Reprinted with permission from Ross MH, Romrell LJ, Kaye GI: *Histology: A Text and Atlas*. 2nd ed. Philadelphia: Lippincott Williams & Wilkins, 1992 p. 277, figs. 1 and 4. **C** Reprinted with permission from Cormack D: *Essential Histology*. 2nd ed. Philadelphia: Lippincott Williams & Wilkins, 2001, p. 250, fig. 10-14. **D** Reprinted with permission from Dellmann HD, Eurell D: *Textbook of Veterinary Histology*. 5th ed. Philadelphia: Lippincott Williams & Wilkins, 1998, p. 89, fig. 5-14. **E, F** Reprinted with permission from Gartner L, Hiatt J: *Color Atlas of Histology*. 3rd ed. Philadelphia: Lippincott Williams & Wilkins, 2000, p. 119, figs. 2 and 4. **G, H** Reprinted with permission from Cormack DH: *Essential Histology*. 2nd ed. Philadelphia: Lippincott Williams & Wilkins, 2001, p. 253, fig. 10-17. **I** Reprinted with permission from Gartner L, Hiatt J: *Color Atlas of Histology*. 3rd ed. Philadelphia: Lippincott Williams & Wilkins, 2000, p.121, fig. 1. **J** Reprinted with permission from Dellmann HD, Eurell J: *Textbook of Veterinary Histology*. 5th ed. Philadelphia: Lippincott Williams & Wilkins, 1998, p. 83, fig. 5-3.

Figure 9-2: A, C, D Reprinted with permission from Cormack DH: *Essential Histology*. 2nd ed. Philadelphia: Lippincott Williams & Wilkins, 2001, p.212, fig. 9-2 and p. 213, fig. 9-3, Plate 9-4 (no page number). **B** Reprinted with permission from Ross MH, Romrell LJ, Kaye GI: *Histology: A Text and Atlas*. 4th ed. Philadelphia: Lippincott Williams & Wilkins, 2003, p. 325, Plate 27, fig. 3. **E, F, G, H, I, J** Reprinted with permission from Damjanov I: *Histopathology: A Color Atlas and Textbook*. Baltimore: Williams & Wilkins, 1996, p. 466, fig. 19-1A; p. 466, fig. 19-1E; p. 467, fig. 19-10; p. 483, fig. 19-25; p. 467, fig. 19-1C; p. 467, fig. 19-1F.

Figure 9-3: A Reprinted with permission from Sternberg SS: *Histology for Pathologists*. 2nd ed. Philadelphia: Lippincott Williams & Wilkins, 1997, p. 290, fig. 5A. **B** Reprinted with permission from Ross MH, Pawlina W, Kaye GI: *Histology: A Text and Atlas*. 4th ed. Philadelphia: Lippincott Williams & Wilkins, 2003, p. 294, fig. 11-10B. **C** Reprinted with permission from Cormack DH: *Essential Histology*. 2nd ed. Philadelphia: Lippincott Williams & Wilkins, 2001, p. 228, fig. 9-23. **D** Reprinted with permission from Dudek RW: *High-Yield Histology*. 2nd ed. Philadelphia: Lippincott Williams & Wilkins, 2000, p. 59, fig. 7-4. **E** Reprinted with permission from Dudek RW: *High-Yield Histology*. 2nd ed. Philadelphia: Lippincott Williams & Wilkins, 2000, p. 60, fig. 7-6.

Figure 9-4: A, C, D, E, F Reprinted with permission from Cormack DH: *Essential Histology*. 2nd ed. Philadelphia: Lippincott Williams & Wilkins, 2001, p. 221, fig. 9-14. **B** Reprinted with permission from Dudek RW: *High-Yield Histology*, 2nd ed. Philadelphia: Lippincott Williams & Wilkins, 2000, p. 58, fig. 7-3. **G** Reprinted with permission from Sternberg SS: *Histology for Pathologists*. 2nd ed. Philadelphia: Lippincott Williams & Wilkins, 1997, p. 272, fig. 47C.

Figure 9-5: A, B Courtesy of Dr. RW Dudek. **C** Reprinted with permission from Dudek RW: *High-Yield Histology*. 2nd ed. Philadelphia: Lippincott Williams & Wilkins, 2000, p. 59, fig. 7-5.

Figure 9-6: A Reprinted with permission from Dudek RW: *High-Yield Histology*. 2nd ed. Philadelphia: Lippincott Williams & Wilkins, 2000, p. 61, fig. 7-7. **B, C** Courtesy of Dr. RW Dudek.

Figure 9-7: A–D Reprinted with permission from Damjanov I: *Histopathology: A Color Atlas and Textbook*. Baltimore: Williams & Wilkins, 1996, p. 477, fig. 19-17B; p. 471, fig. 19-8B; p. 483, fig. 19-27; p. 483, fig. 19-24. **E** Reprinted with permission from Dudek RW: *High-Yield Histology*. 2nd ed. Philadelphia: Lippincott Williams & Wilkins, 2000, p. 204, fig. 29-2.

Figure 10-3: A Reprinted with permission from Damjanov I: *High-Yield Pathology*. Philadelphia: Lippincott Williams & Wilkins, 2000, p. 38, fig. 7-1. **D1, D2, D3, D4** Reprinted with permission from Damjanov I: *Histopathology: A Color Atlas and Textbook*. Baltimore: Williams & Wilkins, 1996, p. 101, figs. 5-5A, B,C, D.

Figure 10-4: A Courtesy of Dr. RW Dudek. **B** Courtesy of Dr. S. Viragh, Postgraduate Medical School, Budapest, Hungary.

Figure 10-5: A, C, D Courtesy of Dr. RW Dudek. **B** Reprinted with permission from Cormack DH: *Clinically Integrated Histology.* Philadelphia: Lippincott-Raven, 1998, p. 134, fig. 5-16.

Figure 10-6: Courtesy of Dr. RW Dudek.

Figure 10-7: Courtesy of Dr. RW Dudek.

Figure 11-3: A, C Reprinted with permission from Stiene-Martin EA, Lotspeich-Steininger CA, Koepke JA: *Clinical Hematology: Principles, Procedures, Correlations.* 2nd ed. Philadelphia: Lippincott, 1998, p. 91, p. 96. **B, D** Courtesy of Jean Shafer, Department of Medicine, University of Rochester, Rochester, NY, Carden Jennings Publishing Co. Ltd., Charlottesville, VA. **D Inset** Reprinted with permission from Stiene-Martin EA, Lotspeich-Steininger CA, Koepke JA: *Clinical Hematology: Principles, Procedures, Correlations.* 2nd ed. Philadelphia: Lippincott, 1998, p. 99.

Figure 11-4: A, B, D Reprinted with permission from Stiene-Martin EA, Lotspeich-Steininger CA, Koepke JA: *Clinical Hematology: Principles, Procedures, Correlations.* 2nd ed. Philadelphia: Lippincott, 1998, p. 95; p. 98; p. 97. **A Inset** Reprinted with permission from Carr JH, Rodak BF: *Clinical Hematology Atlas.* Philadelphia: Saunders, 1999, p. 143. **C** Courtesy of Jean Shafer, Department of Medicine, University of Rochester, Rochester, NY, Carden Jennings Publishing Co. Ltd., Charlottesville, VA.

Figure 11-5: A–D Reprinted with permission from Stiene-Martin EA, Lotspeich-Steininger CA, Koepke JA: *Clinical Hematology: Principles, Procedures, Correlations.* 2nd ed. Philadelphia: Lippincott, 1998, pp. 92-93.

Figure 11-6: A–D Reprinted with permission from Mufti GJ, Flandrin G, Schaefer HE, et al: *An Atlas of Malignant Haematology.* Philadelphia, Lippincott-Raven, 1996, p. 179; p. 225.

Figure 11-7: A, B Reprinted with permission from Mufti GJ, Flandrin G, Schaefer HE et al: *An Atlas of Malignant Haematology.* Philadelphia: Lippincott-Raven, 1996, p. 244; p. 242. **C** Reprinted with permission from Gatter K, Brown D: *An Illustrated Guide to Bone Marrow Diagnosis.* Malden, MA: Blackwell Science, 1997, p. 134. **D** Carr JH, Rodak BF: *Clinical Hematology Atlas,* Philadelphia: Saunders, 1999, p. 143.

Figure 11-8: 3, 4, 5, 6, Reprinted with permission from Gartner L, Hiatt J: *Color Atlas of Histology.* 3rd ed. Philadelphia: Lippincott Williams & Wilkins, 2000, p. 100, figs. 3, 4, 5, 6.

Figure 11-9: Reprinted with permission from Cormack DH: *Clinically Integrated Histology.* Philadelphia: Lippincott-Raven, 1998, p. 43, fig. 3-17J–O.

Figure 11-10: A–I Reprinted with permission from Cormack DH: *Clinically Integrated Histology.* Philadelphia: Lippincott-Raven, 1998, p. 37, fig. 3-11C, D, F, G, H, K; p. 43, fig. 3-17H, I.

Figure 12-1: A Reprinted with permission from Schiffman RJ: *Hematologic Pathophysiology.* Philadelphia: Lippincott-Raven, 1998, p. 16, fig. 1-18. Redrawn from Weiss L: *Cell and Tissue Biology.* Reprinted with permission from Cormack DH: *Clinically Integrated Histology.* Philadelphia: Lippincott-Raven, 1998, p. 58, fig. 3-22A, cropped just a portion. **C, D** Courtesy of Dr. RW Dudek.

Figure 12-3: Courtesy of Dr. RW Dudek.

Figure 13-1: A Redrawn from Takahashi M: *Color Atlas of Cancer Cytology.* 3rd ed. Philadelphia: Lippincott Williams & Wilkins, 2000, p. 375, fig. 17.2A. **B** Redrawn from Ross MH, Romrell LJ, Kaye, GI: *Histology: A Text and Atlas.* 3rd ed. Philadelphia: Lippincott Williams & Wilkins, 1995, p. 343, fig. 13.8. **C** Courtesy of Dr. RW Dudek. **D** Reprinted with permission from Cormack DH: *Essential Histology.* 2nd ed. Philadelphia: Lippincott Williams & Wilkins, 2001, p. 166, fig. 7-8B.

Figure 13-3: A–E Courtesy of Dr. RW Dudek.

Figure 14-1: A Redrawn with permission from Ross MH, Romrell LJ, Kaye GI: *Histology: A Text and Atlas*. 3rd ed. Philadelphia: Lippincott Williams & Wilkins, 1995, p. 350, fig. 13-14. (Based on Weiss L, Tavossoli M: *SEM Hematology* 7:372,1970.)

Figure 15-1: Modified and reprinted with permission from Ross MH, Romrell LJ, Kaye GI: *Histology: A Text and Atlas*. 3rd ed. Philadelphia: Lippincott Williams & Wilkins, 1995, p. 448, fig. 16-7; p. 449, fig. 16-8; p. 450, fig. 16-9.

Figure 16-1: Picture of enterocyte courtesy of Dr. RW Dudek. Picture of Paneth cell Rreprinted with permission from Satoh Y: *J Electron Microsc Tech* 16:69,1990. John Wiley and Sons, Inc.

Figure 16-2: A Reprinted with permission from Fenoglio-Preiser CM: *Gastrointestinal Pathology: A Text and Atlas*. 2nd ed. Philadelphia: Lippincott Williams & Wilkins, 1999, p. 293, fig. 8-38. **B** Reprinted with permission from Damjanov I: *Histopathology: A Color Atlas and Textbook*. Philadelphia: Williams & Wilkins, 1996, p. 197, fig. 8-16A. **C** Reprinted with permission from Yamada T et al: *Atlas of Gastroenterology*. 2nd ed. Philadelphia: Lippincott Williams & Wilkins, 1999, p. 334, fig. 36-10A. **D** Reprinted with permission from Yamada T: *Textbook of Gastroenterology*. Vol 1. 3rd ed. Philadelphia: Lippincott Williams & Wilkins, 1999, p. 1484, fig. 66-17A.

Figure 17-1: A–D Courtesy of Dr. RW Dudek.

Figure 17-2: A–E Courtesy of Dr. RW Dudek.

Figure 18-2: Reprinted with permission from Henrikson RC, Kaye GI, Mazurkiewicz JE: *NMS Histology*. 3rd ed. Philadelphia: Williams & Wilkins, 1997, p. 292, fig. 26-2.

Figure 19-1: (Figure of islet: Reprinted with permission from Henrikson RC, Kaye GI, Mazurkiewicz JE: *NMS Histology*. 3rd ed. Philadelphia: Williams & Wilkins, 1997, p. 368, fig. 33-2.) From Dudek RW: *High-Yield Histology*. 2nd ed.Philadelphia: Williams & Wilkins, 2000, p. 124, fig. 17-1.

Figure 19–3: A, B From Bakerman: Bakerman's *ABC's of Interpretive Laboratory Data*. 4th ed. Scottsdale, AZ: Interpretive Laboratory Data, Inc., 2002, p. 403.

Figure 20-1: A B Reprinted with permission from Cormack DH: *Essential Histology*. 2nd ed. Philadelphia: Lippincott Williams & Wilkins, 2001, p. 343, fig. 14-7A. **C** Reprinted with permission from Dellmann HD, Eurell J: *Textbook of Veterinary Histology*. 5th ed. Philadelphia: Lippincott Williams & Wilkins, 1998, p. 157, fig. 9-16.

Figure 20-3: B Reprinted with permission from Ross MH, Romrell LJ, Kaye GI: *Histology: A Text and Atlas*. 3rd ed. Philadelphia: Lippincott Williams & Wilkins, 1995, p. 587, fig. 18-19. **C** Reprinted with permission from Cormack DH: *Clinically Integrated Histology*. Philadelphia: Lippincott-Raven, 1998, p. 156, fig. 6-13.

Figure 20-5: A, B, C, F From Damjanov I: *Histopathology: A Color Atlas and Textbook*. Baltimore: Williams & Wilkins, 1996, p. 137, fig. 6-10; p. 135, fig. 6-8B; p. 135, fig. 6-7C; p. 137, fig. 6-9C; and p. 137, fig. 6-8B. **D:** Reprinted with permission from Takahashi M: *Color Atlas of Cancer Cytology*. 3rd ed. p. 189, fig. 8-59.

Figure 21-1: (2), (3) Henrikson RC, Kaye GI, Mazurkiewicz JE: *NMS Histology*. 3rd ed. Baltimore: Williams & Wilkins, 1997, p. 331, fig. 29-6; (4),(5) light micrographs of PCT, DCT, and CD are courtesy of Dr. RW Dudek. (7) photograph of kidney sagittal section reprinted with permission from Cormack DH: *Essential Histology*. 2nd ed. Philadelphia: Lippincott Williams & Wilkins, 2001, p. 351, fig. 15-1; (9) EM of thin loop of Henle reprinted with permission from Jennette JC et al: *Heptinstall's Pathology of the Kidney*. 5th ed. Vol 1. Philadelphia: Lippincott Williams & Wilkins, 1998, p. 43, fig. 1-54.

Figure 21-2: A From Dudek RW: *High-Yield Kidney*. Baltimore: Lippincott Williams & Wilkins, 2007:4-3A.

Figure 21-3: From Dudek RW: *High-Yield Kidney*. Baltimore: Lippincott Williams & Wilkins, 2007:4-5.

Figure 21-4: A From Dudek RW: *High-Yield Kidney*. Baltimore: Lippincott Williams & Wilkins, 2007:4-4. **B** From Dudek RW. *High-Yield Histology*. 3rd ed. Baltimore: Lippincott Williams & Wilkins, 2004:21-3B.

Figure 21-5: From Dudek RW: *High-Yield Kidney*. Baltimore: Lippincott Williams & Wilkins, 2007:5-29.

Figure 21-6: From Dudek RW: *High-Yield Kidney*. Baltimore: Lippincott Williams & Wilkins, 2007:8-2.

Figure 21-7: A–D A,B. Courtesy of Dr. RW Dudek. **E–H** From Damjanov I. *Histopathology: A Color Atlas and Textbook*. Baltimore: Williams & Wilkins, 1996, p. 283, fig. 11-14B; p. 288, fig. 11-22A; p. 289, fig. 11-23D; p. 291, fig. 11-24.

Figure 22-1: A Taken from Dudek RW: *High-Yield Histology*. 2nd ed. Philadelphia: Williams & Wilkins, 2000, p. 149, fig. 20-1. **B** Reprinted with permission from Sternberg SS: *Histology for Pathologists*. 2nd ed. Philadelphia: Lippincott Williams & Wilkins, 1997, p. 1060, fig. 21B. **C, E** Reprinted with permission from Sternberg SS: *Histology for Pathologists*. 2nd ed. Philadelphia: Lippincott Williams & Wilkins, 1997, p. 1060, fig. 23A,B **D** Reprinted with permission from Sternberg SS: *Histology for Pathologists*. 2nd ed. Philadelphia: Lippincott Williams & Wilkins, 1997, p. 1065, fig. 28. **F** Reprinted with permission from Sternberg SS: *Histology for Pathologists*. 2nd ed. Philadelphia: Lippincott Williams & Wilkins, 1997, p. 1065, fig. 29.

Figure 23-2: A Reprinted with permission from Sternberg SS: *Histology for Pathologists*. 2nd ed. Philadelphia: Lippincott Williams & Wilkins, 1997, p. 1082, fig. 9.

Figure 23-3: Inset A Reprinted with permission from Sternberg SS: *Diagnostic Surgical Pathology*. Vol 1. 3rd ed. Philadelphia: Lippincott Williams & Wilkins, 1999, p. 536, fig. 9A. **Inset B:** Reprinted with permission from Sternberg SS: *Diagnostic Surgical Pathology*. Vol 1. 3rd ed. Philadelphia: Lippincott Williams & Wilkins, 1999, p. 551, fig. 30A.

Figure 24-2: A Reprinted with permission from Sternberg SS: *Histology for Pathologists*. 2nd ed. Philadelphia: Lippincott Williams & Wilkins, 1997, p. 1096, fig. 7. **B** Reprinted with permission from Sternberg SS: *Histology for Pathologists*. 2nd ed. Philadelphia: Lippincott Williams & Wilkins, 1997, p. 1088, fig. 21. **C** Reprinted with permission from Sternberg SS: *Histology for Pathologists*. 2nd ed. Philadelphia: Lippincott Williams & Wilkins, 1997, p. 1100, fig. 20. **D** Reprinted with permission from Sternberg SS. *Histology for Pathologists*. 2nd ed. Philadelphia: Lippincott Williams & Wilkins, 1997, p. 1100, fig. 22.

Figure 25-3: A Reprinted with permission from Sternberg SS: *Histology for Pathologists*. 2nd ed. Philadelphia: Lippincott Williams & Wilkins, 1997, p. 1108, fig. 1B. **B** Reprinted with permission from Covenhaver, Dounge: *Bailey's Textbook of Histology*. 16th ed. : Lippincott, Williams & Wilkins, 1978, p. 651, fig. 21-19. **C** Courtesy of Dr. RW Dudek. **D** Courtesy of Dr. RW Dudek. **E** Courtesy of Dr. RW Dudek. **F** Reprinted with permission from Sternberg SS: *Histology for Pathologists*. 2nd ed. Philadelphia: Lippincott Williams & Wilkins, 1997, p. 1114, fig. 11. **G** Reprinted with permission from Sternberg SS *Histology for Pathologists*. 2nd ed. Philadelphia: Lippincott Williams & Wilkins, 1997, p. 1114, fig. 12.

Figure 25-4: Courtesy of Dr. RW Dudek.

Figure 25-5: A Reprinted with permission from Sternberg SS: *Diagnostic Surgical Pathology*. Vol 1, 3rd ed. Philadelphia: Lippincott Williams & Wilkins, 1999, p. 614, fig. 43. **C** Reprinted with permission from Sternberg SS: *Diagnostic Surgical Pathology*. Vol 1, 3rd ed. Philadelphia: Lippincott Williams & Wilkins, 1999, p. 609, fig. 33. **D** Reprinted from Dudek RW: *High-Yield Histology*. 2nd ed. Philadelphia: Lippincott Williams & Wilkins, 2000, p. 166, fig. 23-4C.

Figure 26-1: (1), (2) Reprinted with permission from Sternberg SS: *Histology for Pathologists*. 2nd ed. Philadelphia: Lippincott Williams & Wilkins, 1997, p. 942, fig. 23 and fig. 22.(3) Reprinted with permission from Ross MH, Pawlina W, Kaye GI: *Histology: A Text and Atlas*. 4th ed. Philadelphia: Lippincott Williams & Wilkins, 2002, p. 765, fig. 3. (4), (5) Reprinted with permission from Cormack DH. *Clinically Integrated Histology*. Philadelphia: Lippincott Williams & Wilkins, 1998, p. 252, fig. 9-33 and p. 256, fig. 9-37.

Figure 26-2: A–C Reprinted with permission from Sternberg SS: *Histology for Pathologists*. 2nd ed. Philadelphia: Lippincott Williams & Wilkins, 1997, p. 918, fig. 46A,B,C. **D, E** Reprinted with permission from Sternberg SS: *Diagnostic Surgical Pathology*. Vol 2. 3rd ed. Philadelphia: Lippincott Williams & Wilkins, 1999, p. 2396, fig. 1 and p. 2399, fig. 10.

Figure 26-3: (1) Reprinted with permission from Cormack DH: *Clinically Integrated Histology*. Philadelphia: Lippincott Williams & Wilkins, 1998, p. 260, fig. 9-41C. (2), (3) Courtesy of Dr. RW Dudek.

Figure 26-4: (1), (2), (3) Reprinted with permission from Sternberg SS: *Histology for Pathologists*. 2nd ed. Philadelphia: Lippincott Williams & Wilkins, 1997, p. 886, fig. 8; p. 888, fig. 11A; p. 885, fig. 6. (4) Reprinted with permission from Ross M, Pawlina W, Kaye GI: *Histology: A Text and Atlas*. 4th ed. Philadelphia: Lippincott Williams & Wilkins, 2000, p. 750, fig. 22-21.

Figure 26-5: (1), (2), (3) Reprinted with permission from Koss L, Gompel C, and Bergeron C: *Introduction to Gynecologic Cytopathology*. Philadelphia: Lippincott Williams & Wilkins, 1999, p. 39, fig. 6-1; p. 40, fig. 6-4; p. 41, fig. 6-7.

Figure 26-5: A, B Reprinted with permission from Sternberg SS: *Histology for Pathologists*. 2nd ed. Philadelphia: Lippincott Williams & Wilkins, 1997, p. 872, fig. 7 and p. 873, fig. 8. **C–E** Reprinted with permission from Damjanov I: *Histopathology: A Color Atlas and Textbook*. Philadelphia: Lippincott Williams & Wilkins, 1996, p. 327, fig. 13-13, fig. 13-4, fig. 13-2.

Figure 26-6: A Reprinted with permission from Sternberg SS: *Histology for Pathologists*. 2nd ed. Philadelphia: Lippincott Williams & Wilkins, 1997, p. 72, fig. 1. **B, D, E** Reprinted with permission from Ross M, Romrell L, Kaye GI: *Histology: A Text and Atlas*. 3th ed. Philadelphia: Lippincott Williams & Wilkins, 2002, p. 711, fig. 22-35; p. 739, fig. 1, Plate 124; p. 713, fig. 22-37. **C** Reprinted with permission from Cormack DH: *Clinically Integrated Histology*. Philadelphia: Lippincott-Raven, 1998, p. 263, fig. 9-45.

Figure 26-7: A (1) Reprinted with permission from Sternberg SS: *Histology for Pathologists*. 2nd ed. Philadelphia: Lippincott Williams & Wilkins, 1997, p. 872, fig. 7. (2) Reprinted with permission from Koss LG, Gompel C, Bergeran C: *Diagnostic Cytology*. **Figure 26-7B:** (3) Reprinted with permission from Takahashi M: *Color Atlas of Cancer Cytology*, 3rd ed. Philadelphia: Lippincott Williams & Wilkins, 2000, 4th ed. Vol 1. Philadelphia: Lippincott Williams & Wilkins, 1992, p. 397, fig. 11-21B. (3) Reprinted with permission from Takahashi M: *Color Atlas of Cancer Cytology*. 3rd ed. Philadelphia: Lippincott Williams & Wilkins, 2000, p. 92, fig. 6-126A. **B** (1) Reprinted with permission from Koss L, Gompel C, Bergeron C: *Introduction to Gynecologic Cytopathology*. Philadelphia: Lippincott Williams & Wilkins, 1999, P. 39, fig. 6-1. (2) Reprinted with permission from Takahashi M: *Color Atlas of Cancer Cytology*, 3rd ed. Philadelphia: Lippincott Williams & Wilkins, 2000, p. 83, fig. 6-109 and p. 92, fig. 6-126B. **C** Reprinted with permission from Sternberg SS: *Diagnostic Surgical Pathology*. Vol 2. 3rd ed. Philadelphia: Lippincott Williams & Wilkins, 1999, p. 2156, fig. 1B. **D** 24-4. Courtesy of Dr. RW Dudek.

Figure 26-8: A, D Reprinted with permission from Dudek RW: *High-Yield Gross Anatomy*. 2nd ed., Philadelphia: Lippincott Williams & Wilkins, 2001, p. 24, fig. 3-1C,D.

Figure 27-1: A Reprinted with permission from Henrikson R, Kaye G, Mazurkiewicz J: *NMS Histology*. Philadelphia: Lippincott Williams & Wilkins, 1997, p. 393, fig. 36-2. **B** Reprinted with permission from Dudek RW: *High-Yield Histology*. Philadelphia: Lippincott Williams & Wilkins,

2000, p. 183, fig. 25-3. **C–G** Reprinted with permission from Dellmann HD, Eurell J: *Textbook of Veterinary Histology*. 5th ed. Philadelphia: Lippincott Williams & Wilkins, 1998, p. 229, fig. 12-4; p. 232, fig. 12-6.

Figure 27-2: Reprinted with permission from Dellmann HD, Eurell J:, *Textbook of Veterinary Histology*. 5th ed. Philadelphia: Lippincott Williams & Wilkins, 1998, p. 233, fig. 12-7.

Figure 27-5: A, B Reprinted with permission from Cormack DH: *Clinically Integrated Histology*. 2nd ed. Philadelphia: Lippincott-Raven, 1998, p. 272, fig. 9-55. p. 273, fig. 9-56A.

Figure 27-5: C, D Reprinted with permission from Ross M, Pawlina W, Kaye GI: *Histology: A Text and Atlas*, 4th ed. Philadelphia: Lippincott Williams & Wilkins, 1990, p. 710, fig. 21-28B,A.

First figure for Table 27-1. Reprinted with permission from Dellmann HD, Eurell J: *Textbook of Veterinary Histology:* 5th ed. Philadelphia: Lippincott Williams & Wilkins, 1998, p. 233, fig. 12-7.

Second figure for Table 27-1. Reprinted with permission from Dellmann HD, Eurell J: *Textbook of Veterinary Histology,* 5th ed. Philadelphia: Lippincott Williams & Wilkins, 1998, p. 232, fig. 12-6B.

Third figure for Table 27-1. Reprinted with permission from Sternberg SS: *Histology for Pathologists*. 2nd ed. Philadelphia: Lippincott Williams & Wilkins, 1997, p. 1022, fig. 7.

Fourth figure for Table 27-1. Reprinted with permission from Sternberg SS: *Histology for Pathologists* 2nd ed. Philadelphia: Lippincott Williams & Wilkins 1997, p. 1022, fig. 7.

Fifth figure for Table 27-1. Reprinted with permission from Sternberg SS: *Histology for Pathologists*. 2nd ed. Philadelphia: Lippincott Williams & Wilkins, 1997, p. 1022, figure 7.

Sixth figure for Table 27-1. Reprinted with permission from Sternberg SS: *Histology for Pathologists*. 2nd ed. Philadelphia: Lippincott Williams & Wilkins, 1997, p. 1022, fig. 7.

Figure 28-1: A–E Reprinted with permission from Ross MH, Pawlina W, Kaye GI: *Histology: A Text and Atlas*. 4th ed. Philadelphia: Lippincott Williams & Wilkins, 2003, p. 402, fig. 14-2; p. 408, fig. 14-7; p. 431, fig. 1, Plate 42; p. 414, fig. 14-14.

Figure 28-2: A, B Reprinted with permission from Cormack DH: *Clinically Integrated Histology*. Philadelphia: Lippincott Williams & Wilkins, 1998, p. 14, fig. 2-2A,B. **C, D** Reprinted with permission from Damjanov I: *Histopathology: A Color Atlas and Textbook*. Philadelphia: Lippincott Williams & Wilkins, 1996, page 405, fig. 16-3, 16-2.

Figure 29-4: B Reprinted with permissions from Fawcett DW: *A Textbook of Histology*. 12th ed. New York: p. 902. Courtesy of T. Kuwabara. Taken from Dudek RW: *High-Yield Histology*. 2nd ed. Philadelphia: Lippincott Williams & Wilkins, 2000, p. 201, fig. 28-3B.

Figure 30-1: A Reprinted with permission from Copenhaver, Kelly, Wood: *Bailey's Textbook of Histology*. 16th ed. Lippincott Williams & Wilkins, 1978. **B, C left** Reprinted with permission from Dudek RW: *High-Yield Histology*. 2nd ed. Philadelphia: Lippincott Williams & Wilkins, 2000, p. 194, fig. 27-1A,B.

Figure 30-2: Large portion reprinted with permission Dellmann HD, Eurell J: *Textbook of Veterinary Histology*. 5th ed. Philadelphia: Lippincott Williams & Wilkins, 1998, p. 350, fig. 18-5.

Index

Page numbers in *italics* denote figures; those followed by t denote tables; those followed by b denote boxes.

G

H

I